INTERNATIONAL HANDBOOK OF RESEARCH
IN MEDICAL EDUCATION

Kluwer International Handbooks of Education

VOLUME 7

International Handbook of Research in Medical Education

Part Two

Editors:

Geoff R. Norman
McMaster University, Canada

Cees P.M. van der Vleuten
University of Maastricht, The Netherlands

David I. Newble
University of Sheffield, United Kingdom

Section editors:

Geoff R. Norman
McMaster University, Canada

Diana H.J.M. Dolmans
University of Maastricht, The Netherlands

Karen V. Mann
Dalhousie University, Canada

Arthur Rothman
University of Toronto, Canada

David I. Newble
University of Sheffield, United Kingdom

Lynn Curry
CurryCorp, Canada

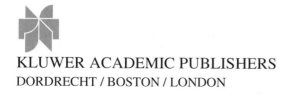

KLUWER ACADEMIC PUBLISHERS
DORDRECHT / BOSTON / LONDON

Library of Congress Cataloging-in-Publication Data is available.

ISBN 1-4020-0466-4

Published by Kluwer Academic Publishers
PO Box 17, 3300 AA Dordrecht, The Netherlands

Sold and distributed in North, Central and South America
by Kluwer Academic Publishers,
101 Philip Drive, Norwell, MA 02061, U.S.A.

In all other countries, sold and distributed
by Kluwer Academic Publishers, Distribution Centre,
PO Box 322, 3300 AH Dordrecht, The Netherlands

Printed on acid-free paper

Printed and bound in Great Britain by MPG Books Limited, Bodmin, Cornwall

Table of Contents

PART TWO

SECTION 5: ASSESSMENT

SECTION 6: IMPLEMENTING THE CURRICULUM

Section 5: Assessment

Introduction

DAVID NEWBLE – SECTION EDITOR
University of Sheffield

Assessment has become a critical area of concern for medical education. It has been recognized by teachers as playing a central role in determining what and how students learn. At the same time the quality of assessment procedures has come under increasing scrutiny not just by the medical profession, but by students, licensing authorities, government bodies, the legal profession, and the community. Long held assumptions have been challenged as traditional forms of assessment frequently have been found to provide less valid and reliable measures than had been assumed. A new level of professionalism is emerging in relation to test development and administration founded upon an increasingly wide and robust research base.

In this section, eight chapters explore some of the key issues in relation to assessment. What becomes apparent is that much of the research on technical aspects of test development has occurred in the North America context. For instance, the prevalence of litigation against licensing institutions has ensured a focus on providing high quality assessments, particularly in relation to levels of reliability, which is rarely matched in other countries. On the other hand, significant innovations have arisen in other parts of the world. The benefit of this has been a global interest in assessment with much sharing of ideas and information, and many examples of productive joint research.

The chapter by Downing deals with the varying test formats which have been developed to test cognitive knowledge. He analyzes the strengths and weakness of both selected response (e.g. MCQs) and constructed response (e.g. essays, written simulations) formats. He precedes these details with a broad overview of the desirable characteristics of all cognitive tests which are also generalizable to other types of assessment discussed in later chapters.

Petrusa, in his chapter on assessing clinical performance, does not attempt to be comprehensive. He starts by mentioning some of the limitations of traditional clinical examinations then looks in detail at structured clinical examinations, particularly those constructed around standardized patients. He features the research looking at many aspects of such SP-based examinations including test reliability, the effect of station length, the reliability of SP portrayal and student factors. He then discusses various aspects of validity including the under-researched area of educational validity – that is the relationship and effect of assessment to student learning. The issue of standard setting for SP-based exams is the next issue tackled,

645

International Handbook of Research in Medical Education, 645–646.
G.R. Norman, C.P.M. Van der Vleuten, D.I. Newble (eds.)
© 2002 *Dordrecht: Kluwer Academic Publishers. Printed in Great Britain.*

one of great importance. Finally the problem of resources to conduct high quality performance-based tests is considered and one strategy for improving efficiency, sequential testing, is considered.

A particularly difficult area of assessment has been the non-cognitive domain covering communication skills, interpersonal skills and attitudes. The latter provides a particular challenge. Cushing describes the various methods being used and there is an evident overlap with issues raised in the previous chapter. However, a much wider range of methods is considered including ratings from tutors, peers, patients and self. The problem of standard setting is again highlighted. The need to assess performance in real-life contexts, in addition to assessing competence in controlled settings, is recognized. This is particularly so in regard to the assessment of attitudes which is best achieved through assessing behaviors in practice. The concept of obtained information from a differing perspective – triangulation – is one approach to improving reliability where single methods of assessment are inappropriate or inadequate.

In recent years the use of computers has assumed an increasingly important place in assessment. Clauser and Schuwirth examine the role of computers in three areas: in delivering tests in standard and adaptive modes, in presenting simulations, and in language processing and virtual reality. Many may be surprised at the extent to which computers are being used in some countries and the added value they may provide. Issues of scoring and standard setting once again are raised.

Turnbull and van Barneveld look specifically at the assessment of performance in the in-training situation. While such assessments may come closest to measuring true performance, current methods are shown to be weak psychometrically. New models and methods are proposed.

As already mentioned, the problem of standard setting becomes a common theme in clinical assessment. The chapter by Norcini and Guille provides an in depth review of the subject. It becomes clear that, while the principles of varying approaches to standard setting can be clearly enunciated, the methods of doing so can be difficult and cumbersome.

The final two chapters, the first by Dauphinee and the second by Cunnington and Southgate, provide comprehensive coverage of licensure and certification and relicensure and recertification. The varying approaches adopted in different countries provide a range of interesting models. There is a growing impression that assessment of competence and performance is becoming more internationalized, one obvious benefit of an increasingly evidence-based approach by medical educational institutions, professional bodies and licensing authorities.

20 Assessment of Knowledge with Written Test Forms

STEVEN M. DOWNING

University of Illinois at Chicago

SUMMARY

Written or computer-based assessment is the most appropriate modality to test cognitive knowledge. Two major classes of written assessment are discussed in this chapter: selected-response and constructed-response formats. Multiple-choice (MCQ), matching and extended matching, true-false, multiple-true false and alternate-choice items are examples of the selected-response format. Long and short essays, very short essays, modified essay questions and written simulations, such as computer simulations, are examples of constructed-response formats. These assessment forms are critically evaluated in terms of their strengths, limitations, appropriateness, efficiency, research basis, psychometric properties, and validity evidence.

INTRODUCTION

This chapter discusses written (and computer-administered) cognitive test forms or formats intended to assess learner achievement. Cognitive assessments are the most common and, arguably, the most important types of evaluation used in medical education settings of all kinds throughout the world. Performance examinations – tests of actual or simulated psychomotor skills or affective behavior – are discussed in other chapters in this section.

Two major types of written cognitive assessments are discussed – selected-response and constructed-response item formats. These names are accurately descriptive of the forms used. Selected-response formats require the examinee to *select* answers from a listing of possible responses; the multiple-choice item form is the most typical example of selected-response, but formats such as the matching and true-false forms are also representative of this format. Constructed-response formats challenge examinees to *produce* responses to more open-ended questions or stimuli. Examples of constructed-response formats include essays – long and short

International Handbook of Research in Medical Education, 647–672.
G.R. Norman, C.P.M. Van der Vleuten, D.I. Newble (eds.)
© 2002 *Dordrecht: Kluwer Academic Publishers. Printed in Great Britain.*

essays and very short-answer essays, modified essay questions and the simulation formats.

The chapter begins with a general discussion of important concerns in testing cognitive knowledge, the generally accepted characteristics of adequate achievement measurement, and the arguments for and against selected-response and constructed-response items. This same structure is carried into a discussion of each particular item format with examples of most item forms.

TESTING COGNITIVE KNOWLEDGE

In order to discuss testing cognitive achievement using written test forms, it is necessary to first operationally define cognitive knowledge in this context. *Cognitive knowledge* includes all learning or achievement that is associated with some theory of mental ability or function. Examples are theories modeled by taxonomies such as described by Bloom (Bloom, Engelhart, Furst, Hill, & Kratwohl, 1956) or information processing models such as discussed by Anderson and Bower (1973) or by cognitive psychology models (e.g., Mislevy, 1993; Snow & Lohman, 1989; Dibello, Roussos, & Stout, 1993). Operationally, cognitive knowledge assessment encompasses all testing intended to measure examinee *mental* learning that is not in the psychomotor or affective domain. Thus, important inferences from test scores are made to some domain of cognitive ability or achievement, rather than some curricular or instructional domain (Millman & Greene, 1989) or some psychomotor (performance) or affective domain.

Tests of cognitive knowledge

Cognitive knowledge is best assessed using written test forms. This bold statement is supported by some eighty years of educational measurement research on objectively scored written examinations. Since almost all cognitive knowledge is verbally mediated, it is of no surprise that verbal (written) assessments are the primary and most desirable forms used to test achievement in this domain. Written test forms, on the other hand, are almost useless as measures of psychomotor or affective skills, abilities, and achievements (with some reservations).

Desirable characteristics of cognitive tests

Cognitive assessments all share a set of desirable characteristics which most educational measurement professionals would agree should be present for adequate assessment of achievement. These desirable characteristics are necessary but not sufficient conditions for good, trustworthy tests of achievement. They are minimum requirements for adequate measurement, but many other attributes may be needed for certain specific types of tests to ensure appropriate inferences from test scores.

Objectivity

Objectivity refers to the characteristic of agreement among content experts that the correct or keyed response is indeed correct or that a constructed answer meets some minimum requirement for credit. Objectivity generally implies that examinee responses can be machine or computer scored since there is little or no subjectivity or judgment involved in deciding whether a particular examinee's answer or response is right or wrong. In its most basic form, objectively scored item formats can be reduced to a set of ones and zeros for each correct and incorrect examinee answer.

Selected-response item formats are most readily and easily objectively keyed. It is much easier for experts to agree on the single-best answer or the most-correct-response out of a set of carefully crafted and edited possible answer options than it is to agree upon a scoring rubric or the minimum essential statements required for a more open-ended constructed-response item.

Constructed-response formats can be objectively scored, but the task is generally much more difficult than with the selected-response formats. Clearly some types of achievement assessment, such as the evaluation of writing skill, require expending the additional effort needed to maximize the objectivity of measurement with constructed-response items.

Measurement properties

All achievement measurements must have certain properties in order to produce test scores that are useful, trustworthy and provide legitimate and accurate inferences. Some of these important properties are: score scales which have adequate validity evidence, are reproducible, and correspond roughly one-to-one with levels of cognitive knowledge attained by examinees.

Some basic definitions of terms may useful:

Test scores

A test score is the quantitative value (the number) or other symbol (a letter) produced by counting the number of correct responses to test questions. Test Score Scales are the set of numbers produced by a group of examinee test scores. Some examples of score scales are: raw score scales which are the simple sum of the number of correctly answered items; transformed scales are raw scores converted into some other metric, such as the percent-correct scale or a standard score scale which is a linear transformation of the raw scores into a scale with the mean and standard deviation of scores set to some arbitrary value.

Validity evidence

The contemporary view of test validity suggests that tests are not valid or invalid, but rather it is the interpretation of test scores and the inferences drawn from those scores that are more or less valid. Evidence is collected, sometimes from many different sources and over a long period of time, to support or refute the claim for the reasonableness of the conclusions drawn from test data or the inferences about examinee achievement in the domain measured or the construct sampled (Messick, 1989; Kane, 1992).

There are direct sources of validity evidence for many achievement tests. The content tested by the questions selected for the examination is the most critical source of validity evidence for most achievement tests. How the content is selected, and in what proportions to the population or domain of interest, are important sources of validity evidence. The qualifications and expertise of the item writers and test constructors may be another source of validity evidence for such examinations. More indirect sources of validity evidence for achievement examinations are statistical relationships of test scores with other measures (such as other tests of similar content) or ratings of clinical performance by independent judges or class rankings.

In general, the more evidence one has to support the intended inferences from test scores (validity evidence), the better. It is not possible to have too much validity evidence to support the specific claims for valid inferences. Also, validity evidence must be constantly updated, as examinees, educational programs, and test questions change and evolve. Validity evidence may have a fairly short shelf life and the more important the consequences of the test scores, the more important it is to update validity evidence.

Reproducibility

Reproducibility refers to the test score characteristic of score and pass-fail decision reliability. Just as with any scientific experiment, the ability to independently reproduce test results and the pass or fail decisions that follow from these scores is critical to the trustworthiness of the test results. Theoretically, a second administration of the same examination to the same examinees (assuming that they have learned or forgotten nothing) should produce about the same test scores, if the test is well constructed. On the other hand, if test results are markedly different on the second administration (we are unable to reproduce the results), one questions the adequacy of the test to measure the content or construct of interest.

Many methods are available to estimate the reproducibility of test scores and the pass-fail decisions resulting from the test scores. For most achievement examinations, an internal-consistency reliability coefficient such as the Kuder-Richardson Formula 20 (Kuder & Richardson, 1937) or the more general formula, Cronbach's Alpha (Cronbach, 1951), is an adequate estimate of score reproducibility. Generalizability Theory (Brennan, 1983) permits parsing more sources of measurement error and may be an appropriate estimate of score reproducibility for many achievement tests.

Pass-fail decision reproducibility is the more important reproducibility, especially for examinations that have serious consequences associated with passing or failing – examinations such as end-of-curriculum tests, licensure and certification examinations or pre-employment tests which must be passed in order to gain employment. Several approaches are used to estimate the reproducibility of pass-fail decisions, but one convenient procedure was suggested by Subkoviak (1988), which uses tabled values associated with the score reliability coefficient and a *z*-score calculated from the passing score on the test and the mean and standard deviation of the test.

Correspondence of test scores with achievement

Cognitive achievement is measured on a continuum of knowledge and skills acquired by the examinee. A fundamental assumption of all testing is that test scores correspond (within measurement error) in a one-to-one fashion with the knowledge attained by the examinee. High scores indicate high mastery of the subject and low scores symbolize low attainment of the content tested. Errors of measurement (low reproducibility) reduce the confidence one has in this one-to-one correspondence, since measurement error introduces noise into the system and clouds one's ability to make appropriate and correct inferences. Low score reproducibility or reliability thus reduces the validity evidence for an examination, since inferences to the domain of interest are made more questionable.

Thus, score and pass-fail reproducibility are an essential source of validity evidence for most tests. "Reliability is a necessary but not a sufficient condition for validity" is an often cited phrase in the educational measurement literature. Test scores must be reliable or reproducible in order to have any chance of being valid but just because tests are reliable does not necessarily mean that they are valid. Another familiar phrase, especially in medical education, is that some testing methods trade off reliability for validity. This is, of course, nonsense if one accepts that reliability is an essential source of a test's validity evidence.

Defensibility

All test scores must be defensible. At a minimum, a teacher must be able to defend the keyed correct answer to students. At the other extreme, a high-stakes licensure or certification agency must be able to defend its test scores and its pass-fail decisions in court.

There are many important aspects to examination defensibility. Some characteristics will be more important than others for certain types of inferences. But the one common thread running through all defensibility arguments for examinations is *validity evidence*. Test validity evidence, as discussed above, refers to all data and information assembled to support or refute the argument for the legitimacy and reasonableness of the inferences made from the examination scores.

Validity arguments (Kane, 1992) supporting inferences for the intended purpose of the test are essential to defending the test scores and their interpretation. Validity evidence is not equivalent or synonymous with issues of test defensibility, rather it is a necessary but not sufficient condition for defensibility.

Score and pass-fail decision *reproducibility or reliability* are also an essential input into test defensibility. These examination traits, as discussed above, are important to test validity arguments and evidence and, thus, are very important to defensibility issues. Since it is not possible to make a strong validity argument for test inferences from unreliable test data that contain much measurement error, it is unlikely that tests with low reliability estimates can be strongly defended.

Due diligence is another component of defensibility and refers to the evidence one assembles to show that great care has been taken to ensure the legitimacy and accuracy of the test scores and their inferences (Norcini & Shea, 1997). Issues such as the thoroughness with which the test content was selected, the expertise of the test item writers, the careful editing and proof-reading of the test before it is administered, the rigor of the standard setting methods, the care with which the examination was scored, and any appeal process for examinee verification of the accuracy of scores all may be components of due diligence, depending on the type of examination and its intended inferences.

How *passing scores* associated with high-stakes examinations are determined is critical to defending the examination. The more important the consequences of passing or failing the examination, the more important and critical is the legitimacy and defensibility of the methods used to determine the passing score. Norcini and Shea (1997) discuss many important aspects of passing score determination.

Passing scores on examinations, especially high-stakes examinations, should be based on a systematic process of collecting the absolute judgments of experts. Such passing scores are non-relative; that is, the passing score is such that all examinees could pass the test or all could fail. The score needed to pass is not based on any distribution of scores from any group of examinees or any norm group external to the examinee sample, but rather is based on a group of content expert judges answering the question: "How much knowledge is enough to pass?"

Many methods of setting absolute standards have been discussed in the literature (e.g., Berk, 1986; Livingston & Zieky, 1982) and are addressed elsewhere in this book. The method proposed by Angoff (1971) remains a popular procedure used to set absolute passing scores on all types of tests – selected-response and constructed-response tests. In Angoff's method and its many modifications by individual users, a group of content-expert judges first discuss and come to a consensus definition of a borderline group of examinees on the test. The borderline group of examinees is a theoretical set of test takers who have an equal probability of passing or failing the examination. Borderline candidates may just barely pass or may just barely fail the test; their knowledge and skills in the content area are just marginally adequate or just below the sufficient-knowledge-to-pass threshold. The Angoff judges systematically review each test item and individually assign a probability estimate of how likely the borderline candidates are to answer the question correctly. The sum of individual standard setting judge's ratings, across all items of the test, is the passing score for the examination.

The Angoff method has been thoroughly researched (e.g., Norcini, 1994) over many years and has been shown to produce highly reliable ratings. While the Angoff method is not without its critics (e.g., Mullins & Green, 1994), this method remains useful to high-stakes examination standard setters because of its practicality of use, its time efficiency, and its reproducibility.

Efficiency

Finally, written tests of cognitive knowledge are efficient. Efficiency, in this context, refers to time and cost efficiency, and ease of test development, administration, and scoring. While efficiency should not be the predominant force in selecting a testing modality, it is an important practical matter.

Written tests, especially objectively scored tests using selected-response items, are very efficient. Their greatest efficiency is associated with the time and cost of scoring. In fact, selected-response item formats were first developed for large-scale US military selection tests which needed to gather test data on large groups of examinees under the pressure of war-time recruitment. Later, optical scanning machines quickly, efficiently, and accurately read test data and produced data files of examinee responses as input to computer scoring software. The costs associated with administering and scoring written test forms are much lower than with any of the constructed-response item formats, which require human readers to produce scores. Other efficiencies are in examination administration, especially for examinees, since much more information can be gathered about student achievement per unit of testing time with written test forms (selected-response) than with other formats, such as the constructed-response formats.

Good selected-response items are difficult to create well and are not as time efficient to write, as are some of the constructed-response formats, such as essays. However, time and cost efficiencies lost in the test development process are more than adequately compensated for in the scoring phase of the testing cycle.

SELECTED-RESPONSE ITEM FORMATS

Selected-response item formats are written or computer-administered test items which require examinees to select rather than produce responses. Examinee responses can be machine-scanned into computer files for objective scoring. The number of choices or options for selected-response items can vary from two to twenty or more, although four or five options is typical for the most common selected-response formats such as multiple-choice.

Various selected-response formats will be discussed in this section: multiple-choice, matching and extended matching items, and true-false and multiple true-false items.

Strengths of selected-response forms

Selected-response formats have many advantages in the measurement of cognitive achievement. These objective written item forms are efficiently computer scored, have very high agreement among content experts on the correctness of the keyed answer, have very strong and desirable educational measurement properties with an extensive research base, and are typically easily defended if their construction has been carefully and systematically carried out. These item forms are efficient in many ways noted above and, if securely maintained in item banks, are reusable, which adds further to their efficiency and their strong measurement properties by permitting statistical equating of test forms.

Objective

Selected-response item formats are objective rather than subjective in their scoring. Objectivity, as discussed above, is an essential characteristic of all good measurement and adds to validity evidence, defensibility, and efficiency of measurement. Part of the objective strength of selected-response item formats is the ability of content experts to agree on the correct or best answer from among the set of possible answers. This is an essential strength of this item form not shared easily with the constructed-response formats.

Strong measurement properties

Selected-response item forms have very strong measurement properties. Validity evidence is frequently more easily gathered for these types of examinations than for constructed-response items. All types of reproducibility estimates (internal consistency, Generalizability Theory analysis) are more readily obtained for these types of tests than for constructed-response tests. Nearly a century of research in educational measurement underpins these item forms, adding much reassurance to the quality of measurement. Measurement theory for these types of tests is well developed and comprises several models from Classical Measurement Theory (e.g., Anastasi, 1982) and Generalizability Theory (e.g., Brennan, 1983) to the statistically stronger Item Response Theory (IRT) models (Lord, 1980). While measurement models and a great deal of research is currently being developed for constructed-response forms, written test forms clearly have the advantage of many years of solid research.

Selected-response item forms are readily defended, as discussed above, if they are carefully crafted, administered and scored. If selected-response items are securely maintained (that is, examinees do not have access to the test questions), some items can be reused from examination to examination. Pretesting or item tryout is also more easily carried out for selected-response items than for constructed-response items, since it is more difficult for examinees to memorize many selected-response items than a few constructed-response items. Reuse of the best test questions adds to efficiency, since it is difficult to produce good selected-response test questions. Further, the reuse of items permits the statistical equating of test forms or passing score standards, so that absolute passing score studies do not have to be repeated for each administration of the examination. Reuse of items, pretesting, and equating are all more challenging for constructed-response items than for selected-response items.

Limitations of selected-response items

There are some limitations to selected-response formats. Some potential negatives associated with these item forms are: the possible cueing of the keyed correct responses, the possibility of random guessing erroneously adding to the score of uninformed examinees, and the relative difficulty of producing good selected-response test items. It is possible to create trivial item content with selected-response items, although this criticism is not limited to this particular item form. Finally, selected-response item forms are currently out of favor and are considered "politically incorrect" by many educators who may overemphasize some of the disadvantages of this item form and overlook many of the advantages.

Cueing and guessing correct answers

Critics of selected-response item forms frequently cite guessing and cueing of correct answers as a major problem for these items forms. If test items are carefully constructed, edited, reviewed and pretested, cueing and random guessing are infrequently major problems and add relatively little measurement error to test scores.

When items are written according to the generally accepted principles of test item writing (Haladyna & Downing, 1989a, 1989b), there is little potential for cueing correct answers such that uninformed examinees mark a correct answer when they do not have the knowledge needed to select the correct answer. Random guessing is also not a major problem with well written test items or on tests composed of sufficient numbers of items to produce reliable measurement. Examinees rarely randomly guess at test answers; examinees do use partial knowledge to eliminate incorrect answers (Ebel, 1972). Especially for high-stakes examinations, examinees are rarely so poorly prepared for tests that they feel the need to randomly guess. One should also remember that the statistical probability of achieving a high score on a short exam through random guessing alone is extremely low (e.g., 70 percent correct out of 30 three-option test items $p = 0.0000356$).

The number of item options is related to the statistical probability of randomly guessing a correct answer. If there are three options, with one correct answer, the probability of randomly guessing the correct answer is 0.33 for that one test item. However, the probability of getting two three-option test items correct through random guessing alone is only 0.11, three correct is 0.04, four correct is 0.01 and five correct is 0.004.

Difficulty of development

Good test questions are difficult and somewhat costly to develop. It is generally much easier and less costly to write essay questions than MCQs, for example. Item writer training is an important aspect of the validity evidence desirable for achievement examinations, as is test editing and review (Downing & Haladyna, 1997). These steps in test development all add to the difficulty and cost of producing good test items.

Trivial content

Critics of selected-response item forms often cite the triviality of the content measured by these test items. While it is certainly possible to write items which test trivial content that may require examinees to merely recall or recognize factual information, it is not inevitable that these items test trivial content. Good item writer training helps greatly to reduce the triviality of content measured and can lead to the production of test items that measure very high levels of the cognitive domain.

Political incorrectness

For many of the reasons cited above (and refuted), selected-response item forms are out of favor with many educators. These item forms have become almost politically incorrect in some circles. There is no question that there are many examples of bad selected-response tests, but it is equally certain that it is possible to produce high-quality selected-response examinations that measure very high levels of the cognitive domain.

There has been a bandwagon effect or movement toward constructed-response and performance examinations, especially in medical education. While these testing modalities can add much information on examinee achievement, they certainly do not and should not attempt to replace written test formats for the efficient measurement of cognitive knowledge.

TYPES OF SELECTED-RESPONSE ITEMS

Multiple-choice questions

Multiple-choice questions are written test questions with a stimulus question (*stem*) and a finite set of possible answers or responses (*options*), which has one or more keyed correct answers.

A multiple-choice question example is given below (Federation of State Medical Boards of the United States and NBME, 1997):

> A 67-year-old man has a nontender lesion on the top of his forehead. He states that he was hit on the head with a bottle 18 months ago and that the lesion bled recently. There are erythematous areas on other parts of his forehead. The lesion is 1 cm in diameter with a rolled-up, darkened border and a translucent, ulcerated center. Which of the following is the most likely diagnosis?
>
> A. Actinic keratosis
>
> B. Basal cell epithelioma
>
> C. Kaposi's sarcoma
>
> D. Melanoma
>
> E. Seborrheic keratosis

Strengths of the multiple-choice question

The multiple-choice question format has all of the general strengths of the selected-response format, as noted above, and only some of the weaknesses. The multiple-choice question format is extremely versatile and is capable of measuring almost all cognitive knowledge and educational achievement efficiently and in a straightforward manner. Higher-order cognitive knowledge, such as judgment, synthesis, and evaluation, can be measured by well-crafted multiple-choice questions (Maatsch, Huang, Downing, & Munger, 1984). This format is familiar to most examinees throughout the world, thus reducing any negative novelty effect for examinees. The responses to multiple-choice questions are easily machine-scanned and computer scored, providing accurate scores quickly and cost-effectively, especially for large-scale examinations. Scoring is completely objective, adding defensibility evidence to the testing process. This item format is perhaps the most well researched of all the written item formats, thus adding support to validity arguments. Multiple-choice questions, like most selected-response item types, are relatively easy to secure, pretest, and reuse on other forms of the examination; therefore, desirable measurement properties are an additional bonus for this format.

Data from multiple-choice questions, like most selected-response tests, are easily assembled into validity evidence. For example, since content-definition methods, such as task or job analysis (e.g., Knapp & Knapp, 1995) are well established, it is relatively straightforward to document the content definition methods used to develop multiple-choice question examinations.

All cognitive examinations are samples of some universe of knowledge or some well specified content domain. Multiple-choice questions allow straightforward sampling of the specified content domain, in fairly exact proportions to some test blueprint. Since each multiple-choice question tests a single specific *testing point,* it reduces the tendency to over- or under-sample certain areas of content.

Defensible passing standards are readily established for multiple-choice questions. Most of the research on standard setting methods has been carried out with multiple-choice questions, so there is added support for defending passing scores on these types of examinations. Multiple-choice questions can be time and cost efficient for both test developers and examinees. Multiple-choice questions maximize information attained about achievement per unit of testing time. The multiple-choice question format is extremely versatile, allowing well trained and experienced item writers to create challenging test questions which sample important aspects of cognitive knowledge.

Limitations of multiple-choice questions

Multiple-choice questions are sometimes criticized for their presentation of non-authentic content. It is sometimes said that patients do not present to the physician with a set of possible diagnoses from which the physician must choose the single correct diagnosis. This criticism should be evaluated in the larger context of all measurement. Tests are, by definition, not real life experiences. Even so-called high-fidelity simulations of clinical encounters are not real life – they are highly structured, standardized imitations of real life. There is a tradeoff between authenticity and measurement. The more authentic or real life the testing environment, the more difficult it is to obtain strong measurement properties for the examination. Some critics say that validity is traded off for reliability, but this criticism is blunted by the fact that validity evidence must include strong evidence for the reproducibility of scores and pass-fail decisions. Other critics argue that multiple-choice questions lack *face validity*. If face validity is defined as the appearance of validity, this argument is completely specious, since the appearance of authenticity or validity is not recognized by any measurement professionals as a type of validity evidence (Downing, 1996).

Good multiple-choice questions are difficult to write. It is especially difficult and challenging to create effective higher-order multiple-choice questions which measure important principles, problem-solving, and synthesis of novel information. The principles of effective multiple-choice question item writing are well documented (e.g., Haladyna & Downing, 1989a, 1989b). Training of item writers is an important source of test validity evidence (Downing & Haladyna, 1997) and may lead to more effective test questions.

Verbal ambiguity is a potential problem with all selected-response questions including the multiple-choice question format. Careful editing, review and pretesting of items can largely eliminate this potential problem. Cueing of correct answers and guessing were discussed above as general potential difficulties with all selected-response formats. If items are carefully written, edited, reviewed and tried out, these problems can be eliminated or greatly reduced. Traditionally, multiple-choice questions have four or five total options, with one option keyed as the correct response. There is some controversy about the number of options to use, but the research suggests that for high-ability examinees, three options is ideal (Lord, 1977). For all types of examinations, it is rare that more than three options are actually chosen by more than a small proportion of examinees (Haladyna & Downing, 1993). While it is true that more options lower the probability of randomly guessing the correct answer, there is little evidence that random guessing is an important strategy used by examinees, at least on higher-stakes tests. More options do tend to increase the reproducibility estimates for examinations, but there is little gain in reliability for typical examinations by adding more than about four or five options. The best advice to item writers is: Use as many options as makes sense for the particular test item. And there is no necessity (in most cases) that multiple-choice questions have the same number of options.

Matching and extended matching items

Matching and extended matching items have several stimulus prompts, with a finite set of possible answers (option list) to which the stimulus prompts must be matched.

Traditional matching items typically contain short stimuli that must be matched to brief statements (such as diagnoses); all stimuli and options are related concepts or conditions. Extended matching items (Case & Swanson, 1993) are typically longer, more complex matching sets, containing clinical vignettes as the stimuli which must be matched to a long list of possible diagnoses or treatments, all of which are related in some logical manner.

Traditional matching items

A matching item example is given (ACOG, 1994):

Each of the patients described below has symptoms of urinary urgency, frequency, and dysuria. Each has a midstream urine culture showing fewer than 10^6 colony-forming units per milliliter. For each of the numbered patients (1-2), select the most likely cause from the list of conditions (A-E).

A. Low-count bladder bacteriuria

B. Chlamydial urethritis

C. Urethral instability

D. Urethral diverticulum

E. Bacterial infection

1. A 36-year-old woman with symptoms for 2 years; additional symptoms include postvoid dribbling and dyspareunia.

2. A 20-year-old college student with pyuria and the gradual onset of symptoms over a period of 2-3 weeks. She acquired a new sexual partner one month ago.

Strengths of the matching item

Many of the strengths of the multiple-choice question are shared by matching items. Traditional matching items may be efficient for testing comparisons and related concepts and principles across broad content topic areas.

These items are fairly straightforward to write and edit. It is important that all options relate to some common concept or theme and that there are more stimuli than options, so that examinees cannot attain correct answers by eliminating options.

Limitations of the matching item

Matching items tend to measure lower-level cognitive knowledge, such as recall or recognition of facts. It is difficult, but not impossible, to write traditional matching items that measure higher-order cognitive knowledge. Since the focus of matching questions must necessarily be narrow (e.g., a set of related treatments for a specific diagnosis) and the items must pose classic presentations so that examinees can make correct distinctions, there is a tendency for this item type to test recall-recognition type information. Oversampling of test content may also be problematic, especially if large numbers of matching items are used on the examination. Since matching item sets must contain related concepts, it is certainly possible to test more extensively in some areas than the test blueprint requires. If some areas are oversampled, other content areas must necessarily be undersampled, thus reducing the test's validity evidence.

Extended matching items

An extended matching item example is given below (Case & Swanson, 1996):

A. Acute leukemia
B. Anemia of chronic disease
C. Congestive heart failure
D. Depression
E. Epstein-Barr virus infection
F. Folate deficiency
G. Glucose 6-phosphate dehydrogenase deficiency
H. Hereditary spherocytosis
I. Hypothyroidism
J. Iron deficiency
K. Lyme disease
L. Microangiopathic hemolytic anemia
M. Miliary tuberculosis
N. Vitamin B_{12} (cyanocobalamin) deficiency

For each patient with fatigue, select the most likely diagnosis.

1. A 19-year-old woman has had fatigue, fever, and sore throat for the past week. She has a temperature of 38.3 C (101 F), cervical lymphadenopathy, and splenomegaly. Initial laboratory studies show a leukocyte count of 5000/mm^3 (80% lymphocytes, with many lymphocytes exhibiting atypical features). Serum aspartate aminotransferase (AST, GOT) activity is 200 U/L. Serum bilirubin concentration and serum alkaline phosphatase activity are within normal limits.

2. A 15-year-old girl has a two-week history of fatigue and back pain. She has widespread bruising, pallor, and tenderness over the vertebrae and both femurs. Complete blood count shows hemoglobin concentration of 7.0 g/dL, leukocyte count of 2000/mm^3, and platelet count of 15,000/mm^3.

Extended-matching items are a variation and extension of the traditional matching question format. Extended-matching items have four essential components: a common theme of related concepts, a lead-in, a list of options which are usually lengthy, and two or more item stems.

Strengths of extended matching

This format encourages item stems that provide more detail (e.g., clinical scenarios) and usually contain a long option list. Case and Swanson (1989) show that this format is more difficult than multiple-choice questions, with higher item discrimination, and higher reliability estimates. Extended-matching items are best used for diagnostic questions, but are also used for testing management decisions. Because of the extensive clinical stems and patient situations presented in these items, they may measure higher levels of the cognitive domain than the traditional matching item.

Item authors appear able to produce large numbers of these items fairly easily (Case & Swanson, 1993).

Limitations of the extended-matching item

Over- and undersampling of content may be the most important potential difficulty of this item type, as with the traditional matching item. Also, attempts by item authors to take complete advantage of the longer option list may lead them to create questions that make trivial distinctions.

True-false and multiple true-false items

True-false items are short propositions, which must be answered as either *true* or *false*, and require the absolute truth or falsity of the propositions.

True-false items: True-false items are rarely used in medical education tests, but perhaps they should be reconsidered for some types of examinations. True-false items can be written to be very effective and challenging types of test questions that measure higher-order verbal knowledge (Ebel, 1972).

A true-false example is given below:

On a 100 item true-false examination, the probability of a student scoring 70 percent correct by random guessing alone is 0.0035.

Strengths of true-false

The true-false item is a very straightforward test of cognitive knowledge. Well written true-false items can test higher levels of the cognitive domain and can be very challenging to examinees. Long true-false tests (composed of 100 or more well written items) tend to be very reliable and may well discriminate between high and low scoring examinees. These items are extremely cost and time efficient, both for examinees and item writers. More information can be collected per unit of testing time with true-false items than with typical four- or five-option multiple-choice questions.

Limitations of true-false

Critics point to many limitations of true-false items. For example, true-false items may tend to test trivial content, if written by inexperienced item writers. This format, however, does not demand triviality of content; with training and experience it is possible (but difficult) to produce higher-level true-false items. Random guessing of correct answers can be problematic for short true-false examinations. But, since the probability of randomly guessing the correct answer for a single true-false item is 0.50, it is highly improbable that an examinee could receive a high score on a 100-item true-false test through random guessing alone. Some examinees believe that true-false tests measure only lower-level knowledge that is trivial; this belief, supported in fact or not, can be problematic for the use of this item format. Finally, it is very difficult to create good true-false items that measure important knowledge at a level that is appropriate to the examinees. Much training and experience is needed to create good true-false tests; there may be more art than science involved in the skills needed to create these items.

Alternate-choice items

Alternate-choice items are test questions with a stimulus and two response options, only one of which is true.

Alternate-choice items are similar to true-false items in that they have only two possible answers. They may also be thought of as a variant of the multiple-choice question with only two possible responses.

An example of an alternate-choice item follows (Ebel, 1982):

The items used in a criterion-referenced test are (1) distinctly different from (2) quite similar to those used in a norm-referenced test.

Strength of the alternate-choice item

The alternate-choice item does not require absolute judgments of truth or falsity, as does the true-false item, and may therefore reduce some potential ambiguity of true-false items (Ebel, 1982). The alternate-choice item may be more efficient than the typical four- or five-option multiple-choice question, since more scorable units can be obtained per unit of testing time than with multiple-choice questions. Alternate-choice items may also be somewhat more adaptable to higher-level cognitive measurement than some true-false items. Ebel (1981) stated *"there is no element of verbal knowledge, no mental ability, no achievement in cognitive learning that cannot be tested by using alternate-choice items"* (p. 3).

Alternate-choice items tend to be more reliable than true-false items and may discriminate high and low achievers slightly better (Ebel, 1981, 1982).

Limitations of alternate-choice items

Many of the potential difficulties of the true-false item format also pertain to the alternate-choice format. The potential for a guessing effect is present, if few alternate-choice items comprise a test, but this is not a problem if sufficient numbers of alternate-choice items are used. Beliefs about the triviality of content, as with true-false items, persist, although there is little or no empirical evidence to suggest that this is an inherent flaw of the alternate-choice item type.

Multiple true-false items

Multiple true-false items contain a stimulus (the stem) followed by a finite set of answers (options) each of which must be responded to as *true* or *false*.

An example of a multiple true-false item follows (Downing, Baranowski, Grosso, & Norcini, 1995):

Which of the following favor(s) the diagnosis of Eaton-Lambert syndrome over myasthenia gravis?

A. *Thymic hyperplasia*

B. *Normal extraocular muscle function*

C. *The presence of circulating acetylcholine receptor antibodies*

D. *An increasing response of a muscle to repetitive voluntary movements*

Strengths of multiple true-false

Examinees must respond *true* or *false* to each option of the *multiple true-false* item. These items produce many scorable units per question and therefore produce efficient information about examinee achievement. Most timing studies (e.g., Frisbie, 1992) show the ratio of multiple true-false items to multiple-choice questions answered per minute ranges from about 2.3 to 3.4.

Many of the strengths of the multiple-choice question and matching item forms may also pertain to the multiple true-false item format. Multiple true-false items tend to be more reliable than comparable multiple-choice questions, when the reliability estimates are adjusted for equal amounts of testing time (Frisbie, 1992). These items tend to be more difficult than multiple-choice questions in some studies (e.g., Kreiter & Frisbie, 1989). Validity studies using multiple true-false items are sparse, but Frisbie and Sweeney (1982) showed that multiple true-false items and multiple-choice questions measure about the same cognitive knowledge. Albanese, Kent, and Whitney (1977) found that multiple true-false items predicted GPA (student grade point average) about as well as other formats, such as multiple-choice questions.

Limitation of multiple true-false items

As with matching and extended matching formats, the multiple true-false format may tend to oversample content. It is also difficult to appropriately combine multiple true-false scores with scores from other formats (such as multiple-choice questions) because of the differences in time needed to complete multiple-choice questions and multiple true-false items. In one study (Downing, Grosso, & Norcini, 1994), criterion-related validity coefficients were lower for multiple true-false items than for comparable multiple-choice questions. Multiple true-false items also tend to measure lower cognitive levels than some multiple-choice questions. For example, Downing, Baranowski, Grosso, and Norcini (1995) showed that 40% to 80% of multiple true-false items were classified as measuring knowledge, rather than synthesis or judgment, on subspecialty certification examinations in Internal Medicine.

CONSTRUCTED-RESPONSE ITEM FORMATS

Constructed-response examinations require the examinee to create responses rather than select answers from lists of possible answers. Constructed-response tests comprise many different formats, ranging from the traditional long and short essay examinations to very high-fidelity computer simulations.

Strengths of constructed-response forms

The greatest perceived strength of constructed-response item forms is that examinees must supply answers to questions rather than select those answers from a predefined list. Examinee responses are non-cued and this is generally believed to be a more complex and authentic examinee task than recognizing correct answers. Further, it is generally held that constructed-response forms measure higher-order cognitive tasks and do this more easily than selected-response formats. The research evidence for this perceived advantage of constructed-response over selected-response is sparse, but nevertheless, constructed-response is typically thought to require different skills than selected-response formats (Bennett, 1991).

Some types of constructed-response formats, such as long and short essays, are much easier to write than most selected-response formats. For all essay-type formats, there is no need to devise a list of plausible distractors or to write a lengthy stem giving a long patient history or clinical situation.

Limitations of constructed-response forms

It is difficult, inefficient, and costly to score constructed-response answers objectively and in a reproducible manner. Thus, it is difficult to create constructed-response examinations that have as strong measurement properties as selected-response tests. Since it is a great deal more difficult and costly to obtain reproducible examinee scores from constructed-response formats, validity evidence for these formats is harder to obtain. It may be harder to defend constructed-response examinations than typical selected-response tests.

In order to score written constructed-response examination answers reliably, it is generally necessary to use multiple independent readers or raters and to use their average ratings of the essay answers as the examinee score. Interrater agreement is an important aspect of score reproducibility for these tests (e.g., Ebel, 1951). Essay raters must be well trained and calibrated, using standard or model answers to questions, and their rating performance must be monitored over time, especially for large-scale, standardized constructed-response tests. Model or sample correct answers make explicit the range of correct and incorrect answers. This rating process is, therefore, expensive and time consuming, often requiring expert judgment from content experts in the discipline tested, further adding to the cost and complexity of the constructed-response rating process.

While there is much research and development underway in the area of computer scoring of open-ended constructed-response test questions (e.g., Martinez & Bennett, 1992; Kaplan, 1992), there may be no practical way to computer-score high-stakes, written constructed-response tests such as essays at this time.

It is also difficult to adequately sample a large cognitive domain with some types of constructed-response items. For example, if only a few long essays are used in a test, it is likely that the universe of cognitive knowledge will be inadequately sampled.

It should be noted that selected-response formats were developed, in large measure, to compensate for the real limitations of constructed-response formats. There is little research evidence that constructed-response forms measure anything very different from selected-response formats. Typically, constructed-response and selected-response formats correlate highly, especially when both measures are corrected for the attenuation due to unreliability of both measures (Downing & Norcini, 1998). Thus, the perceived advantage of constructed-response over selected-response is somewhat questionable for many testing settings, especially for large-scale, standardized, and high-stakes examinations.

TYPES OF CONSTRUCTED-RESPONSE ITEMS

Long and short essays

Long essay examinations typically consist of a few open-ended essay questions which require lengthy written responses from examinees. Short essay tests generally consist of many essay questions which require short written answers, consisting of a sentence or two. Very short essays may have a stem question similar to an multiple-choice question and require the examinee to give a brief written answer. Very short essays are a variant of the short essay format. Tests composed of short essays are, in general, preferable to long essay tests.

Strengths of long and short essay questions

The greatest advantage of all essay-type examinations is that they require examinees to produce written responses to open-ended questions in a completely non-cued format. Educators consistently believe that producing responses is a more complex, higher-order cognitive task than recognizing correct answers from a list and that this is a more real-life or authentic task and is therefore better.

It is possible to evaluate the thought or reasoning processes which examinees use to answer open-ended essay questions or, at least, this is often cited as an advantage of essay questions over selected-response items. It may indeed be possible to evaluate the logic or the reasoning processes which examinees use to arrive at their answers, but it is a very difficult task to score this factor objectively. For lower-stakes tests, such as classroom-type quizzes, it may be quite reasonable to attempt to give some type of partial credit to examinee logic or reasoning, even if their answer is not completely correct. Essay readers, however, must accept some subjectivity in this type of scoring and realize that the reproducibility of their scores may be low.

Currently, written essay-type responses are about the only way to assess examinee writing skills. So, if the objective of the test is to measure writing ability or skill, essay-type, open-ended *production* tests are about the only format available. A computer may be used to record and at least partially score such writing tests, but human readers of these essay writing tests will most likely be required, at least for higher-stakes examinations.

Limitations of long and short essay questions

There are many limitations to long and short essay examinations and the key to their effective use must be that the advantages should outweigh the disadvantages for a specific testing purpose.

Essay-type tests are difficult, costly, and inefficient to score reliably. For any high-stakes essay testing, multiple raters must be used and the mean ratings from multiple independent raters are used as examinee scores. Raters must be well trained, model answers to essay questions must be used, and rater performance must be monitored. Interrater reliability is an important source of reproducibility evidence, since rater error is a primary source of measurement error for these types of examinations. Reading essays is time intensive and costly, since professional content experts must often be employed to do essay reading, at least for higher-stakes examinations.

It is difficult to adequately sample a large, complex cognitive domain, especially with long essay examinations, since the sampling of content is very limited by using only a few questions. This sampling inadequacy may lead to reduced validity evidence for the examination.

Both long and short essay tests minimize the information gained about examinee achievement per unit of testing time. Since production of written responses takes examinees considerably longer than completing selected-response item responses, much less information is gained about cognitive achievement in the domain than with typical selected-response tests.

Defensible passing standards may be more difficult to establish for essay-type or open-ended tests than for selected-response tests. Methods for setting defensible absolute passing scores for selected-response examinations are well established and well researched; such methods are more tedious and less well researched for constructed-response tests.

It is generally more difficult to defend constructed-response test scores than it is selected-response scores. Constructed-response scores are more subjective, by definition, than selected-response scores, since human readers are involved in making judgments about the adequacy of examinee answers. The necessity for multiple independent essay readers, the training and tracking of rater performance, and the use of model answers all are aimed at reducing the subjectivity of constructed-response ratings.

Modified essay questions

Modified essay questions are clinical problem-solving exercises in which a patient clinical vignette is presented, with short essay-type questions interspersed throughout. Patient history and clinical data are revealed gradually throughout the exercise, with more open-ended, short essay-type questions spread throughout the case.

Modified essay questions have some similarities with Patient Management Problems (PMPs) which are highly structured written simulations of problem-solving cases (McGuire & Babbott, 1967).

Strengths of modified essay questions

Modified essay questions have most of the strengths of the short-essay format, plus this item form is a type of mini-simulation in that the short-essay questions are imbedded in a clinical case. The modified essay question format has been shown to be fairly reliable (Feletti, 1980; Norman, Smith, & Powles, 1987). Modified essay questions and multiple-choice questions are moderately correlated (Irwin & Bamber, 1982) and also have been shown to predict clinical evaluations (Stratford & Pierce-Fenn, 1985).

Limitations of modified essay questions

The limitations of the modified essay question format are the same as those noted for the long and short essays. In addition to the difficulty of scoring and the content sampling problems of all essays, examinees may look forward in the test books to gain information or change previous answers, after more data are revealed. Computer administration of modified essay questions could solve this problem. Also, the lack of statistical independence of questions within modified essay question cases may reduce the psychometric quality of these examinations.

SIMULATION FORMATS

Simulation formats present stimuli with varying degrees of fidelity to real life or with varying authenticity. These types of examinations require examinees to gather data, make decisions and judgments or take actions that are somewhat similar to real life decisions and actions.

All test formats are simulations. Selected-response items are low-fidelity simulations of real life, while the simulation formats, such as the National Board of Medical Examiner's *Primum Computer-based Case Simulations* (CCS) (Federation of State Licensure Boards of the United States and NBME, 1999) is a high-fidelity computer simulation of actual patient encounters.

Tests are not and should not be real life. All tests strive to elicit maximum behavior from examinees. It is very difficult to elicit maximum or the best behavior from non-standardized stimuli in real life and it is almost impossible to score and interpret the meaning of such tests carried out in real-life settings (such as live patient examinations). Since the inherent difficulty of real-life cases varies so widely, and the settings in which these real-life cases are found vary greatly, it is almost impossible to objectively score real-life tests, using real patients or real stimuli in natural settings. While these types of examinations may feel and look authentic and valid, it is extremely difficult to assemble defensible validity evidence for real-life examinations. For this reason, for example, most medical specialty boards in the United States have abandoned the bedside oral examination, though they are still commonly found in other parts of the world.

Strengths of simulation questions

The greatest strength of simulations is their requirement that examinees interact with more realistic problems and attempt to solve those problems in a manner that reflects real life more closely than many selected-response tests. This may also be their greatest limitation and impose the greatest measurement burden on the format.

The higher the fidelity of the simulation, the more like real life the test is and the more authentic the examination seems. The test has the *feel* of validity, but it may be very difficult to assemble real validity evidence for these types of examinations and to defend their scoring.

With the simulation formats, it is possible to creatively score examinee responses, especially with computer-administered simulations. Partial credit can be given for various paths through the problem-solving exercise and various types of novel scoring can be carried out to attempt to assess and evaluate various aspects of examinee problem-solving behavior.

Limitations of simulation questions

Despite their intuitive appeal as measures of more real-life problem solving, there are many difficulties and challenges to the simulation formats.

These formats are very difficult and costly to create, especially the higher-fidelity computer simulations of complex problem solving. They are also difficult to score fairly, accurately, reproducibly, and defensibly.

Human problem-solving behavior is a complex process, so its measurement and evaluation is necessarily a complex enterprise. This very complexity leads to enormous challenges for creating realistic and accurate simulations and presents difficulties in scoring fairly and defensibly, especially for high-stakes examinations. Since these tests are not scored as *correct* or *incorrect,* but rather as partially correct, depending on the type of problem exercise and the scoring rubrics being used, it is difficult to produce reliable scores that accurately reflect examinee skill or ability in the content area being sampled.

Case specificity may also reduce the reliability and validity evidence for this type of measurement. Because of this phenomenon, many cases must be used to fully assess the cognitive domain of interest. The development, administration, and scoring of many cases adds to the cost and overall inefficiency of this format for the assessment of cognitive knowledge.

The psychometric theory of simulation measurement is in its infancy, compared to the theoretical framework and research base of selected-response testing. This too tends to reduce somewhat the confidence one places on simulation measurement, especially for higher-stakes tests.

RECOMMENDATIONS FOR FUTURE RESEARCH

Computer-administered testing of all types is the future of the assessment of knowledge. Thus, the research agenda should be directed toward computer testing.
- Research and development on delivery systems for all types of computer-based testing.
- Research on new selected-response item forms that use the full power of the computer.
- Research on computer scoring of constructed-response item forms.
- Research on computer simulation formats that are designed using cognitive or problem-solving theory.
- Research on psychometric theory specifically directed toward computer testing.

GUIDELINES FOR PRACTITIONERS

The following points summarize suggestions to practitioners:
- Use objectively scored selected-response items wherever possible.
- Use well written and edited multiple-choice questions wherever possible.
- The number of options for multiple-choice questions need not always be four or five; three options are sufficient in many cases.
- Use computer-based selected-response tests where feasible.
- Avoid constructed-response formats for high-stakes testing unless there are resources available to support a large-scale research and development effort.
- Use constructed-response formats sparingly if you wish to efficiently assess cognitive knowledge.

REFERENCES

ACOG. (1994). *Prolog, Gynecology* (3rd ed.). Washington: DC: Author.

Albanese, M. A., Kent, T. H., & Whitney, D. R. (1977, November). A comparison of the difficulty, reliability, and validity of complex multiple-choice, multiple response and multiple true-false items. Paper presented at the AAMC annual conference on Research in Medical Education, Washington, DC: American Association of Medical Colleges

Anastasi, A. (1982). *Psychological testing* (5th ed.). New York: Macmillan.

Anderson, J. R., & Bower, G. H. (1973). *Human associative memory*. Washington, DC: V.H. Winston.

Angoff, W. H. (1971). Scales, norms, and equivalent scores. In R. L. Thorndike (Ed.), *Educational measurement* (pp. 508-600). Washington, DC: American Council on Education.

Bennett, R. E. (1991). *On the meanings of constructed-response*. Princeton, NJ: Educational Testing Service.

Berk, R. A. (1986). A consumer's guide to setting performance standards on criterion-referenced tests. *Review of Educational Research, 56,* 137-172.

Bloom, B. S., Engelhart, M. D., Furst, E. J., Hill, W. H., & Kratwohl, D. R. (1956). *Taxonomy of educational objectives*. New York: Longman.

Brennan, R. L. (1983). *Elements of generalizability theory*. Iowa City, IA: ACT.

Case, S. M., & Swanson, D. B. (1996). *Constructing written test questions for the basic and clinical sciences*. Philadelphia, PA: National Board of Medical Examiners.

Case, S. M., & Swanson, D. B. (1989, April). Evaluating diagnostic pattern: A psychometric comparison of items with 15, 5, and 2 options. Paper presented at the annual meeting of the American Educational Research Association, San Francisco, CA.

Case, S. M., & Swanson, D. B. (1993). Extended-matching items: A practical alternative to free-response questions. *Teaching and Learning in Medicine, 5,* 107-115.

Cronbach, L. J. (1951). Coefficient alpha and the internal structure of tests. *Psychometrika, 16,* 297-334.

Dibello, L. V., Roussos, L. A., & Stout, W. F. (1993). Unified cognitive/psychometric diagnosis foundations and application. Paper presented at the annual meeting of the American Educational Research Association, Atlanta, Ga.

Downing, S. M. (1996). Test validity evidence: What about face validity? *CLEAR Exam Review, 7,* 31-33.

Downing, S. M., & Haladyna, T. M. (1997). Test item development: Validity evidence from quality assurance procedures. *Applied Measurement in Education, 10,* 61-82.

Downing, S. M., & Norcini, J. J. (1998). Constructed response or multiple choice: Does the format make a difference for prediction? In T.M. Haladyna (Chair*), Constructed response or multiple choice: A research synthesis. Symposium conducted at the annual meeting of the American Educational Research Association,* San Diego, CA.

Downing, S. M., Baranowski, R. A., Grosso, L. J., & Norcini, J .J. (1995). Item type and cognitive ability measured: The validity evidence for multiple true-false items in medical specialty certification. *Applied Measurement in Education, 8,* 189-199.

Downing, S. M., Grosso, L. J., & Norcini, J. J. (1994, April). Multiple true-false items: Validity in medical specialty certification. Paper presented at the annual meeting of the National Council on Measurement in Education, New Orleans, LA.

Ebel, R. L. (1951). Estimation of the reliability of ratings. *Psychometrika, 16,* 407-424.

Ebel, R. L. (1972). *Essentials of educational measurement.* Englewood Cliffs, NJ: Prentice-Hall.

Ebel, R. L. (1981, April). Some advantages of alternate-choice items. Paper presented at the annual meeting of the National Council on Measurement in Education, Los Angeles, CA.

Ebel, R. L. (1982). Proposed solutions to two problems of test construction. *Journal of Educational Measurement, 19,* 267-278.

Federation of State Medical Boards of the United States and the National Board of Medical Examiners. (1999). *USMLE: Computer-based testing: Bulletin of information.* Philadelphia, PA.

Federation of State Medical Boards of the United States and the National Board of Medical Examiners. (1997). *USMLE Step 2: General instructions, content description, and sample items.* Philadelphia, PA: Author.

Feletti, G. I. (1980). Reliability and validity studies on modified essay questions. *Journal of Medical Education, 5,* 933-941.

Frisbie, D. A. (1992). The multiple true-false format: A status review. *Educational Measurement: Issues and Practice, 11,* 21-26.

Frisbie, D. A., & Sweeney, D. C. (1982). The relative merits of multiple true-false achievement tests. *Journal of Educational Measurement, 19,* 99-105.

Haladyna, T. M., & Downing, S. M. (1989a). A taxonomy of multiple-choice item-writing rules. *Applied Measurement in Education, 2,* 37-50.

Haladyna, T. M., & Downing, S. M. (1989b). Validity of a taxonomy of multiple-choice item-writing rules, *Applied Measurement in Education, 2,* 51-78.

Haladyna, T. M., & Downing, S. M. (1993). How many options is enough for a multiple-choice test item? *Educational and Psychological Measurement, 53,* 999-1010.

Irwin, W. G., & Bamber J. B. (1982). The cognitive structure of the modified essay question. *Medical Education, 16,* 326-331.

Kane, M. (1992). An argument-based approach to validity. *Psychological Bulletin, 112,* 527-535.

Kaplan, R. M. (1992). Scoring natural language free-response items – A practical approach. *Proceedings of the 33rd Annual Conference of the Military Testing Association* (pp. 514-518).

Knapp, J. E., & Knapp, L. G. (1995). In J. C. Impara (Ed.), *Licensure testing: Purposes, procedures, and practices* (pp. 93-116). Lincoln, NE: Buros Institute of Mental Measurements.

Kreiter, C. D., & Frisbie, D. A. (1989). Effectiveness of multiple true-false items. *Applied Measurement in Education, 2,* 207-216.

Kuder, G. F., & Richardson, M. W. (1937). The theory of the estimation of test reliability. *Psychometrika, 2,* 151-160.

Livingston, S. A., & Zieky, M. J. (1982). *Passing scores: A manual for setting standards of performance on educational and occupational tests*. Princeton, NJ: Educational Testing Service.

Lord, F. M. (1977). Optimal number of choices per item – A comparison of four approaches. *Journal of Educational Measurement, 14,* 33-38.

Lord, F. M. (1980). *Applications of item response theory to practical testing problems*. Hillsdale, NJ: Lawrence Erlbaum.

Maatsch, J. L., Huang, R. R., Downing, S. M., & Munger, B. S. (1984). The predictive validity of test formats and a psychometric theory of clinical competence. *Proceedings of the 23rd Conference on Research in Medical Education*. Washington, DC: Association of American Medical Colleges.

Martinez, M. E., & Bennett, R. E. (1992). A review of automatically scorable constructed-response item types for large-scale assessment. *Applied Measurement in Education, 5,* 151-169.

McGuire, C. H., & Babbott, D. (1967). Simulation technique in the measurement of problem solving skills. *Journal of Educational Measurement, 4,* 1-10.

Messick, S. (1989). Validity. In R. L. Linn (Ed.), *Educational measurement* (3rd ed., pp. 13-104). New York: American Council on Education and Macmillan.

Millman, J., & Greene, J. (1989). In R. L. Linn (Ed.), *Educational measurement* (3rd ed., pp. 335-366). New York: American Council on Education and Macmillan.

Mislevy, R. J. (1993). Foundations of a new test theory. In N. Frederiksen, R. J. Mislevy, & I. Bejar (Eds.), *Test theory for a new generation of tests,* (pp. 19-39). Hillsdale, NJ: Lawrence Erlbaum Associates.

Mullins, M., & Green, D. R. (1994). In search of truth and the perfect standard-setting method: Is the Angoff procedure the best available for credentialing? *CLEAR Exam Review, 5*(1), 21-24.

Norcini, J. J. (1994). Research on standards for professional licensure and certification examinations. *Evaluation and the Health Professions, 17,* 160-177.

Norcini, J. J., & Shea, J. A. (1997). The credibility and comparability of standards. *Applied Measurement in Education, 10,* 39-59.

Norman, G. R., Smith, E. K. M., & Powles, A. C. P. (1987). Factors underlying performance on written tests of knowledge. *Medical Education, 21,* 297-304.

Snow, R. E., & Lohman, D. F. (1989). Implications of cognitive psychology for educational measurement. In R. L. Linn (Ed.), *Educational measurement* (3rd ed., pp. 263-332). New York: American Council on Education and Macmillan.

Stratford, P., & Pierce-Fenn, H. (1985). Predictive validity of the modified essay question. *Physiotherapy Canada, 37,* 356-359.

Subkoviak, M. J. (1988). A practitioner's guide to computation and interpretation of reliability indices for mastery tests. *Journal of Educational Measurement, 25,* 47-55.

21   Clinical Performance Assessments

EMIL R. PETRUSA
Duke University School of Medicine

SUMMARY

Evaluation of clinical performance for physicians in training is central to assuring qualified practitioners. The time-honored method of oral examination after a single patient suffers from several measurement shortcomings. Too little sampling, low reliability, partial validity and potential for evaluator bias undermine the oral examination. Since 1975, standardized clinical examinations have developed to provide broader sampling, more objective evaluation criteria and more efficient administration. Research supports reliability of portrayal and data capture by standardized patients as well as the predictability of future trainee performance. Methods for setting pass marks for cases and the whole test have evolved from those for written examinations. Pass marks from all methods continue to fail an unacceptably high number of learners without additional adjustments. Studies show a positive impact of these examinations on learner study behaviors and on the number of direct observations of learners' patient encounters. Standardized clinical performance examinations are sensitive and specific for benefits of a structured clinical curriculum. Improvements must include better alignment of a test's purpose, measurement framework and scoring. Data capture methods for clinical performance at advanced levels need development. Checklists completed by standardized patients do not capture the organization or approach a learner takes in the encounter. Global ratings completed by faculty hold promise but more work is needed. Future studies should investigate the validity of case and test-wise pass marks. Finally research on the development of expertise should guide the next generation of assessment tasks, encounters and scoring in standardized clinical examinations.

International Handbook of Research in Medical Education, 673–709.
G.R. Norman, C.P.M. Van der Vleuten, D.I. Newble (eds.)
© 2002 *Dordrecht: Kluwer Academic Publishers. Printed in Great Britain.*

INTRODUCTION

The assessment of clinical competence is a key step in assuring that health-care providers have sufficient knowledge and skills to carry out their professional responsibilities in a competent and safe way. Techniques for assessing clinical competence have evolved dramatically over the last 15 years. In particular, techniques have been developed to measure the dynamic doctor-patient relationship while at the same time assessing the learner's clinical performance. First called pseudo-patients (Barrows & Bennett, 1972), then simulated patients and now referred to as standardized patients (Anderson, Stillman, & Wang, 1994), these people, typically laypersons, are able to accurately portray problems of real patients such that advanced practitioners are unable to tell the difference between standardized and real patients (Rethans, Drop, Sturman, & Van der Vleuten, 1991; Gallagher, Lo, Chesney, & Christianson, 1997). A relevant sample of clinical challenges, portrayed by standardized patients and organized in an efficient circuit, may be wedded with modern measurement characteristics to produce a credible and high-quality assessment of clinical performance.

While SP-based examinations have increased in use, the time-honored method of oral examination remains the preferred assessment approach in many countries. With variations, the typical oral examination includes an experienced faculty examiner who observes a learner workup one real patient. When a history and physical examination are complete, the learner presents his or her findings, a differential diagnosis and the rationale for this list. The examiner, who may or may not have observed the history and physical examination, then asks a series of questions to probe the learner's understanding of signs and symptoms and pathophysiology as well as clinical reasoning and conclusions. Variations on this general scheme are called *viva voce* or oral examinations. From a measurement perspective and from the literature on clinical performance, there are major limitations to the traditional oral examination. Very different patients for different examinees, limited number of patient workups for each examinee and usually only one examiner undermine the measurement quality of the oral examination. In the last twenty years an approach has been developed to overcome almost all of these limitations. This chapter will focus on the variations of this new approach and key research findings regarding its measurement and educational characteristics. A number of excellent and more thorough reviews of standardized patients and SP-based examinations have been published (Van der Vleuten & Swanson, 1990; Colliver & Williams, 1993; Vu & Barrows, 1994; Van der Vleuten, 1996). The reader is directed to these reviews for additional understanding of the research supporting these methods.

In general, the new approach typically consists of several patients who have been trained to portray their case in the same manner for each examinee. This training is intended to have each portrayal be as standardized as possible for each examinee. Patients may actually have the disease or clinical problem they are portraying or they may simulate them. Patients, real or simulators, who have been through training to produce consistent portrayals, are called standardized patients (SPs). Most variations of this approach have patients learn checklists of observable behaviors that are expected from examinees that the SPs or observers complete after the examinees finish the tasks of each station. Examples of the kinds of clinical challenges that may occur in a station are to interpret an X-ray, to attach leads for an electrocardiogram to a person, to describe a medical instrument and its purpose, to intubate a manikin and to instruct an SP mother about breastfeeding. These clinical challenges are arranged in a circuit for efficient administration (Harden, Stevenson, Downie, & Wilson, 1975; Harden & Gleeson, 1979). Examinees are assigned a starting point on the circuit and then all move clockwise or counterclockwise for their next station. Time allowed for each station is usually the same for everyone in the circuit. Examinees are signaled when to begin the next station. As an example, with a circuit of 12 stations each up to 15 minutes in length, 12 examinees' clinical performance would be evaluated on 12 different clinical challenges in approximately three hours. Oral examinations typically allow 60 to 90 minutes for the examinee to do the history and physical examination and then present to the examiner. An examinee's clinical performance could be evaluated with two patients in this approach in three hours. Developers of this new approach with all the variations must provide evidence that the new approach is better than established methods that purport to evaluate the same thing. This chapter reviews key evidence about the measurement and educational features of this multi-station approach for evaluating clinical performance.

Before presenting this evidence, a brief overview of measurement characteristics will be described. Primary among these measurement concepts are reliability and validity. Following this section, methods for setting pass/fail marks for cases and for a whole examination will be reviewed. Throughout these sections the consistency (or more accurately the lack of consistency) between models of clinical performance, materials in the examination, scoring and selection of measurement characteristics will be highlighted. Recommendations for important new research are addressed within each section.

GENERAL ISSUES IN ASSESSMENT AND MEASUREMENT

The two primary criteria on which tests, measurements or assessments are evaluated are reliability and validity. Reliability refers to the consistency of results. This consistency may be between two observers marking the same interaction (inter rater reliability), between two ratings of an interaction by the same observer at two different times (intra rater reliability), or between observed performance and an estimate of future performance (test reliability). There are several accepted approaches to estimating test reliability (Guilford, 1965; Linn, 1989). Challenges in an evaluation may be divided into two groups (e.g., first half-second half or odd-even). The correlation between scores on the two halves provides an estimate of test reliability. Another approach is to estimate test reliability from the proportion of cases or challenges answered correctly. More recently generalizability theory is the preferred framework for estimating test consistency (Brennan, 1983). The major advantage of generalizability theory is that components of the assessment exercise are identified and their separate contributions to the total variance in scores are quantified. This separation of components allows for more precise refinement or better interpretations of the data.

A body of evidence, not a single calculation, should establish the validity of an assessment procedure, the degree to which an examination measures what it claims to measure. Evidence may bear on the quality of predictions of future performance, whether that future performance is on the same assessment or on different tasks (predictive validity). If relationships between the assessment outcomes and other features of the concept being assessed (e.g., "if clinical performance improves with more education, then learners earlier in the educational process would be expected to score lower than more advanced learners") are empirically supported, then the assessment is said to have "construct validity". A third type of validity, concurrent validity, is claimed if strong relationships can be demonstrated between an assessment and other assessments administered at the same time. Educational validity may be claimed if there is alignment of learning opportunities with tasks and challenges in the assessment. For example if clinical performance is conceptualized as *a set of skills,* e.g., relationship, communication, history taking, physical examination, ordering diagnostic studies and an assessment and follow-up plan, then these *skills* ought to be the focus of the test. However, if clinical performance is conceptualized as "adequately addressing the patient's problem(s)", the focus ought to be the *complete encounter* as the unit of measurement. For the skills concept of clinical performance, validity of the examination rests with whether these skills are the focus of challenges and the units of measurement. For the second concept, however, validity would not rest with separate skill, but rather with the quality of the full encounter. Certainly "skills" are part of this full encounter, but are considered *interwoven* with clinical knowledge, clinical judgment and the ability to communicate with the patient.

Can both concepts of clinical performance be "correct"? Yes, but not for the same level of expertise. Excellent work by Elstein and colleagues clearly demonstrated that experienced clinicians are continuously considering convergent and divergent historical and physical examination information that bears on the diagnoses they are entertaining at a given point in the workup (Elstein, Shulman, & Sprafka, 1972). Further, measurement research with patient management problems rejected a "skills" orientation for evaluating performance due to the non-independence of items within skills and skills within problems (Yen, 1993). Both of these lines of research used advanced clinical tasks, addressing a "patient's" problem. It is conceivable that, at much lower levels of expertise, all that is expected is the skill of structuring history questions, for example. Does the learner ask the seven key questions about the chief complaint? Does she use open-ended questions early in the encounter? Are his questions unitary or does he string together three or four options as he asks the question? These evaluation questions focus on the *process* of taking a history and far less on how a learner directs the content of her questions, based on the patient's responses. If these evaluation questions are used with more advanced learners, but more advanced learners would be expected to invoke clinical knowledge and reasoning to guide the content and organization of their history questions while also using appropriate "skill" in conducting the medical interview, then the construct validity of the assessment is compromised. Thus, the validity of a clinical performance examination must be judged in the context of its purpose, the nature of performance expected from those being evaluated and the alignment of an examination's materials and scoring with the purpose and nature of expected performance. The quality of this alignment is one of the shortcomings of published work on clinical performance examinations. We will return to this issue of what ought to be evaluated at increasing levels of expertise later in this chapter. Now we will consider the frame of reference or the types of comparisons that may be made with examination results and the implications these frames of reference have for selection of various kinds of psychometric characteristics for the examinations.

Two types of comparisons might be desired from a clinical performance examination. One is the comparison of test takers to one another. A common use for this comparison is to determine the highest score so that an award may be given. This is called a norm-referenced framework. Another comparison is each test taker's performance with an expected performance. An example is where the expected performance is 70% of actions with a given patient. Every test taker's performance is compared with this number. All could accomplish more actions; all could accomplish less. This is called a criterion-referenced framework.

The index for reporting the reliability of an examination is different for these two frames of reference. The psychometric index for the consistency of a norm-referenced test is a generalizability coefficient. As mentioned earlier, whether actually measured or estimated, the reliability of a test will be higher when test taker scores are spread widely and where some test takers perform relatively well on most patient cases while others perform relatively poorly. For criterion-referenced comparisons, the consistency of classification is of interest. How consistently (reliably) are test takers classified as scoring above or below an expected level? This consistency may be indexed by a dependability coefficient, a phi coefficient or kappa. With the focus on classification, spreading test taker scores is no longer desired. An extreme example is where every test taker accomplishes 100% of expected actions. A good outcome occurs, there is no spread of scores, test reliability is zero and classification is perfect. In evaluating the measurement quality of a standardized clinical performance examination, first one must understand the intended frame of reference to determine whether the appropriate index of reliability or consistency is reported and then evaluate the size of the index.

How high does a generalizability or classification index have to be?

The general answer is "the higher the better". There is no absolute cut off for acceptable indices. As an index approaches 1.00, variability in the intended comparisons approaches zero. Licensing and certification tests have generalizability coefficients of 0.90 and above. Most reported indices of reliability for structured clinical examinations range from 0.50 to 0.75, with an occasional report of 0.90. Early work on the reliability of multiple station examination is shown in Table 1. There are steps to increase the reliability. One is to increase the number of cases in a clinical examination, but there are practical limits to the administrative time and cost of any examination. An interesting line of research investigated the impact of varying the length of time at a given station. By shortening the length of cases, more cases could be added to the examination without increasing administrative time.

In our experience, administering 20 cases of 30 minutes each proved too much time and cost for the North Carolina Medical Schools Consortium to continue. Twenty cases of 30 minutes each was determined from the literature indicating that it is the total amount of testing time, about 10 hours, that is most important in achieving a highly consistent or reliable result (Van der Vleuten & Swanson, 1990). However, without dedicated space, the schools had to take three evenings to administer the 20 cases to 20 students. With a class of 160, 24 evening sessions are needed to get all students through the test. Six weeks of testing by staff personnel who still had regular jobs during the day were too much. The following year, the Consortium limited the test to 15 cases of 25 minutes each, administered in two evenings. Shortening the length of time at stations would allow more stations in a given time period. Research on the impact of various station lengths is discussed below.

Validity

Research aimed at the validity of clinical performance examinations has typically taken one of two tacks. Either learners at different levels of education (e.g., clerkship students and advanced residents) are compared, or performance scores are correlated with other evaluations. In the first strategy, residents are expected to perform better than medical students; in the second, low correlations are interpreted as evidence that the clinical examination "measures something different".

Results have shown that indeed residents perform better on some components such as physical examination and assessment and plans; that is, they achieve a higher percent of expected results (Petrusa, Blackwell, & Ainsworth, 1990; Stillman et al., 1991b). Residents' interviewing skills actually are poorer than students' (Petrusa, Blackwell, & Ainsworth, 1990). Correlations between scores on clinical examinations and locally developed tests or faculty ratings from a month of interactions are all in the 0.20 to 0.35 range, slightly higher when disattenuated. Both strategies need critical analysis.

Table 1. Reliability indices from early studies of SP-based examinations

Study	Actual Test Time	Number of SP Cases	Level of Students	Number of Students	Index
Newble & Swanson (1983)	0.5-1.0 hrs	3 to 5	6th (final) year	429	0.31*
Vu et al. (1992)	11 hrs	17	4th (final) year	405	0.62*
Shatzer, DaRosa, Colliver, & Barkmeier (1993) A 5 mins. 10 mins 20 mins. B 5 mins 10 mins	3.5 hrs 2 hrs	11 11 11 8 8	2nd year 2nd year	15 23	0.62 0.82 0.77 0.52 0.60
Shatzer, Wardrop, Williams, & Hatch (1994) 5 mins 10 mins	1.5 hrs	12	3rd year	36 36	0.77 0.43
Stillman et al. (1990) Data gathering Interviewing	3.25 hrs 4.25 hrs	13 17	4th year	311	0.68 0.88
Petrusa, Guckian, & Perkowski (1984)	1.5 hrs	10	3rd year	343	0.26-0.50
Matsell, Wolfish, & Hsu (1991)	1.5 hrs	10	4th year	77	0.12-0.69
Rutala, Witzke, Leko, & Fulginiti (1990)	4.8 hrs	16	4th year	76	0.94**
Rutala, Witzke, Leko, Fulginiti, & Taylor (1990)	4.8 hrs	18	3rd year	74	0.74
Cohen, Rothman, Ross, & Poldre (1991)	5 hrs	28	4th year	36	0.74***
Mann, MacDonald, & Norcini (1990)	1.5 hrs	5 (of 15)	4th year	89	0.07

* From weighted variance components of multiple classes.
** Mosier methods for estimating composite reliability (Mosier, 1943).
*** Reliability for criterion-referenced tests (Suboviak, 1976).

Content sampling

The number of clinical challenges presented to a learner directly affects reliability and validity of the test. This is easily understood when thinking about testing knowledge. A single question, even an essay question, would never be sufficient to judge the adequacy of someone's medical knowledge. Similarly, a single patient is insufficient to judge the adequacy of clinical performance. There are a number of extraneous and unpredictable variables that could affect the performance (Swanson & Norcini, 1989). For example the patient could be a poor historian or have multiple diseases where signs and symptoms may relate to more than one disease, i.e., a complex patient. The learner may not have had firsthand experience with a similar patient problem. Further, if the observer has not had training, he may have personal biases, like "history is 80% of the workup" or "warmth" is the most important nonverbal behavior for the provider to exhibit. This observer will mark quite differently from another who has different views of appropriate patient care. If one or more of these extraneous factors influences the learner's performance or the marking unsystematically, the results will not be as valid an indicator of capability. Further, if this learner's performance will be compared with that of another learner who saw a different patient, the comparison will be less valid.

Research in the early 1970s on clinical problem solving and clinical reasoning clearly demonstrated that the diseases seen shape a physician's expertise. Clinicians will perform better on problems within their area of practice than on problems rarely, if ever seen (Elstein, Shulman, & Sprafka, 1972). "Better" means fewer questions and maneuvers, the eventual diagnosis in the differential earlier and more rapidly arriving at the single most likely diagnosis (Norman, 1985). For example a nephrologist would demonstrate expert performance working with patients with kidney diseases. However when this subspecialist is given problems in cardiology, performance is much less than expert. The reverse situation is also true, that the cardiologist would demonstrate expert performance for cardiology problems but only average performance for kidney problems (Kassirer & Gorry, 1978). This is called "content specificity". A valid performance examination is one in which challenges are sampled from the entire range.

Definitions of performance tests

Multiple station examinations of clinical performance have had a variety of names. The objective structured clinical examination or OSCE was the name given to a multistation examination by Harden and colleagues in the late 1970s (Harden, Stevenson, Downie, & Wilson, 1975; Harden & Gleeson, 1979). This examination had 10 stations each with a different clinical challenge to the student. The range of clinical challenges included interpreting a chest X-ray, educating a patient about diabetic foot care, describing the use of a surgical instrument and critiquing a videotape of an emergency. Each station was 5 minutes. Ten students could be evaluated on 10 clinical challenges within 90 minutes. From this early description of a multiple station examination, the term "OSCE" often is assumed to have only 5-minute stations. Casual use of terminology has blurred this assumption.

More recently tests of clinical performance are composed entirely of patient-based challenges. Encounter lengths have ranged from 5 to 30 minutes or more. Some test developers claimed 15-30 minutes was more valid because it closely approximates what happens in the real situation. Empirical results are not quite so clear. The reliability and generalizability coefficients reported by researchers using a 5-minute or a 15-minute station length have been very similar (see Table 1).

RELIABILITY OF DATA FROM SP-BASED EXAMINATIONS

The reliability or consistency of data from SP-based tests is crucial for accurate interpretation of results. A number of factors can influence reliability of performance tests (Swanson & Norcini, 1989). Consistency of case portrayal, recording behavior by the SP or other observer, marking of answers and student performance from case to case are the major ones. Research on the reliability or consistency of these is reviewed next.

SP portrayal and marking

Reliability of standardized patients' portrayal of cases is central to a claim that these tests are indeed standardized, i.e. that the same case is made available to every student. One large-scale study (Tamblyn, Klass, Schnabl, & Kopelow, 1991) investigated the accuracy of SPs' portrayals where accuracy was defined as the proportion of important clinical data (history, physical exam, affect) given by the SP when an appropriate occasion for such arose. Results supported the claim of standardization. The majority of SPs were between 75% and 90% accurate over multiple encounters. Where accuracy was below 80%, the cases usually involved simulation of physical findings or required special affect. One-third of the inaccuracies were correctable with further training. SP accuracy was not different with different trainers. Careful monitoring of SP portrayal is prudent, especially where SPs simulate physical findings.

Research on the impact of using several different SPs to portray the same case supports this high level consistency. In a comprehensive multi-station SP-based examination for final year students, of twenty-three cases where multiple SPs were used, nine had significant differences in scores derived from checklists, but only six were different when all of the cases' scores were analyzed (Colliver, Robbs, & Vu, 1991). Four cases had differences in the number of students classified as pass or fail. These differences were not detectable in total test scores or overall pass/fail rates. These differences would be predicted on the basis of chance alone. That is, the likelihood of obtaining at least 6 of 23 significant differences would be expected from random variation. Although this study did not investigate portrayal separately from differences in marking, the implication is that portrayal variation is minimal and does not affect scores on the overall test scores.

It is conceivable that multiple, repeated encounters by a single SP could decrease the consistency of portrayal and/or marking due to fatigue or mental interference from prior encounters. Studies on data from large numbers of students found no systematic decrement when one SP repeated the portrayal multiple times. Data from five years of testing (Colliver, Steward, Markwell, & Marcy, 1991) where several SPs performed as many as 70 portrayals for one class were analyzed. Between 13 and 18 SPs portrayed and marked all 70 students in a given year. Consistency of portrayal and marking early and late in the 15 days of testing each year were compared to find evidence of fatigue. Generalizability of checklist scores did not decrease from the first to the fifth cohort for any of the classes, nor did unexplained variance, an indication of measurement error. In a related study with the same data set (Colliver, Vu, Markwell, & Verhulst, 1991), checklist data were analyzed for trends over the fifteen examination days. A decrease might occur if standardized patients and/or students became tired. However, there was no systematic increase or decrease in mean checklist scores over the five groups of students. Again, variation in SP portrayal was not evident in the students' performance scores.

Another approach for analysis of changes in SP marking is comparison of SP ratings about the quality of the doctor-patient relationship with checklist performance to yield a more sensitive measure of the co-influence of the SP and the content of the case (Abramowicz, Tamblyn, Ramsay, Klass, & Kopelow, 1990). Preliminary analysis showed that statistical adjustments could increase the precision and hence the reliability of checklist portions of these examinations. However, this approach treats checklist items as independent, a dubious assumption (see section on Reliability of Total Test Scores below).

Other potential sources of bias in portrayal and marking

Conceivably gender, ethnicity, or use of non-native language might systematically influence marking and/or portrayal by SPs. Two studies found no effect for gender (Colliver et al., 1990; Colliver, Marcy, Travis, & Robbs, 1991). Data from approximately 150 students on 26 cases in two medical school classes were analyzed for same and cross gender pairings of students and SPs. Generally, performance of male and female students was not significantly different. Scores on cases portrayed by male SPs were 3.6 percentage points higher than female portrayals. However, women students performed about 2.7 points higher with women SPs than men students. There was no difference for men and women students with male patients. Although the overall differences in mean scores are relatively small, these might be important under a criterion-referenced framework. Authors hypothesized that the content of the cases may have favored one gender or the other. For example, with obstetrics cases, women students may relate better to women problems than men students do. This was addressed directly in a subsequent study.

Despite statistically significant student gender-by-SP gender interactions in a combined analysis of six medical school classes from one institution, no interaction was significant within any single class. Authors concluded that to the extent that gender interactions occur they are very weak effects. Male students performed only

0.02 points higher than women students with male SPs, while women students performed an average 0.72 points higher than men students with female SPs. On a case-by-case basis, there were equal occurrences where male students performed better and where women students performed better with both male and female SPs. There was no significant difference in performance between men and women students for the entire set of cases. Women students performed significantly better on six cases, while men performed better on five. Overall, there does not seem to be a substantial impact of student and SP gender on case scores or overall test scores. Neither study investigated gender differences for particular skills such as interviewing or interpersonal relationship where women might be expected to do better. No studies with medical students were identified that investigated race, ethnic origin or native language.

Outside the health professions literature, the field of interpersonal relations, perceptions, and reactions is rich with interesting and educationally useful research relevant to understanding and evaluating the doctor-patient relationship (Roloff & Miller, 1987). An example is the influence of affective responses, by SPs and by students, on each other, and whether this response correlates with changes in SPs' and/or students' performance. SPs' affective responses to some students might result in more false positive or false negative marking. Students may respond negatively to SPs portraying cases that physicians generally find difficult. The type of role portrayed by the SP, and whether that influences the accuracy of portrayal and/or marking, should be studied. For example, if SPs portray a difficult patient, do they mark more generously, especially for communication and relationship dimensions?

Another aspect of these clinical performance examinations that deserves attention is where SPs portray patients from different socioeconomic levels. If SPs rate the quality of the doctor-patient relationship by how the SP felt, the SP's values, experience with doctors, and general quality of interpersonal sensitivity are likely to influence the nature of those judgments. If people are recruited from a narrow socioeconomic or interpersonal sensitivity range, which is more likely if no real physical findings are needed, their judgments may be biased to the ways in which this group views interpersonal and doctor-patient relations.

To conclude, consistency of SPs' portrayal is very good, exceeding 90% of intended actions. Portrayal of physical findings and affective cues is less accurate, but may be corrected with additional training. Multiple repetitions by the same SP have a very small impact on case scores, but none on the total test scores. Gender of SPs and students does not seem to result in any systemic bias.

Small differences in percent scores do not influence generalizability coefficients, but may be important in pass/fail determinations. New research should focus on ethnicity issues, to investigate both bias and real differences that ought to occur. Background of SPs tends to be narrower than the population of patients; the influence of this should be investigated, especially where perceptions and reactions to the encounter from the patient's perspective are included in the evaluation of students. Finally, some attention should be given to determining when a therapeutic relationship is established, what behaviors are associated with higher ratings and whether a therapeutic relationship can be established in time frames typically allotted to SP encounters. A therapeutic relationship "goes beyond establishing rapport to relieving suffering" (Cassell, 1990).

Reliability of performance within cases

A number of studies have reported the reliability of skills evaluated in SP-based tests. Skills of history taking, physical examination and patient education may be evaluated within one case or with several cases. In general, the reliability of skill scores is lower than that of the test scores. Interviewing or communication scores sometimes are the exceptions to this conclusion (Petrusa, Guckian, & Perkowski, 1984; Petrusa, Blackwell, & Ainsworth, 1990). However, these studies need critical review on two important issues regarding the conceptualization and measurement of skills within cases. One issue has to do with the alignment of the construct of clinical performance being evaluated and analysis of skill data. The other pertains to the dependent relationship among skill scores evaluated within any case that has a clinical problem.

If clinical performance is conceived as "care for a patient", as would be appropriate near the end of medical school, the unit of analysis should be the case score. Artificial dissection of skills with these cases is inaccurate and misleading because early actions with the SPs tend to influence later actions and because this dissection belies the "care for the patient" concept. For example, if, while taking a history, a student does not consider an appropriate range of potential diagnoses, he or she may neglect to ask some questions on the checklist. Without this historical information the student may limit the physical examination maneuvers. Without historical and physical data the student's assessment and plan likely would not be as comprehensive as expected, based on the scoring of performance with the case. This is called cumulative error, and has been a problem in developing scoring rules for patient management problem and other case-based tests (Berner, Hamilton, & Best, 1974; Elstein, Shulman, & Sprafka, 1978; Yen, 1993).

However, for skill-oriented courses, such as interviewing or physical examination courses, students are learning techniques without having to decide which techniques to use. SP based evaluations in these courses should align with the course goals and pose challenges where students need only demonstrate the range and technical quality of interviewing process or physical examination maneuvers. Instructions for students and the design of the challenges should be consistent with these course goals. Of course, if these preclinical courses do emphasize a focused approach to a patient's complaint, then the clinical performance examination should have similarly structured challenges with scoring consistent with the concept of clinical performance being taught and evaluated.

To summarize, the reliability of skill scores tends to have lower reliability than full test scores because they are measured less frequently in an exam. Conceptual and measurement ambiguity occurs when skills are artificially dissected within cases where the unit of analysis should be the integrated and orchestrated performance for the case as a whole. Clinical performance examinations should be constructed so its challenges and scoring are consistent with the educational goals, the construct of performance expected, measurement frame and corresponding indices of consistency for the course or curriculum.

Reliability of total test scores

Van der Vleuten and Swanson (1990) summarized reliability data for total tests, using case scores as the unit of analysis. All reports were less than the proposed benchmark of 0.80 (Norcini, 1999). They recommended use of generalizability theory for conceptualizing and computing reliability. The vast majority of subsequent research has followed this recommendation. Table 1 summarizes reported reliability indices from early studies of SP-based examinations all of which fall short of the 0.80 benchmark. The next several sections will explore possible explanations. Issues mentioned in the previous section regarding the alignment between data reported in the studies, the purpose of the SP test and its measurement framework are pertinent for data in Table 1. Most of these reliability indices reflect a norm-referenced perspective (generalizability coefficients). This index does not include differences in case difficulty. The indices would be lower if case difficulty was included. In addition to the measurement framework other factors that might reduce reliability of total test scores are student fatigue, length of encounters and placement of the pass/fail mark.

Changes in student performance over the course of a multi-station examination

Over several hours or days of testing, students may tire and not put forth their best effort. Scores on cases near the end of the exam would be lower. Several research groups have investigated this possibility. The general design of these studies is to analyze case scores based on the order in which they were encountered. Of course, each student begins at a different place in a circuit of cases, but every student has a "first, second, third, etc. case". Scores for all cases encountered first are compared with scores for cases encountered second, third, etc. Petrusa (1987) found no change in mean case scores throughout a circuit of 17 cases lasting 3.5 hours in a medicine clerkship. Each case was 10 minutes and each case score combined checklist data with answers to questions that followed each encounter. In contrast, Ross, Syal, Hutcheon, and Cohen (1987) found a significant and substantial (one standard deviation) *increase* in average scores from the first to the last case in a 16-case, 90 minute, final test in an introduction to clinical medicine course. Case length was 5 minutes for either a brief history or physical examination of the cardiovascular or pulmonary system. Authors offered several possible explanations for this improvement including students' increasing familiarity with the format, a reduction in their anxiety and their more efficient use of time. One additional possibility is that, since only cardiovascular and pulmonary system cases were used, after the first few cases, students may have remembered more of their routine examinations for these systems and to incorporate them for the remainder of the test.

No fatigue or practice effect was found in a 16-case SP exam for senior medical students (Lloyd, Williams, Simonton, & Sherman, 1990). Each case was 18 minutes long with the whole test lasting approximately 5 hours. Correlations of case order and case score for 73 students revealed only two statistically significant correlations – one positive and one negative. Authors offered a unique hypothesis. They suggested that student and SP fatigue might have canceled each other. If students were tiring in the last part of the examination and their performance decreased but patients, also tiring, gave students more benefit of the doubt later in the exam, this could result in no net change of scores. To evaluate this hypothesis, independent ratings of videotaped performance on cases early and late by rested observers could be compared with marks from the original SPs to determine whether fatigue affected marking. A similar comparison could be made for student performance.

Length of student-SP encounter

Changing the time allowed for cases or stations might increase test reliability if more cases are added. However, if time for tasks is too short, students may not be able to complete their work in a way that shows they know what they are doing. Under a norm-referenced framework, if most all students begin their tasks in a similar way, but cannot finish, performance scores would be very similar (little spread) which would reduce test reliability. For evidence about balancing content sampling without unduly truncating performance opportunity, we can look to three studies that systematically varied station length and evaluated the impact. From a purely empirical perspective, Van der Vleuten and Swanson (1990) calculated the relationship between length of stations and the reported test reliability for the studies they reviewed. They found no correlation. Their interpretation was that shorter encounters compensated completely by allowing more cases, whereas tests with longer encounters had fewer cases but apparently obtained more information from each encounter. Later this possibility was studied experimentally.

In the first of a series of studies with clinical performance data from SP-based examinations in an introduction to clinical medicine (ICM) course and surgery clerkship, researchers had faculty observers use different color ink to mark student performance for three different intervals during any given encounter (Shatzer, Wardrop, Williams, & Hatch, 1994). The final examination consisted of five 20-minute, history-only encounters with SPs. Performance was tracked for the first 5 minutes, then the second 5 minutes and finally for the last 10 minutes. Norm-referenced generalizability coefficients were 0.52, 0.62 and 0.54. for the three intervals. Ten-minute encounters appeared to be slightly better for spreading student performance. However, variance among cases was 3.31, 5.29 and 7.84, respectively, indicating case scores (percent of items achieved) became more varied as students had more time with patients.

There are many important questions about patterns of examinee performance that should be answered. How do students understand the task of seeing SPs? Are they approaching patients as if in a walk-in clinic? Do students take instructions seriously even when explicitly told to establish a good relationship with each patient? Is there sufficient time to meet the challenges or are cases built with an idealistic expectation of performance? Do students demonstrate a more similar pattern of performance as they gain more clinical experience? Do SPs reveal signs and symptoms more easily if they perceive that a student has little idea about what to do? Do some students perform most of the critical actions early, while others eventually perform them only if allowed a sufficiently long amount of time with patients? If there is evidence that even a small number of students can meet the challenges, then exploration of educational and learner characteristics might reveal factors that are preventing the majority of students from achieving this level of performance. Do more experienced students perform the majority of important actions earlier than less experienced students? If so, then shorter cases at more advanced levels could be used. Do patterns of performance change when psychosocial issues are part of a case? Do case instructions, checklists and scoring policies at different medical schools influence patterns of performance differently, even though the cases are intended for students at the same educational level?

In a follow-up study students knew prior to the encounters that the maximum time with the ICM cases was either 10 or 20 minutes (Shatzer, Wardrop, Williams, & Hatch, 1994). In addition to total percent correct for each case, items were clustered for history, chief complaint, review of systems, past medical and social history and personal information. The pattern of questions from these clusters was analyzed at 5, 10 and 20 minutes for 20-minute encounters and at 5 and 10 minutes for the 10-minute encounters. Generalizability coefficients were 0.62, 0.81 and 0.77 for 20-minute cases and 0.52 and 0.60 for 10-minute ones. These coefficients indicate that student performance was more consistent (more reproducible) for the 20-minute encounters, especially when analyzed midway through the allowable time, than 10-minute encounters at the end. Apparently students accelerated their performance for the 10-minute cases. Students asked 68% of all questions in the first 5 minutes of 10-minutes cases, but only 57% of all questions were asked in the first 5 minutes of 20-minute encounters. However, when allowed more time, these preclinical students achieved an average of 50% compared to only 38% for 10-minute cases. Clearly the length of time allowed for cases influences not only how students decide to structure the encounter, but also the overall quality of their performances.

In the third study the content of cases was counterbalanced with the time for the encounter. Six of the 12 cases in an SP-based exam given at the end of the first surgery clerkship were 10 minutes, while the other six were 5 minutes (Shatzer, DaRosa, Colliver, & Brakmeier, 1993). In the second clerkship rotation encounter times were reversed. When computed from same-length cases in both clerkships, the generalizability coefficient for 5-minute encounters was 0.77 and was 0.43 for 10-minute encounters. Similarly to the previous studies for short stations, students apparently did relatively similar things as tracked by the checklists early in the encounters but did different things when they had longer with each case. One explanation might be that all students used the first half of allowed time to focus directly on the chief complaint or reason for the encounter. If sufficient additional time remained, what students did with that time changed depending upon the student and the case. Performance on the written portion of cases was essentially identical: 72.6% for 5-minute encounters and 72.7% for the same cases seen in 10 minutes.

Collectively, these three studies have mixed results and different implications for case or station length depending on whether the evaluation is conducted under a norm-referenced or a domain-referenced perspective. From a norm-referenced point of view, 5-minute encounters appear to be the most efficient length. However, from a mastery point of view, performance on 10- and perhaps 20-minute cases is better.

While Van der Vleuten and Swanson's (1990) recommendation that the primary criterion for determining station length should be the task or challenge presented to the student, the (mis)*match* of challenges in SP-based tests and those in typical clinical activities is an important factor in interpreting examination results. Most clerkship programs allow students a relatively long time (e.g., an hour or more) to work-up patients in the hospital. Further, the expected performance is a complete history and physical examination. Obviously this does not prepare students for focused workups in an examination. One wonders how well students would do if the educational tasks were the same as those in the performance examinations.

VALIDITY OF SP-BASED EXAMINATIONS

In general "validity" refers to the veracity of measurement; the degree to which it measures was it is purported to measure. The most compelling evidence for validity of clinical performance examinations is their "face" validity or the degree to which clinical challenges in the examination look real. Studying concurrent validity is easiest since its source are correlations of the performance examination with other available evaluation tools, such as ratings from supervisors, locally developed tests and licensure tests. Construct validity is at the heart of the matter. This calls for a detailed description of what clinical performance is, and assurance that the examination materials and scoring are consistent with this concept. Next one would hypothesize about the factors that might cause this concept to change in some way. Finally, one would identify naturally occurring factors or design a specific study to test the hypotheses. However, good evidence of concurrent and construct validity for Standardized Patient-based tests is difficult to find. Presently, the only other measure of clinical performance is ratings from upper level residents and/or faculty members. The validity of these ratings is suspect. Research and experience consistently find that faculty instructors rarely, if ever, directly observe students' interactions with patients (Maxwell, Cohen, & Reinhard, 1983; Mattern, Weinholtz, & Friedman, 1984; Stillman, Haley, Regan, & Philbin, 1991). Therefore, the data upon which their ratings of clinical skills are based are not similar to those evaluated in clinical examinations. Another ubiquitous problem with validity studies is that most are correlational, often using too few data points. These shortcomings are evident in the published literature about clinical performance examinations' validity.

After Van der Vleuten and Swanson (1990) reviewed purported evidence of concurrent and construct validity from a number of large-scale trials of SP-based examinations, they recommended that correlation studies of validity not be done. Many of these studies correlated scores from the SP-based examinations with other convenient variables such as ratings of students by faculty and upper level residents, ratings from clerkship directors and scores on local or national written examinations. Typically only moderate relationships with these other measures are found either because the actual relationship is not very strong or because the two measures being correlated are not highly reliable themselves. Despite these difficulties, authors continue to interpret the correlation coefficients as supporting the validity of SP exams. When correlations are small, authors often interpret this as indicating that SP exams measure something different from the other measures. When correlations are high, writers claim that SP-based exams are as good as written exams in identifying top students. A sample of these studies is briefly reviewed here to illustrate the difficulty with correlation studies.

In a study of construct validity, Stillman et al., (1990) correlated variables from an SP exam given to fourth year medical students with their NBME Part 2 scores[5] and clerkship grades. Within the clinical examination itself data gathering scores (history, questions and physical examination maneuvers) correlated with interviewing technique at 0.58. Data gathering and interviewing correlated with Part 2 scores, 0.28 and 0.06, respectively. All coefficients were disattenuated (the expected correlation coefficient when all test scores were perfectly reliable) for their less-than-perfect reliability. Correlations between data gathering variables and clerkship grades ranged from 0.21 to 0.35, while interviewing scores with clerkship grades ranged from 0.20 to 0.43. In another construct validity study with data from an internal medicine clerkship it was hypothesized that SP-based examination scores would increase from the second to the fourth rotations (Petrusa, Perkowski,

---

[5] The National Board of Medical Examiners (NBME) is the agency that develops the licensure examinations used in the United States. There were three "Parts", a basic science, a basic clinical science and a management oriented part. Subsequently, three "Steps" of the United States Medical Licensing Examination (USMLE) replaced these three examinations.

& Guckian, 1984); more clinical experience should result in higher performance. No statistically significant increase was found. Apparently educational activities in other specialties' clerkships that occurred between the second and fourth rotations did not contribute to that learned during the internal medicine clerkship, at least as measured with the performance exam.

Construct validity was also studied by comparing performance of third year medical students with first and second year residents (Petrusa, Blackwell, & Ainsworth, 1990). Again, the notion was "more clinical experience should result in better performance" but now measured in years rather than a few months. Upper level residents did do better identifying and describing physical findings, listing differential diagnoses and outlining management plans. There were no significant differences between students and residents for interviewing style or history taking. There was a trend of *lower* interviewing scores for upper level residents.

In a different approach to study construct validity, Cohen, Rothman, Ross, and Poldre (1991) compared faculty observers' global ratings of foreign medical graduates' performance in an examination with checklist scores also completed by faculty. Some observers remained at their SP stations and rated consecutive examinees on "approach" and "attitude toward the patient". Other faculty observers stayed with given examinees as they moved through three sets of five cases and then rated approach and attitude for performance across all five cases. Data were obtained from an SP exam used to select applicants for a pre-internship program (Rothman, Cohen, Dirks, & Ross, 1990). The same research design was used again in the exit exam taken after the pre-internship program. Ratings by faculty who observed examinees over five cases were the criterion against which to test ratings of that examinee by other observers at the various cases. Results from both studies were similar. The generalizability index for "general approach" was 0.76 and 0.77 for "attitude toward patients". Consistency of global ratings was lower than that for checklists, suggesting faculty may be using different criteria and/or expected levels of performance in judging approach and attitude. Another facet of construct validity of the global ratings was studied by comparing ratings about the same examinees in the entrance and exit examinations. To increase statistical power, data were obtained from both the 1989 and 1990 groups. Not surprising, ratings were significantly higher in the exit exam. Correlations between global ratings and total test scores derived from checklists were 0.82 and 0.78 for "approach to the patient" and 0.56 and 0.34 for "attitude toward the patient" for cohorts in 1989 and 1990. Correlations between ratings at individual stations with those made after five cases were statistically significant for both approach and attitude. However, intra-class correlations for these ratings were 0.49 and 0.47, respectively indicating that use of the global ratings, as the criterion to judge other facets of the multi-station examination, is premature.

Validity of case scores

Curiously, no research has addressed the validity of case scores in SP-based tests. In researching this validity, known differences between novices and experts in medical practice must be addressed as well. Other research (Elstein, Shulman, & Sprafka, 1978; Kassirer & Gorry, 1978) has shown that experts are more efficient in solving medical problems, especially within their area of expertise. If experts are included in the validity studies, their scores, especially scores derived from checklists, are likely to be *lower* than those of medical students. If performance of experts is lower than for novices with SP cases in these exams, then the notion that "more clinical experience should yield higher scores" must be rejected until reasonable explanations can be found. One likely explanation would be that the scoring of performance with cases is spurious. Simply changing the interpretation of case scores to "lower scores mean better performance" obviously would be wrong. Within the student population it is likely that some students are more advanced than others. Careful research is needed to discern the validity of checklists and their scoring. The educational utility of checklists must also be considered when judging their validity.

Checklists are extremely useful for specific, structured feedback to students. It is much more useful for a student to hear that he "did not auscultate the carotid arteries when examining a patient with chest pain" than to hear "your physical examination was marginal". One resolution is to have clinician observers complete both a checklist and a set of ratings for a student's performance. A related solution is to use clinicians as SPs. Retired faculty, physician assistants and nurse practitioners could portray patients across the life span. One of the first questions to answer here would be can these people be consistent in their repeated portrayals and, at the same time, be reliable in remembering specific actions and patterns of organization of each examinee.

The most important limitation of checklists completed by laypersons is that they do not capture the coherence or implicit logic of a student's approach with a particular patient. Clinicians are able to observe patterns in students' performance with a patient. These patterns of behavior indicate which differential diagnoses she is pursuing. If the pattern has questions from several different diagnoses intermingled, the clinician observer interprets this as "shot gunning". This implicit logic or organization of approach to the patient is a necessary and central feature to evaluate in higher levels of clinical performance. A number of recent studies have demonstrated that global ratings of these meta-level variables yield as high or higher reliability coefficients than checklists, whether completed by standardized patient or faculty observer. It is tempting to speculate that a major cause of "content specificity" is actually an artifact of the measurement tool. This is an excellent area for more research.

Educational validity

Less commonly discussed or investigated, but as important as construct and criterion validity, is the educational validity of an assessment tool. Educational validity for a standardized clinical examination occurs when there is alignment of cases and challenges in the examination with those during the students' clinical education. Educational validity is improving, but slowly. Whether in introductory clinical skills courses or the clinical clerkships, students are expected to conduct a complete history and physical on patients assigned to them. During the clerkships, assignment of patients to students is rotational without much concern for any clinical curriculum. For hospitalized patients often the diagnosis is already known. Rarely are students able to reason from the historical and physical data they obtain from a patient. Accuracy of students' data collection, if addressed at all, is judged by comparing a student's report of findings with what the intern and resident found. Without direct observation, no one knows the students' patterns of behavior and thus their reasoning skills during data collection. Further, establishing a good relationship with a patient is almost never observed for students whether they are in the hospital or the clinic. This is not to say that poor relationships are acceptable, only that no one observes or assesses this facet of students' clinical performance. The only time doctor-patient relationship becomes an issue is if the student does something to upset or offend a patient. Any expectation that these kinds of learning activities help develop good diagnostic skills seems unrealistic.

Clinical education should be structured to facilitate students achieving a high level of performance, at least on a specified group of patient problems. Usually students are assigned to clinical locations for a fixed period of time (for example 12 weeks) without much concern for the types of problems they encounter, the amount of prior information students are allowed to have, the implicit logic of data collection patterns and the quality of doctor-patient relationship. Residents may receive much of this over the course of 3 to 5 years of supervised practice. Regardless of whether this is a valid assumption for residents it does not apply to the education of students. The implicit educational philosophy for students seems to be that "allowing them exposure to the major specialties of medicine and participation on the health-care team" is sufficient. Clinical performance examinations, especially developed from a domain or criterion referenced framework, are in conflict with this philosophy. Developers will need continually to artificially adjust case scoring and test pass/fail rules in order to keep the fail rate at an acceptable level. Resolving this conflict of philosophies about clinical education and evaluation of medical students is one of the major challenges for medical education worldwide.

There is growing evidence from psychology and human performance research indicating that repeated practice with constructive feedback for the kinds of situations that will eventually be faced in life is necessary to achieve competent or expert levels of performance (Ericsson & Charness, 1995). No studies have ever shown any substantial increase in scores or pass rates on standardized clinical performance examinations taken by students during medical school. One study did show a specific improvement in performance for a structured neurology curriculum. This will be discussed later.

DETERMINING PASS MARKS FOR CASES AND TESTS

The practice of medicine is competency based; it is evaluated from a criterion-referenced framework. Clinical practice is evaluated on the basis of what was done, how well it was done and whether there was a positive or negative outcome for a patient. A recent report by the Institute of Medicine (1998) in the United States indicates that there are between 3% and 5% errors for hospitalized patients. Of these, between 40% and 60% were judged avoidable. Further, approximately 25% of these avoidable errors resulted in negative consequences for patients. It is the actions of clinicians (and the health care teams) that determine whether an error occurs. Performance in standardized clinical exams, especially near the end of medical school, should be judged the same way. Researchers in medical education have studied a number of methods for setting pass marks for cases and whole tests that are consistent with the evaluation framework used with actual practice.

A standard is defined as the level of performance (score) that separates important categories of performance (Glass, 1978; Hambleton & Powell, 1993). For example, a standard could separate "minimally unacceptable" from "minimally acceptable" or "passing performance" from "failing performance" or "just barely excellent" from "just less than excellent". The labels chosen for each category reflect the purpose and judgment of those using the test results. What is good enough? Just as with interpretations of reliability and validity, our concept of clinical performance, including the notion of "good enough" is key to a valid interpretation of an examinee's performance. Concepts of clinical performance may be relative to a level of education or may be more absolute as in "standard of care".

Setting a standard or a pass mark requires judgment. Faculty members bring a myriad of implicit and explicit concepts, values and experiences to a standard setting task. These may relate to their notion of what education ought to emphasize, what clinical performance should look like in learners at a given level of education and his or her particular views on how to best approach a particular patient in the examination. The following section describes studies in which different strategies and techniques were used to minimize any one person's biases to establish a specific score that separates passing from failing.

Research on strategies for determining pass/fail marks for cases and SP-based tests has increased dramatically since the Van der Vleuten and Swanson (1990) review where they could find no studies about pass marks in clinical examinations. Early work applied techniques developed for multiple-choice tests, such the modified Ebel method, the Angoff methods, reference groups and contrasting groups (Norcini, 1992; Linn, 1989). Techniques and their resulting pass marks applied to cases are summarized in Table 2. Table 3 summarizes approaches for setting a test-wise pass mark.

Table 2. Approaches for setting case pass marks

Study	Population(s)	Approach	Case Pass Mark
Vu, Barrows, March, Verhulst, Colliver, & Travis (1992)	4th (final) year	Author judgment	Minimal percent score
Norcini et al. (1992)	PGY1s (FMGs)	Protocol judgment	Continuous scale – Avg % score of "Fail" group; Dichotomous scale – Avg % score of "Fail" group then 1 or 0
Poldre, Rothman, Cohen, Dirks, & Ross (1992)	PGY 1s FMG "ineligible"	Critical elements	All critical elements for a given case
Stillman et al. (1991)	PGY 1 through 4	Modified Ebel Reference Group	[not reported] Standard score of 400
Rothman, Poldre, Cohen, & Ross (1993)	PGY 1s FMG "ineligible"	Global judgment from MD observer, then contrasting groups	Avg. of points of overlap for SP & written scores

In one of the earliest studies, three approaches were compared for setting a test-wise pass mark for an SP exam given to residents in internal medicine (Stillman et al., 1991b). Investigators used the modified Ebel method, the reference group method and the contrasting groups approach. All had been previously developed for written examinations. For the first method, physician judges classified each item for a given case as essential, important, indicated, or noncontributory. Items in the first category were assigned three points, those in the second category two points, one point for those in the third and zero points for those in the noncontributory category. Next judges discussed characteristics of a hypothetical borderline resident and then estimated the number of items in each category that the borderline resident likely would perform. This estimate was then multiplied by the weight associated with that category. These were summed and divided by the total number of weighted points available for each checklist. Finally this number was converted to a percent.

Results from several judges were averaged to determine a pass/fail score for a given case. For the whole test the pass mark was set at the average of case pass scores. With this modified Ebel method the proportion of 240 first, second, and third and fourth year residents who would have passed the full test was 79%, 86%, and 95%, respectively.

The second method used one group of test takers as the reference group to which all other examinees would be compared. Third and fourth year internal medicine residents were chosen as the reference group. Their percent scores for each SP case were normalized to a mean of 500 and a standard deviation of 100. A linear transformation placed all other examinee scores on this scale. All cases used a pass/fail score of 400, one standard deviation below the mean of the reference group. This pass mark also was applied to content items (history, physical examination and assessment) and interview scores. The percent of residents passing content items was 59, 58, 68 and 78 for first, second, third and fourth year residents, respectively. Pass rates for interviewing scores were 62, 72 and 80 (third and fourth year residents combined), respectively. Note that all residents in the reference group did not pass. These pass rates are considerably lower than those obtained with the modified Ebel approach.

Finally the contrasting groups methods was applied to the data. Typically, using other information, two groups are identified. One is considered "masters", with the other being non-masters. Both groups take the test and distributions of their scores are plotted. The case (or test) pass mark is that score that maximally separates the two groups. Pass rates for content items were 41% for first year residents and 63% for third and fourth year residents. Similar rates were obtained for interviewing scores. With only 63% of the "mastery" group passing, it was decided that the pass mark was unacceptably high. Performance for the two groups was expected to be more different than actually occurred.

In another study with post-MD examinees, a contrasting groups approach also was used, except that judges focused on items within cases and avoided the concept of "borderline examinee" (Poldre, Rothman, Cohen, Dirks, & Ross, 1992). Instead, eight judges indicated items within a case that they considered "critical and essential" for minimally competent performance on that case, i.e., a clinically referenced pass mark. The pass/fail score for each case was the sum of these items. These pass/fail scores were adjusted so that at least 80% of current interns (master group) would pass each case. These scores were then used in a 23-case SP-based examination to evaluate foreign medical graduates seeking residency positions. Sixty-seven foreign-trained graduates and a random sample of 36 interns 2 weeks into the year took the examination. Interns were the "master group" and the 43 foreign medical graduates not selected for residency positions were the "non-master group". The number of cases passed by the two groups was plotted and the point of maximum discrimination determined. The test pass mark was passing 17 of the 23 cases. Five interns (14%) would have failed the test. For 100% of the interns to pass, the test pass mark would have to be 16 cases passed. With this mark,

Table 3. Approaches for setting a test pass mark

Study	Population(s)	Approach	Pass Mark	Results % Passing	Consistency
Stillman et al. (1991)	Int. Med PGY 1,2,3&4	Avg of case pass marks	Avg case pass level	79, 86, 95%	Not reported
		Reference group	-1sd from standard score of 500	Content: 59, 58, 68% Interview: 62, 72, 80%	
	PGY 1 vs 3&4	Contrasting groups		Content: 41% v. 63%	
Poldre, Rothman, Cohen, Dirks, & Ross (1992)	PGY 1s FMG "ineligible"	Critical elements, then contrasting groups	16 of 23 cases	PGY 1s – 100% FMGs – 52%	Not reported
Norcini et al. (1992)	PGY 1s (FMGs)	Judged Angoff estimates	Contin – 54.8% Dichot – 5.6 (of 8) cases	100% 91%	0.97 0.77
Rothman, Poldre, Cohen, & Ross (1993)	FMG applicants	Empirical Angoff estimates	Contin – 54.6% Dichot – 15.4 (of 29) cases	81% 79%	0.64 0.58

52% of the "non-masters" would have passed. As with the previous study, the proportion of non-masters who would have passed was deemed unacceptably high.

A consortium of medical schools that administers the same set of SP cases to all students at all schools evaluated an approach that would create a clinical standard of performance for each of their SP cases (Morrison & Barrows, 1994). In general the approach was to ask clinical faculty members to identify "critical actions" for each case. Faculty judges were instructed to select those items that, if not done, would constitute either malpractice or a complete missing of the essence of the patient's problem. In other words, judges were to establish a clinically-based pass mark for each case. From one to three clinical faculty members identified checklist items, laboratory studies and post-encounter questions that had to be done or answered correctly. Authors were interested in the number of medical students who had achieved minimal clinical competence for each case and the set of 11 cases. For the purposes of this study, authors assumed that the educational goal was to have all students perform at least at a minimally clinical level on all 11 cases. The pass mark for the set of 11 cases was manipulated and the number of students who would pass was calculated. Results are shown in Table 4. If the pass mark for the 11 cases were set at "failing zero cases", less than 1% of the students would have passed the set and would have been labeled clinically competent (operationally defined as passing the set of 11). If the set's pass mark was lowered to "fail no more than 3 of 11" (27% of the cases), half of the students would be classified as "clinically competent". If the set pass mark was "fail no more than 6 of 11 (55%) cases", one interpretation of the results was "after 1 year of required clinical training (clerkships), 85-90% of medical students (n = 350) were performing at minimally acceptable clinical performance for about half of the cases". This interpretation seems very positive – only 1 year of clinical work and 85% of the class is performing at a minimal standard of care expected of practicing physicians for half of the cases in a standardized clinical performance examination. It is even more amazing given the near random assignment of patients to students. It is not out of the realm of possibility that a *prescribed* clinical curriculum (e.g., Des Marchais, 1993), composed of real, standardized, computer-based and paper patients, would

Table 4. Percent of students passing a test with various pass marks

Pass test with X failed cases	0	1	2	3	4	5	6	7	8	9
Percent of students failing	0.6	4.5	17.6	27.5	23.2	14.7	8.2	2.8	0.6	0.3
Cumulative %	0.6	5.1	22.7	50.1	73.4	88.1	96.3	99.2	99.7	100

result in 100% of students performing at least minimally competently for a domain of patient problems from which a sample was evaluated in a standardized clinical examination.

RELIABILITY AND VALIDITY OF PASS MARKS

Reliability and validity of these and other approaches to setting case and test pass marks are areas of important and urgently needed research. How much agreement is there between faculty judges about critical actions or borderline performance? How much agreement is there between faculty from research-intensive and more clinically oriented medical schools? What is the nature of differences between generalists and sub specialists in pass mark-setting exercises? From a validity perspective, it is important to know what differences occur when pass marks are set from case materials compared with those based on direct observation of performance without benefit of checklists. Qualitative work, such as interviewing clinician judges who have participated in checklist-based and observation-based procedures to illuminate their thinking and judgment, is central to the validity of pass marks. Do midlevel practitioners, such as physician assistants, derive the same pass mark as physicians, thus providing a less expensive source of judgments? Two studies that directly address the question of validity of pass marks illustrate the kinds of work needed.

Norcini et al. (1992) had judges determine minimally acceptable clinical performance for each of eight cases for evaluation of foreign medical graduates' readiness to enter residency training in the United States. Examinees were allowed 15 minutes with each SP who recorded history and physical examination actions on a checklist. After each encounter examinees had 7 minutes to answer questions about findings, differential diagnoses and management plans for that patient. The eight cases were administered to 131 first year internal medicine residents in their fourth to seventh month of their residency program. All were expected to pass this examination. To establish case pass marks, program directors who had developed the cases, sorted a sample of examinees' performances for each case based on checklist data and post-encounter answers into one of two categories. The two categories were either "at least minimally acceptable clinical care" or "less than acceptable clinical care". The average percent score of all protocols categorized as unacceptable became the case pass mark. This score was then used to categorize all remaining case protocols not directly examined by judges.

The test pass mark was established using a modified Angoff approach. After sorting examinee protocols, judges briefly discussed the concept of "borderline examinees" and then estimated the proportion of 100 such borderline examinees that would pass each case. Estimations for each of the eight cases were added and then rounded to the nearest integer. This was the number of cases that must be passed to pass the whole test. The consistency and reproducibility of these pass marks were evaluated using a continuous scale score, percent correct, and a dichotomous score, pass/fail for each case.

Performance on cases was typical of other SP-based tests where average case scores (percent of items done) varied considerably. Case scores ranged from 66% to 82% with a mean of 75%. For dichotomous scoring (i.e., passing = 1 and failing = 0), the mean case scores ranged from 0.74 to 0.99. With continuous scores, protocols classified as acceptable were at least one standard deviation higher than those classified as inadequate. With dichotomous scoring, the proportion of borderline candidates estimated to pass a given case ranged from 0.40 to 0.85 with a mean of 0.70. The test pass mark for continuous scores was 54.8% and all interns would have passed. Under dichotomous case scoring, with a test pass mark of 5.56 cases (70% of 8.0), 91% would have passed.

This study raises interesting research questions. How many examinees, classified as failing a case, had higher percent scores than those classified as passing? The answer is both clinically and educationally meaningful. Would judgments be more similar if based on direct observation? A variation on the holistic judgment approach would be to interview judges about actions in the paper summaries and on the videotape that influenced their sorting, so called "policy capturing". Regression analysis could be used to determine the influence of items identified through these procedures on the precision of the classifications. Finally, as Norcini et al. (1992) indicated, the relatively low number of inadequate performances explicitly reviewed affected the classification precision for protocols not actually reviewed by judges. With a larger number of inadequate protocols, their mean score would have been a more stable estimate to use for those not actually reviewed. Although resource intensive, future studies of case scoring and pass/fail determination should use all available examinees to obtain the most stable estimates. If more faculty members were available, the number of protocols each would review would be far less. Protocol review will require faculty to review performance on each new case to establish the case pass mark. Similarly, each new grouping of cases will need to have a test pass mark established. Comparative studies using various equating approaches are needed, preferably involving large datasets from collaborating schools.

Another study also used a contrasting groups design, but with direct observation and an empirical procedure for estimating the number of borderline candidates who would pass each case. Data came from a 29-case OSCE given to 70 foreign medical graduate applicants to a program to prepare them for residency training (Poldre, Rothman, Cohen, Dirks, & Ross, 1992). Faculty physicians observed examinees at each SP station and other physicians scored examinees' written responses. All were asked to judge whether each examinee's performance or answers were minimally acceptable (pass) or not (fail). Plotting the score distributions of two groups and locating the point of overlap determined the pass mark for the SP component of each case. "Masters" were all current residents in training and "non-masters" were those foreign medical graduates not selected for the pre-internship program. Similar judgments were made and plotted for the written components of each case. The mean of the two points of overlap (SP component and written component) was the case cut score. The mean of these case cut scores was taken as the test-wise cut score on the continuous scale.

"Borderline" examinees were empirically derived by identifying 5 examinees with test scores just above the test-wise cut score and another five with scores just below. Performance of these 10 examinees was examined for each case. The proportion of these 10 examinees that scored above each case cut score became the estimate of borderline examinees that would pass each case. The sum of these proportions for the 29 cases produced the test-wise pass mark.

Results were similar for both approaches but somewhat lower for the dichotomous scoring. Alpha coefficients for the full tests were 0.86 for continuous and 0.79 for dichotomous scoring. Test-wise pass marks were 54.6% on the continuous scale and 15.4 (of 29) cases on the dichotomous scale. Pass rates were 81.4% and 78.6% respectively. Agreement and kappa coefficients were 0.86 and 0.64 for continuous scoring and 0.81 and 0.58 for dichotomous scoring. Twelve examinees (17%) were classified as "fail" by both approaches.

SEQUENTIAL TESTING

Developing and administering a 15 case standardized patient examination to a medical school class of 150 is resource intensive. There will be 2250 student-SP encounters. One strategy for reducing resources is to test in two steps. Sequential testing is where a relatively short test is given to all students to determine those highly likely to pass a longer test. Those with sufficiently high scores are excused from further testing since the accuracy of classifying them would not be substantially improved if they took additional cases. A much smaller group of examinees continue to take additional cases. The overall number of encounters is reduced, yet those students whose performance might be marginal are afforded a larger number of cases on which to base their final classification. The potential error for misclassification is much smaller.

Several authors have recommended sequential testing (Van der Vleuten & Swanson, 1990; Colliver & Williams, 1993), but relatively few studies have examined the consequences of sequential testing with actual data. The two studies described here both are retrospective in that a full test of cases was administered to all examinees and then possible screening tests were created from those results. One study used data from the first day of testing as the screening test and evaluated classification errors based on actual outcomes of the full, 3-day test. The other study also used data from a full test to create retrospectively four screening tests and then evaluated their predictive accuracy and financial savings.

Colliver, Mast, Vu, and Barrows (1991) used data from six cases administered on the first day of a three-day test to approximate a screening and evaluated its predictive utility for reducing the total number of cases that would have to be administered. SP encounters were 20 minutes with another 20 minutes available to answer additional questions. Each case author determined the minimal number of points needed to pass each case. The pass/fail mark for the whole test was the mean of all minimal points for the cases. For the screening test two pass marks were evaluated for classification accuracy against the actual outcomes from the full test. One was + 0.5 standard error of measurement (SEM) above the mean case pass level (HIGH) and the other was simply the mean case pass level (LOW). Based on a six-case performance relative to these two pass marks, students were classified as "masters" or "non-masters". This classification was compared with pass/fail results from the full test. The pass mark for the full 18 case test was −1.29 SEM from the mean case pass level. This downward adjustment was chosen to minimize false-negative classifications (being classified as "non-master" when performance was actually at the "master" level). With the HIGH screening test pass mark, 66% of the class (46 students) would have been excused from further testing and no one in this group failed the full test. Of the remaining 24 students who would have taken the additional 12 cases, five (21%) ultimately failed the full examination.

This procedure then was applied to data from six medical school classes at that school, a total of 404 students. With the HIGH pass mark for the screening test, 228 students (56%) would have been excused from further testing. Only one student in this group (less than 0.5%) eventually failed the full examination. Of the 176 students who would have been given the full examination, 25 (14%) ultimately failed the full examination.

For the LOW screening pass mark, 73% of the class would have been excused with only one student subsequently failing the full test; a pass error rate of 2%. Of the 19 students who would have failed the screening test, four ultimately failed the full examination. For six classes combined, four of 275 students (1.5%) who would have been excused after the first day eventually failed the long test. Twenty-two (17%) of the 129 students who would have had to take the remaining cases, ultimately failed the full examination.

With the HIGH screening test pass mark the total number of student-SP encounters would have been reduced by 44% with a pass error of 0%. The LOW screening cut point would have reduced the number of encounters by 49% with a pass error of 2%. Cases used on day one were not specially selected for their predictive value of the full examination outcome. Saving nearly half of the encounters of the full administration is substantial, but the saving must be evaluated against the rate and type of misclassification as well as the reduction in information available as feedback to some students.

Cases from a performance examination given to more than 350 medical students at four schools in a consortium were used to retrospectively create four different screening tests from a set of 13 cases (Petrusa, Hales, Wake, Harward, Hoban, & Willis, 2000). All four schools administered the same cases to their students who had just completed the year of required clerkships. SP encounters were 15 or 20 minutes with post-encounter times of 10 and 5 minutes, respectively. Case pass marks were based on critical actions deemed necessary to avoid malpractice by a practicing physician. Passing 10 of 13 cases was the test pass mark. Strategies for selecting the four screening test cases were (1) cases with the best pass/fail consistency with the full test, (2) those that correlated best with the total number of cases passed, (3) four cases representing a sample from the range of case-to-total correlations and (4) those with the best case-to-total correlations. Financial savings and classification errors were compared.

Cases that correlated highest with total number of cases passed was the best screening test. "Best" was determined by the least number of false positives, i.e., students categorized as "pass" when performance was actually "fail". Also, there would have been a 0% false pass rate with this screening test. This error-free classification came at the price of more total encounters. This screening test would have allowed only a 27% savings. It is not surprising that increasing the precision resulted in less financial savings. The screening test that would have resulted in the largest financial savings also would have allowed 5% false pass classifications. For 350 students, 17 would have been passed inappropriately. When viewed from the perspective of a national screen of 15,000 fourth year students in the United States, 750 young physicians would have been inappropriately classified as having the skills when they actually did not.

IMPACT OF PERFORMANCE EXAMINATIONS ON EDUCATION

There is considerable evidence that educational tests have a major influence on the behavior of learners and instructors (Frederiksen, 1984). Tests give specific indications about what the faculty believe is important for students to learn. Evidence of this influence for SP-based tests is provided from a number of studies. Newble and Jaeger (1983) asked students to identify which type of evaluation, given at the end of the year, had had the most influence on their study habits. Prior to instituting an SP-based examination, students reported that multiple-choice tests had the greatest influence. However, for three years when the SP-based examination was part of the evaluation system, the proportion of students that reported the multiple choice examination as the most influential fell from 87% to 61%. This is exactly the amount of *increase* reported for the influence of the clinical examination. Over that same three-year period, clinical examination mean scores increased from about 63% to greater than 70%. Ward ratings had a parallel increase but scores on the multiple-choice test did not change. This indicates that the clinical examination not only had a strong influence on students' study habits, but also resulted in a substantial increase not only for exam performance, but also during their ward work. In a follow-up study, this influence continued to increase. After seven years, the proportion of students that rated the clinical exam a strong influence on their study behavior changed from about 50% to over 80% while their reported influence of the multiple-choice tests declined (Newble, 1988).

Stillman, Haley, Regan, and Philbin (1991) surveyed fourth year students about the number of times faculty and upper level residents observed them doing patient workups. Prior to the administration of a comprehensive, SP-based test the proportion of students reporting zero or one observation by a faculty member was 70% and by residents was 35%. Subsequently, the proportion reporting five or more faculty observations increased from 10% to 45% and five or more resident observations increased from 25% to 80%.

In another study data from an SP-based examination provided direct and specific evidence for the effectiveness of a structured clinical curriculum (Anderson et al., 1991). A medical school with neurology clerkships at several hospitals was interested in whether better educational outcomes for students would result from better clinical education. One hospital consistently received higher ratings from students. This hospital provided students with a structured clinical curriculum on the workup of several neurological patients. In the SP-based exam, students from this hospital performed significantly better on the four neurology cases, two regarding mental status and two assessing motor and reflex functions, than did students from the other neurology placements. What makes their performance so compelling is that these students did *not* have higher SP examination scores; nor did they rate the SP exam more favorably.

Additional evidence of a positive effect of structured education was provided in a study where faculty members gave students feedback for two minutes following every four-minute encounter with a patient during a clinical performance examination (Hodder, Rivington, Calcutt, & Hart, 1988). Impact of this feedback was evaluated against two other conditions, one where students were allowed to continue their workup of each patient for an additional two minutes and another where students were able to review their performance with each patient. Performance on subsequent cases increased more than 25% after the two-minute feedback, but not for the other two conditions. Structured teaching can have a dramatically positive effect on students' performance.

SUMMARY, CONCLUSIONS AND FUTURE DIRECTIONS

If one of the purposes of evaluation of professional performance is to assure that future performance is likely to be of a certain quality, then a sufficiently large sample from the variety of challenges that will confront the professional should be in the evaluation. Further, evaluators must have sufficient knowledge and experience to judge that performance. Selecting a patient from those available in a hospital as the one challenge on which to judge a clinician's level of performance, even if that performance is judged by a well prepared evaluator, is simply too limited a sample on which to base predictions of future performance. The oral examination, or *vive voce,* is just such an evaluation event. A single patient assigned to one examinee whose interaction with that patient might or might not be directly observed by the examiner, is simply insufficient information to predict the examinee's performance with different patients.

The multiple-station examination, with some or all of the stations containing patients, overcomes many of the limitations of the oral examination approach and has potential for a more solid basis on which to predict future performance of examinees. Tasks and challenges should be selected from the range of challenges that examinees are expected to address. Dimensions of performance, important to the quality of the performance, are specified in advance and used by any examiners. Often an expected level or quality of performance is also delineated prior to observing any examinee performance. These examinations must be judged by core concepts in the evaluation of performance, consistency/reliability and validity. Usefulness and practicality are just behind reliability and validity as criteria for judging evaluation methods.

Multiple-station examinations have many more components where consistency and validity must be determined than do oral examinations. Adequacy of the sample of challenges, consistency of patient portrayal, consistency when more than one person portrays the same patient, consistency of marking performance of examinees, the influence of patient and examinee gender, validity of the dimensions used for marking, test reliability and/or classification consistency and the validity of classifications have all been the focus of research on multiple-station examinations over the last 25 years. The quality and consistency of portrayal, by one or more persons, whether trained by one or different trainers, has been quite high with any detectable variation having little or no impact on the examinee's total score. Careful monitoring of the intensity and accuracy of affective cues is indicated. Marking by patients or observers also has been quite high. Coefficients of inter-rater agreement are typically 0.90 or higher. Ratings of interpersonal qualities and general communication skills are much more reliable than scores from checklists of history or physical examination actions. Moderate test reliability (e.g., 0.45-0.75) of these examinations has been attributed to variation in content of the different challenges, so called "content specificity". This concept was identified in research from the early 1970s, well before the multiple-station examination was developed. An interesting line of recent research has looked at "global ratings" made by clinical observers with mixed results (e.g., Keynan, Friedman, & Benbassat, 1987; Swartz, et al., 1999). The notion is that checklists, by their very nature, are content specific and thus may limit the correlation between performances on different cases simply as an artifact of the data forms. More global features of performance, such as "approach to the problem" and "attitude toward the patient", certainly could be evaluated for any problem and any patient without reference to specific actions, such as "checked bilateral patellar reflexes". Interrater reliability of these global ratings has been only modest, but total test reliability seems promising.

Global features versus specific actions of clinical performance relates to the validity of these examinations as well as reliability. More work is needed regarding scoring of performance. Research indicates that experts are more efficient in their patient workup actions than non-experts. From a strictly "checklist perspective" the expert should not get a "poorer" score. Scoring of performance with patient cases has always been interpreted as "more points equals better performance". However, if an expert worked through a case from one of these examinations, fewer points would mean better performance. This author suspects that there are some students who, for any variety of reasons, are nearer to expert for particular problems than their peers. Their performance in a clinical examination should be "better" than their peers. More work needs to be done with data collection and scoring in performance examinations to be sure that better performance has a better score. The more central issue concerning validity is the stated purpose and specific concept of clinical performance that the examination is supposed to evaluate. In early clinical skills courses often the expected performance is simply a demonstration of a list of actions, e.g. cardiovascular examination, items in the Family History. Later, faculty expect learners to exercise judgment about which questions to ask and what maneuvers to perform, to recognize and describe abnormal findings and to synthesize patient data into a prioritized list of possible causes of the signs and symptoms. A clinical examination for the former should use checklists to record the completeness of performance as well as the technical accuracy of actions. The latter performance must address the organization of performance, its modification in light of new information, as well as the meaning given to the obtained data. Using a checklist from the skills course to evaluate performance in the second would not capture all of the important dimensions of expected performance, resulting in a less valid assessment.

In the absence of earlier data about the learner's technical capability of actions, it seems reasonable to try to capture that aspect of performance even in examinations of more advanced performance. If a medical school is building its first multiple-station clinical performance examination, and it will be used near the end of the final year, checklists seem reasonable. The school wants to know what was done and not done by each student. However, if the school already had evidence about students' technical accuracy and selection of actions for particular problems, the examination in the final year could focus on different features of performance such as the structure and content of each student's assessment or rationale for the diseases and their priority in the differential diagnosis. Several medical schools around the world have the opportunity to experiment with changes in the data collected about performance at progressive levels of training.

Another important line of research on the validity of performance examinations is the validity of pass marks, particularly for patient-based cases (Jaegar & Tittle, 1980; Livingston & Zieky, 1982; Berk, 1986; Hambleton & Powell, 1993). Again the concept of performance being assessed is central to this validity question. Is the acceptable quality of clinical performance for cases going to be that of a practitioner, or is it something different, something created to match the educational tasks that students perform? This validity issue in turn relates to the goals of the educational program for which a clinical performance examination is the outcome evaluation tool. It should be clear that the validity of clinical performance examinations is defined not only by the materials and data within the test, but also by the educational goals for performance and the nature of that performance. Misalignment of any of these aspects undermines the validity of the examination as used in that context.

Standardized patient-based examinations have advanced our understanding about how to evaluate components of clinical performance. They are feasible, relatively reliable and valid, and useful in providing data unavailable from other sources (Kassebaum, 1990). More development should focus on capturing meta-level features of clinical performance such as organization, efficiency and integration of questions, physical examination maneuvers and comments to the patient. Validity of data capture, scoring and pass marks needs immediate investigative attention. This knowledge will help improve the quality and utility of data derived from multiple-station, standardized patient-based clinical performance examinations and advance the science of clinical performance assessment.

REFERENCES

Abrahamowicz, M., Tamblyn, R. M., Ramsay, J. O., Klass, D. K., & Kopelow, M. L. (1990). Detecting and correcting for rater-induced differences in standardized patient tests of clinical competence. *Academic Medicine, 65*, S25-S26.

Allen, S. S., Bland, C. J., Harris, I. B., Anderson, D., Poland, G., Satran, L., & Miller, W. (1991). Structured clinical teaching strategy. *Medical Teacher, 13*, 177-184.

Anderson, D. C., Harris, I. B., Allen, S., Satran, L., Bland, C. J., Davis-Feickert, J. A., Poland, G. A., & Miller, W. J. (1991). Comparing students' feedback about clinical instruction with their performances. *Academic Medicine, 66*, 29-34.

Anderson, M. B., Stillman, P. L., & Wang, Y. (1994). Growing use of standardized patients in teaching and evaluation in medical education. *Teaching and Learning in Medicine, 6*, 15- 22.

Barrows, H. S., & Bennett, K. (1972). The diagnostic (problem solving) skill of the neurologist: experimental studies and their implications for neurological training. *Archives of Neurology, 26*, 273-275.

Berk, R. A. (1986). A consumer's guide to setting performance standards on criterion-referenced tests. *Review of Educational Research, 56*, 137-172.

Berner, E. S., Hamilton, L. A. & Best, W. R. (1974). A new approach to evaluating problem-solving in medical students. *Journal of Medical Education, 49*, 666-671.

Brennan, R. (1983). *Elements of generalizability theory.* Iowa City, IA: American College Testing Program.

Cassell, E. J. (1990). *The nature of suffering and the goals of medicine.* New York: Oxford University Press.

Cater, J. I., Forsyth, J. S., & Frost, G. J. (1991). The use of the objective structured clinical examination as an audit of teaching and student performance. *Medical Teacher, 13*, 253-257.

Cohen, D. S., Colliver, J. A., Marcy, M. S., Fried, E. D., & Swartz, M. H. (1996). Psychometric properties of a standardized-patient checklist and rating-scale form used to assess interpersonal and communication skills. *Academic Medicine, 71*, S87-89.

Cohen, R., Rothman, A. I., Poldre, P., & Ross, J. (1991). Validity and generalizability of global ratings in an objective structured clinical examination. *Academic Medicine, 66*, 545-548.

Cohen, R., Rothman, A. I., Ross, J., & Poldre, P. (1991). Validating an objective structured clinical examination (OSCE) as a method for selecting foreign medical graduates for a pre-internship program. *Academic Medicine, 66*, S67-S69.

Colliver, J. A., & Williams, R. G. (1993). Technical issues: test application. *Academic Medicine, 68*, 454-460.

Colliver, J. A., Marcy, M. L., Travis, T. A., & Robbs, R. S. (1991). The interaction of student gender and standardized-patient gender on a performance-based examination of clinical competence. *Academic Medicine, 66*, S31-S33.

Colliver, J. A., Markwell, S. J., Vu, N. V., & Barrows, H. S. (1990a). Case specificity of standardized-patient examinations: Consistency of performance on components of clinical competence within and between cases. *Evaluation in the Health Professions, 13,* 252- 261.

Colliver, J. A., Mast, T. A., Vu, N. V., & Barrows, H. S. (1991). Sequential testing with a performance-based examination using standardized patients. *Academic Medicine, 66,* S64-S66.

Colliver, J. A., Morrison, L. J., Markwell, S. J., Verhulst, S. J., Steward, D. E., Dawson-Saunders, E., & Barrows, H. S. (1990b). Three studies of the effect of multiple standardized patients on intercase reliability of five standardized-patient examinations. *Teaching and Learning in Medicine, 2,* 237-245.

Colliver, J. A., Steward, D. E., Markwell, S. J., & Marcy, M. L. (1991). Effect of repeated simulations by standardized patients on intercase reliability. *Teaching and Learning in Medicine, 3,* 15-19.

Colliver, J. A., Vu, N. V., Marcy, M. L., Travis, T. A., & Robbs, R. S. (1993). The effects of examinee and standardized-patient gender and their interaction on standardized-patient ratings of interpersonal and communication skills. *Academic Medicine, 2,* 153-157.

Colliver, J. A., Vu, N. V., Markwell, S. J., & Verhulst. S. J. (1991). Reliability and efficiency of components of clinical competence assessed with five performance-based examinations using standardized patients. *Medical Education, 25,* 303-310.

Des Marchais, J. E. (1993). A student-centered, problem-based curriculum: 5 years' experience. *Canadian Medical Association Journal, 148,* 1567-1572.

Elstein, A. S., Shulman, L. S., & Sprafka, S. A. (1978). *Medical problem-solving: an analysis of clinical reasoning.* Cambridge, MA: Harvard University Press.

Ericsson, K. A., & Charness, N. (1994). Expert performance: its structure and acquisition. *American Psychologist, 49,* 725-747.

Frederiksen, N. (1984). The real test bias: Influences of testing on teaching and learning. *American Psychologist, 39,* 193-202.

Gallagher, T. H., Lo, B., Chesney, M., & Christensen, K. (1997). How do physicians respond to patient's requests for costly, unindicated services? *Journal of General Internal Medicine, 12,* 663-668.

Glass, G. V. (1978). Standards and criteria. *Journal of Educational Measurement, 15,* 237-261.

Guilford, J. P. (1965). *Fundamental statistics in psychology and education.* New York: McGraw-Hill, 486-489.

Hambleton, R. K., & Powell, S. (1993). A framework for viewing the process of standard setting. *Evaluation in the Health Professions, 6,* 3-24.

Harden, R. M., & Gleeson, F. A. (1979). Assessment of clinical competence using an objective structured clinical examination (OSCE). *Medical Education, 13,* 41-54.

Harden, R. M., Stevenson, M., Downie, W. W., & Wilson, G. M. (1975). Assessment of clinical competence using objective structured examination. *British Medical Journal, 1*(5955), 447-451.

Hodder, R. V., Rivington, R. N., Calcutt, L. E., & Hart, I. R. (1988). The effectiveness of immediate feedback during the objective structured clinical examination. *Medical Education, 23,* 184-188.

Jaegar, R. M., & Tittle, C. K. (Eds.) (1980). *Minimum competency testing: Motives, models, measures and consequences.* Berkeley, CA: McCutchan.

Kassebaum, D. G. (1990). The measurement of outcomes in the assessment of educational program effectiveness. *Academic Medicine, 65,* 293-296.

Kassirer, J. P., & Gorry, G. A. (1978). Clinical problem-solving: A behavioral analysis. *Annals of Internal Medicine, 89,* 245-255.

Kohn, L. T., Corrigan, J. M., & Donaldson, M. S. (Eds.) (1999). *To err is human: building a safer health system.* Committee on Quality of Health Care in America, Institute of Medicine. Washington, D.C.: National Academy Press.

Linn, R. L. (Ed.) (1989). *Educational measurement,* London: Collier Macmillan.

Livingston, S. A., & Zieky, M. J. (1982). *Passing scores: a manual for setting standard of performance on educational and occupational tests.* Princeton, NJ: Educational Testing Service.

Lloyd, J. S., Williams, R. G., Simonton, D. K., & Sherman, D. (1990). Order effects in standardized patient examinations. *Academic Medicine, 65,* S51-S52.

Matsell, D. G., Wolfish, N. M., & Hsu, E. (1991). Reliability and validity of the objective structured clinical examination in pediatrics. *Medical Education, 25,* 293-299.

Mattern, W. D., Weinholtz, D., & Friedman, C. P. (1984). The attending physician as teacher. *New England Journal of Medicine, 237,* 1129-1132.

Maxwell J. A., Cohen, R. M., & Reinhard, J. D. (1983). A qualitative study of teaching rounds in a department of medicine. *Proceedings of Annual Conference on Research in Medical Education, 22*, 192-197.

Morrison, L. J., & Barrows, H. S. (1994). Developing consortia for clinical practice examinations: The Macy Project. *Teaching and Learning in Medicine, 6*, 23-27.

Mosier, C. L. (1943). On the reliability of a weighted composite. *Psychometrika, 8*, 161-168.

Newble, D. I. (1988). Eight years' experience with a structured clinical examination. *Medical Education, 22*, 200-204.

Newble, D., & Jaeger, K. (1983). The effects of assessments and examinations on the learning of medical students. *Medical Education, 17*, 165-171.

Newble, D. L., & Swanson, D. B. (1983). Psychometric characteristics of the objective structured clinical examination. *Medical Education, 22*, 325-334.

Norcini, J. J. (1990). Equivalent pass/fail decisions. *Journal of Educational Measurement, 27*, 59-66.

Norcini, J. J. (1992). Approaches to standard setting for performance-based examinations. *Proceedings of the Fifth Ottawa Conference on the Assessment of Clinical Competence.* Dundee, Scotland, 33-37.

Norcini, J. J. Jr. (1999). Standards and reliability in evaluation: when rules of thumb don't apply. *Academic Medicine, 74*, 1088-1090.

Norcini, J., Stillman, P., Regan, M. B., Haley, H., Sutnick, A., Williams, R., & Friedman, M. (1992). Scoring and standard-setting with standardized patients. Presented at the annual meeting of the American Educational Research Association, San Francisco, CA.

Norman, G. (1985). Objective measurement of clinical performance. *Medical Education, 19*, 43-47.

Petrusa, E. R. (1987). The effect of number of cases on performance on a standardized multiple-stations clinical examination. *Journal of Medical Education, 62*, 859-860.

Petrusa, E. R., Blackwell, T. A., & Ainsworth, M. A. (1990). Reliability and validity of an objective structured clinical examination for assessing the clinical performance of residents. *Archives of Internal Medicine, 150*, 573-577.

Petrusa, E. R., Blackwell, T. A., Carline, J., Ramsey, P. G., McGaghie, W. C., Colindres, R., Kowlowitz, V., Mast, T. A., & Soler, N. (1991). A multi-institutional trial of an objective structured clinical examination. *Teaching and Learning in Medicine, 3*, 86-94.

Petrusa, E. R., Hales, J. W., Wake, L., Harward, D. H., Hoban, D., & Willis, S. (2000). Prediction accuracy and financial savings for four screening tests of a sequential test of clinical performance. *Teaching and Learning in Medicine, 12*, 4-13.

Petrusa, E. R., Guckian, J. C., & Perkowski, L. C. (1984). A multiple station objective clinical evaluation. *Proceedings of the Twenty-third Annual Conference on Research in Medical Education, 23*, 211-216.

Petrusa, E. R., Richards, B., Willis, S., Smith, A., Harward, D., & Camp, M.G. (1994). Criterion referenced pass marks for a clinical performance examination. Presented at the annual meeting of the Association of American Medical Colleges, Washington, DC.

Poldre, P. A., Rothman, A. I., Cohen, R., Dirks, F., & Ross, J. A. (1992). Judgmental-empirical approach to standard setting for an OSCE. Presented at the annual meeting of the American Educational Research Association, San Francisco, CA.

Rethans, J. J., Drop, R., Sturmans, F., & Van der Vleuten, C. (1991). A method for introducing standardized (simulated) patients into general practice consultations. *British Journal of General Practice, 41*, 94-96.

Reznick, R., Smee, S., Rothman, A., Chalmers, A., Swanson, D., Dufresne, L., Lacombe, G., Baumber, J., Poldre, P., & Levasseur, L. (1992). An objective structured clinical examination for the licentiate: report of the pilot project of the Medical Council of Canada. *Academic Medicine, 67*, 487-494.

Roloff, M. E., & Miller, G. R. (1987). *Interpersonal processes. New directions in communication research.* Newbury Park, CA: Sage Publications.

Ross, J. R., Syal, S., Hutcheon, M. A., & Cohen, R. (1987). Second-year students' score improvement during an objective structured clinical examination. *Journal of Medical Education, 62*, 857-858.

Rothman, A. I., Cohen, R., Dirks, F. R., & Ross, J. (1990). Evaluating the clinical skills of foreign medical school graduates participating in an internship preparation program. *Academic Medicine, 65*, 391-395.

Rothman, A., Poldre, P., Cohen, R., & Ross, J. (1993). Standard setting in a multiple station test of clinical skills. Presented at the annual meeting of the American Educational Research Association.

Rutala, P. J., Witzke, D. B., Leko, E. O., & Fulginiti, J. V. (1990). The influence of student and standardized-patient genders on scoring in an objective structured clinical examination. *Academic Medicine, 66*, S28-S30.

Rutala, P. J., Witzke, D. B., Leko, E. E., Fulginiti, J. V., & Taylor, P. J. (1990). Student fatigue as a variable affecting performance in an objective structured clinical examination. *Academic Medicine, 65,* S53-S54.

Shatzer, J. H., Wardrop, J. L., Williams, R. G., & Hatch, T. F. (1994). The generalizability of performance on different-station-length standardized patient cases. *Teaching and Learning in Medicine, 6,* 54-53.

Shatzer, J. H., DaRosa, D., Colliver, J. A., & Barkmeier, L. (1993). Station-length requirements for reliable performance-based examination scores. *Academic Medicine, 68,* 224-229.

Stillman, P. L., Haley, H. L., Regan, M. B., & Philbin, M. M. (1991a). Positive effects of a clinical performance assessment program. *Academic Medicine, 66,* 481-483.

Stillman, P. L., Regan, M. B., Swanson, D. B., Case, S., McCahan, J., Feinblatt, J., Smith, S. R., Williams, J., & Nelson, D. V. (1990). An assessment of the clinical skills of fourth-year students at four New England medical schools. *Academic Medicine, 65,* 329-326.

Stillman, P., Swanson, D., Regan, M. B., Philbin, M. M., Nelson, V., Ebert, T., Ley, B., Parrino, T., Shorey, J., & Stillman, A. (1991b). Assessment of clinical skills of residents utilizing standardized patients. A follow-up study and recommendations for application. *Annals of Internal Medicine, 114,* 393-401.

Subkoviak, M. J. (1976). Estimating reliability from a single administration of a mastery test. *Journal of Educational Measurement, 13,* 265-276.

Swanson, D. B., & Norcini, J. J. (1989). Factors influencing the reproducibility of tests using standardized patients. *Teaching and Learning in Medicine, 1,* 158-166.

Swartz, M. H., Colliver, J. A., Bardes, C. L., Charon, R., Fried, E. D., & Moroff, S. (1999). Global ratings of videotaped performance versus global rating of actions recorded on checklists: a criterion for performance assessment with standardized patients. *Academic Medicine, 74,* 1028-1032.

Tamblyn, R. M., Klass, D. J., Schnabl, G. K., & Kopelow, M. L. (1991). The accuracy of standardized patient presentation. *Medical Education, 25,* 100-109.

Van der Vleuten, C. P. M. (1996). The assessment of professional competence: developments, research and practical implications. *Advances in Health Sciences Education, 1,* 41-67.

Van der Vleuten, C. P. M., & Swanson, D. B. (1990). Assessment of clinical skills with standardized patients: state of the art. *Teaching and Learning in Medicine, 2,* 58-76.

Vu, N. V., & Barrows, H. S. (1994). Use of standardized patients in clinical assessments: recent developments and measurement findings. *Educational Researcher, 23,* 23-30.

Vu, N. V., Barrows, H. S., March, M. L., Verhulst, S. J., Colliver, J. A., & Travis, T. (1992). Six years of comprehensive, clinical performance-based assessment using standardized patients at the Southern Illinois University School of Medicine. *Academic Medicine, 67,* 43-50.

Williams, R. G., Barrows, H. S., Vu, N. V., Verhulst, S. J., Colliver, J. A., Marcy, M., & Steward, D. (1987). Direct, standardized assessment of clinical competence. *Medical Education, 21,* 482-489.

Yen, W. M. (1993). Scaling performance assessments: Strategies for managing local item dependence. *Journal of Educational Measurement, 30,* 187-213.

22   Assessment of Non-Cognitive Factors

ANNIE CUSHING

Barts and The London, Queen Mary's School of Medicine and Dentistry

SUMMARY

The array of instruments and methods designed to assess communication skills, interpersonal skills and attitudes in undergraduate and postgraduate settings are reviewed. The literature points to an emerging evidence base for those elements in the doctor-patient interaction which should be assessed. Some instruments have undergone psychometric testing, mostly inter-rater reliability, but few have been tested for internal consistency or validity.

Communication and interpersonal skills are observable whilst attitudes are complex and have an emotional, intellectual and behavioral component. Attitudes in all their complexity can be explored in learning settings which provide feedback but methods reported for summative assessments are confined to either observed behavior in simulated surgeries, Objective Structured Clinical Examinations (OSCE) and real consultations, or to written examinations covering ethical principles, reasoning and psychosocial issues.

In addition to generic instruments described in the chapter, issue-specific guides have been designed for particular clinical situations. There is, however, a lack of instruments to assess empathy and especially non-verbal behaviors. Research reveals knowledge of clinical content to be a confounding variable and testing to date has not identified generalizable communication and interpersonal skills independent of clinical content. This has implications for the range and number of test cases needed. Recent studies are reported which indicate shorter testing times with more reliable global assessment instruments. The latter are now preferred over detailed checklists which produce negative effects on learning behavior and triviality of measurement.

Assessment may be from tutors, standardized patients, real patients, peers or self. Large numbers of ratings by real patients are needed to achieve reliability with faculty assessors. The importance of developing self-assessment skills is discussed but little research was found on improving such skills. Despite good reliability and lower costs with assessments made by standardized patients, faculty are still preferred in high stakes exams because of greater credibility. The various approaches to standard setting for pass/fail decisions are described. However,

International Handbook of Research in Medical Education, 711–755.
G.R. Norman, C.P.M. Van der Vleuten, D.I. Newble (eds.)
© *2002 Dordrecht: Kluwer Academic Publishers. Printed in Great Britain.*

there are no predictive validity studies of actual patient outcome to define a level of competency. Standard setting remains a difficult issue for every type of assessment including medical interviewing.

Despite problems in achieving reliability, assessment in real life clinical contexts enables judgements to be made of performance as distinct from competence. Guides in assessing professional behavior with clear explicit behavioral descriptors for attitudes in daily clinical practice have been reported. Assessment of non-cognitive factors needs to be an integral part of the educational process and not just summative assessment. Methods appropriate to postgraduate assessment and audit are also reviewed. Triangulation in assessments helps to corroborate findings and increase the reliability of judgements.

A number of instruments and methods have been developed for this complex and challenging area of assessment. Further research will enable educators to build upon advances already made.

INTRODUCTION

Non-cognitive factors in this chapter will be defined as those components of professional competence that relate to communication skills, interpersonal skills and attitudes. These elements fundamentally affect the practice of medicine in the interaction with patients, relatives, colleagues and other members of the health care team. Novack (1999) has pointed out that somewhere along the way, as scientific discovery and the possibilities it offers has burgeoned, the humanistic aspect of medicine and the therapeutic aspects of the clinical encounter have been lost. Enlightened teachers and practitioners have always emphasized and written about the therapeutic relationship (Balint, 1972; Engel, 1977). What then has prompted the resurgence of interest in the doctor-patient relationship? There is mounting evidence linking elements of the consultation to diagnosis, informed consent, concordance with treatment, coping with illness, satisfaction, complaints, litigation and health outcome (Levinson, 1997; Stewart et al., 1999; Simpson et al., 1991). In essence they are key components of the doctor-patient relationship and good medical practice.

Ironically it may well be the scientific advances themselves that are driving some of the present changes. Science has brought with it enormous possibilities together with more complex decision making and ethical dilemmas that pose particular challenges in the clinical encounter. Access to information has also increased markedly. Societal expectations have changed and prompted calls for greater involvement of patients in understanding their illness and decisions over their care. There is now too much research data to ignore and evidence based medicine has begun to include the doctor-patient relationship as a component of effectiveness (Stewart et al., 1999). With an organized approach to the therapeutic aspects of the doctor-patient relationship the result will be medical care that is both more scientific and more humanistic (Novack, Epstein, & Paulsen, 1999). This requires educators to define a set of core skills and attitudes, to implement a curriculum, deliver a learning experience which fulfills these objectives and to use valid and reliable assessment methods to ensure they have been achieved.

It is really only in the last decade or so that medical schools and licensing bodies have seriously taken this on board. In Canada and the USA in 1994, some 39 out of 142 schools required students to pass an Objective Structured Clinical Examination which contained tests of communication and interpersonal skills, in order to graduate (Anderson, Stillman, & Wang, 1994). The creation of consortia for professional exams has enabled sharing of resources, research and expertise. This can help to reduce costs and develop a database of valid and reliable cases and assessment instruments to test core clinical skills and professional behaviors (Morrison & Barrows, 1994). Such assessments are used, although less commonly, in other parts of the world including the United Kingdom and Australasia (Newble & Wakeford, 1994). Competency in these areas of professional practice is still not tested in all countries and all schools in their qualifying examinations.

Assessment has two main purposes. Formative assessment is a vital part of shaping learning by providing feedback and identifying areas of strengths, weaknesses and plans for improvement. As Pololi (1995) points out, we shall be failing as educators if it is only at the end of a long course that we realize students have not attained a minimum acceptable standard. Assessment in the learning context does not demand a high level of psychometric rigor although it must focus on important and relevant educational goals (Case, 1997). Indeed, as Kurtz and colleagues (1998) stress, it is important for the method of assessment to mirror the method of instruction so that instruments for assessment and learning match. Assessment can be from self, peers, real patients, simulated patients and tutors. The development of a practitioner motivated to continue learning, to possess insight, to request feedback and to recognize his or her own shortcomings and learning needs is embodied in recommendations on medical education such as that of the General Medical Council in the United Kingdom (1993). Self-assessment skills and personal awareness are, therefore, a particular area of importance in medical education.

The other essential purpose of assessment is to ensure students progress and graduate with an acceptable level of competence to practice and that they maintain their competency as tested through re-certification mechanisms. These high stakes summative exams must fulfill the psychometric requirements of validity, reliability and accuracy, in addition to being feasible in terms of cost and time.

Assessments of non-cognitive interactional behaviors and attributes present considerable challenges. One of these is how to avoid deconstructing complex processes and trivializing them down to checklists of preferred behaviors in artificial contexts, to the extent that they have no real meaning in terms of professional practice and patient care. Inappropriate reductionism is in danger of arising because of the need for rigorous observation of things which are difficult to assess. It has been argued that this is already occurring and that reliability in measurement is winning out over validity (Marinker, 1997).

This chapter will attempt to answer the following questions:

- What specifically are we trying to assess and is there a consensus on this?
- What criteria do assessment methods need to fulfill?
- What assessment guides, instruments and methods exist?
- What research has been carried out on these assessment instruments?
- Can and should non-cognitive factors be assessed independent of clinical content?
- How is a level of competency in this area defined and how are standards set?
- How important is context, with respect to both environment and clinical content, when assessing non-cognitive factors?

WHAT TO ASSESS?

A starting point must be how educators define the set of non-cognitive factors that the curriculum aims to deliver and assess. This must be based on first defining what is considered to be "good" patient-doctor interactions. Over the years ideas and evidence have been derived from:

- theoretical and conceptual models, e.g. the biopsychosocial model of health and health care, behavioral science, counseling theory and concepts of therapeutic relationships (Engel, 1977; Levenstein et al., 1989; Davis & Fallowfield, 1991),
- clinical practice-based studies involving observation, analysis of interactions and definitions of effective consultations (Korsch & Negrete, 1972; Byrne & Long, 1976; Tuckett, 1985; Pendleton, 1984; Ley, 1988) and
- research findings which indicate a relationship between specific aspects of communication and outcomes including satisfaction, compliance and, most recently and importantly, health status (Stewart et al., 1999; Simpson et al., 1991; Levinson & Roter, 1995; Levinson et al., 1997; Davis & Fallowfield, 1991).

This body of knowledge is drawn together in what is generally called the Biopsychosocial model of medicine and its associated clinical method of Patient-Centred Medical Interviewing (Levenstein et al., 1989). Excellence in communication is now recognized as founded on a more active role for patients, leading to mutuality in the doctor-patient relationship and resulting in better health outcomes (Stewart & Roter, 1989, p. 19). Patient-centered medical interviewing encompasses communication skills, interpersonal skills and attitudinal aspects of the relationship. A further term, history taking skills, is often to be found in the literature.

Is there an evidence base for what should be incorporated into assessment? Is there a consensus in the literature on a defined set of communication, interpersonal skills and attitudes to test for?

Some of the theoretical and analytical frameworks for the consultation have been devised by experts from observation of consultations. This was done prior to research evidence on outcome. These frameworks may present functions or tasks within a consultation and specify skills that help to achieve these functions, providing guides for feedback and learning (Bird & Cohen-Cole, 1990; Pendleton et al., 1984). Other approaches incorporate a time line and interactional structure to the consultation with different activities being the focus at different times (Byrne & Long, 1976). Identifying what it is that recognized exemplary physicians do in their consultations is another approach to defining desirable behaviors in the clinical encounter (Marvel et al., 1998).

More recently some authors have supported the inclusion of items in their guides by reference to the research evidence on outcome. They have included individual skills that have been shown to constitute effective doctor-patient communication (Silverman et al., 1998).

Roter (1989) reviewed existing studies and applied a meta analysis technique to identify patterns and to investigate the relationship of these to outcomes. This methodology represents a consensual validation of the resulting groupings which, one can then assume, have both content and face validity. In 61 studies using 28 instruments, over 200 communication skills process variables were identified. These could be grouped into six categories: information giving, information seeking, social talk, positive talk, negative talk and partnership building. They also differentiated between socioemotional and task-oriented domains. They found significant relations between patient satisfaction, recall and compliance with all of the six categories of physician behavior. Their groupings were consistent with prior conceptual work in the field (Parsons, 1951; Bales, 1965; Bloom, 1983; Ben-Sira, 1980). The relationship between task domain and socioemotional domain was interesting. They noted that when doctors provide more medical information (task domain) they speak with an interested voice (socioemotional domain). Similarly, proficient or active advice giving is interpreted by patients as being interested and caring. Hence, a positive inference is made about the doctors' motivation for engaging in this task behavior.

The reviewers were struck, moreover, by the fact that so many authors devised their own schemes to analyze interactions rather than use previously developed schemes, and they recommended that future efforts be aimed at refining existing instruments rather than development of new measures.

Other reviewers have found an overlap in assessment instruments. Ovadia, Yager, and Heinrich (1982) investigated eight instruments used to assess medical interviewing and found many common items in five of the eight instruments, although each instrument had at least one item not mentioned in any of the others.

Stewart et al. (1999) note a striking similarity in the key findings on effective doctor communication from a review of the studies of malpractice, adherence and patient's health outcome. They identify four common and important dimensions of the communication process together with behaviors, which fulfill these evidence-based guidelines.

* Clear information provided to the patient.
* Mutually agreed upon goals.
* An active role for the patient.
* Positive affect, empathy and support from the doctor.

Petrusa et al. (1994) developed an instrument of doctor-patient relationship and communication by reviewing the literature, identifying 64 items which were then condensed to 15 items which were split into two domains; socioemotional component (interpersonal) and communication component. Schnabl et al. (1991) used factor analysis to reveal three domains from the checklist which pertain to (1) sensitivity and rapport, (2) involvement of patient, (3) providing explanations. Interestingly, but perhaps not surprisingly, these match those identified by Stewart et al. (1999). The latter, however, also include aspects of effective history taking which specifically involve exploring the patient's understanding, concerns, expectations and perceptions of the impact of the problem on function and feelings.

Clinicians' sensitivity to non-verbal cues is of particular importance given the research findings of its strong relationship with patients feeling understood. Physicians' abilities to express emotions non-verbally and detect and respond to patients' non-verbal communication have been shown to correlate with satisfaction and attendance (DiMatteo et al., 1980, 1986). Despite its importance Boon and Stewart (1998) point out the lack of assessment instruments which specifically focus on non-verbal behavior.

Another approach to identifying a set of competencies is that of Sanson-Fisher and Cockburn (1997) who advocate defining the clinical communication tasks which students need to be proficient in. They present seven criteria by which to select clinical issues that are appropriate foci for communication skills courses. Issues must be common, associated with a high disease burden, influenced by improved skills, cost-effective as a means of dealing with the issue, acceptable in routine practice and acceptable to patients. Relevance is deemed highly important in order for the skills to be maintained in post-training medical practice. They include communication for various health behavior change situations, recovery from medical interventions and breaking bad news as particular tasks that fit these seven criteria. In this way they attempt to define the "curriculum" and the test set.

Hence, there would appear to be considerable similarities in how and what experts in the field are incorporating into their models and guides for good communication.

Mostly the models and frameworks described above do not constitute assessment instruments as such, but provide guides for specific descriptive feedback and discussion in training. There is a need for formative methods and feedback guides to match summative assessment instruments so that expectations are congruent and made explicit to learners (Kurtz et al., 1998, p. 176).

Whilst there is undoubtedly overlap between history taking skills, communication skills, interpersonal skills and attitudes, it is worth considering the distinctions in their meaning and the implications for design of assessment of each domain.

History taking skills

There is a difference between communication and interpersonal skills and the traditional interpretation of what were termed history taking skills. The latter both in terms of learning and assessment have historically focused on the content of a particular clinical problem rather than on the process of a consultation. Typically the question asked of history taking skills would be "Did the student ask the patient about X or did the student explain Y?" i.e. the more technical and content items. The assessment here focuses on how accurate and complete is the information that is obtained from or given to the patient. They are easy to assess. Assessment of the student's history taking skills will be dependent on content knowledge about the clinical case in question. History taking may of course include relevant psychosocial information (e.g. "Did the candidate ask about social support at home") as well as biomedical data but the focus is still content.

Communication and interpersonal skills

These are linked, commonly grouped together and specifically relate to the process. They can be observed and assessed. They tend to be distinguished in that communication is about behaviors or techniques that facilitate accurate exchange and understanding. Items here might include use of clear language and checking understanding.

Interpersonal skills are behaviors that attend to the affect in the relationship and promote rapport, trust and acceptance. They facilitate exchange of information and understanding. An example would be the use of empathic statements or non-verbal responses which help to establish a therapeutic relationship. Empathic communication has received particular attention given its relationship to outcome (Stewart et al., 1999.) Clinicians' sensitivity to non-verbal cues and their non-verbal response influences outcomes in a positive way (DiMatteo et al., 1980, 1986). Suchman et al. (1997) provide a helpful definition and empirically derived model of verbal empathic communication in medical interviews by describing the specific behaviors and patterns of expression associated with verbal expressions of emotion. Empathy occurs when patients feel listened to, understood and acknowledged.

Attitudes

Attitudes are the emotional and intellectual predisposition which are the result of our efforts to make sense of, organize, predict and shape our reactions to the world (Sears et al., 1991). In the United Kingdom, the General Medical Council's recommendations on medical education state: *"Attitudes of mind and behaviour that befit a doctor should be inculcated, and should imbue the new graduate with attributes appropriate to his/her future responsibilities to patients, colleagues and society in general"* (General Medical Council, 1993, p. 23).

They are complex, serve individuals in a variety of ways, are fundamental to a sense of self and variably resistant to change. They are shaped by early socialization, professional socialization and experiences. They may change but can also form a filter or resistance in the face of new evidence or demands when the threat experienced is too great. Hence attitudes are described as having an affective (feeling), cognitive (thought) and behavioral (action) component (Sears et al., 1991). They may be manifest in behaviors and are linked to underlying beliefs and values about which a person has feelings, either positive or negative. In this way they constitute an emotional and intellectual predisposition to behave in particular ways in response to specific circumstances.

For this reason the attitudes of medical students or doctors could lead to inappropriate behavioral responses and, therefore, must be within the remit of medical education. For example, a student or doctor may believe that the psychosocial aspects of illness and its management are not important. Alternatively he or she might have difficulties with patients' addictive or sexual behaviors. This could result in failing to both identify important information needed for diagnosis of the patient's problem, and failing to understand social and cultural beliefs and circumstances in negotiating decisions and plans for the patient's care. A clinician may also not fully respect a patient's autonomy and be less likely to share decision-making. Korsch (1989) has pointed out that patients want more information and a more active role in doctor-patient communication with implications for a more egalitarian relationship. Thus, being aware of the judgmental and ethical implications of the communication process is an important area of study.

The behavioral components of appropriate professional attitudes have been defined, for example, by the General Medical Council in the United Kingdom in its document *Duties of a doctor* (General Medical Council, 1998). These duties, of course, relate to interactions between qualified practitioners and their patients (see Table 1). Undergraduate students have a different role with respect to their interactions with patients than the physicians responsible for a patient's care, although some of the duties illustrated in the General Medical Council document do still apply. The question also arises as to whether it is possible to identify a set of attitudes to assess medical students' interactions with patients, staff and colleagues. A recent Consensus Statement (1998) on a national medical ethics curriculum has been published in the United Kingdom which covers the content and knowledge domain.

Table 1. General Medical Council's *Duties of a doctor*
(General Medical Council, 1998)

- Make the care of your patient your first concern.
- Treat every patient politely and considerately.
- Respect patients' dignity and privacy.
- Listen to patients and respect their views.
- Give patients information in a way they can understand.
- Respect the rights of patients to be fully involved in decisions about their care.
- Keep your professional knowledge and skills up to date.
- Recognize the limits of your professional competence.
- Be honest and trustworthy.
- Respect and protect confidential information.
- Make sure that your personal beliefs do not prejudice your patients' care.
- Act quickly to protect patients from risk if you have good reason to believe that you or a colleague may not be fit to practice.
- Work with colleagues in the ways that best serve patients' interests.

In all these matters you must never discriminate unfairly against your patients or colleagues. And you must always be prepared to justify your actions to them.

Some guides have been produced for professional behavior of students in the clinical encounter covering for example communication skills, responsibility, respect, self-awareness and self-evaluation (Bienenstock et al., 1994). The ethical concerns that students experience during their undergraduate studies have been identified from case studies and relate to learning on patients, dealing with evaluation pressures, personal development, sexuality and economic health care issues (Hundert et al., 1996). The hidden curriculum of expected attitudes, the difficulties that students have in gauging how they are doing in this respect and the different perspectives that might exist for students and their clinical teachers regarding attitudes and behaviors is expounded in a fascinating piece of research by Hundert et al. (1996). In this study the student's recognition that he was failing, but his lack of understanding about why, arose from a lack of clearly articulated expectations about what constituted appropriate behavior. Ethics teachers refer to the development of moral character, integrity and other personal attributes which come within the remit of education (Miles et al., 1989). The power of the informal curriculum, the process of socialization throughout the medical course and the context of learning have been highlighted (Hundert et al., 1996). It has been pointed out that the medium is the message, in that the learning method should mirror the attributes it is attempting to develop in doctor-patient interactions (Bird et al., 1993). The educational process itself needs to model appropriate attitudes in order to demonstrate an internal consistency, i.e. the teacher/student relationship mirrors the doctor/patient relationship. This fundamentally means empowering the students, understanding and helping them to understand their experience and offering expertise to further their effectiveness in their tasks. As medical education shifts toward more student-centered methods so there may be greater congruence between the students' experience of interaction with teachers and the interactions with patients which are being advocated. Groupwork offers the opportunity not only to undertake a task (content learned) but also to reflect on how people worked with each other in the group. This starts to address working with colleagues and the effect of behaviors and attitudes on others. The move toward problem based learning in many curricula has already begun to highlight changes in learning beyond cognition or knowledge domains and offers the possibility to research its influence on non-cognitive factors of communication and interpersonal skills.

Reflective awareness and explicit discussion of underlying attitudes, feelings, thoughts and ethical dilemmas are within the remit of the teaching and learning process. Providing students with feedback on the effect of their behavior helps to guide their learning on professional attitudes and behavior. Some authors argue for the primacy of skills based learning. Whilst acknowledging the vital importance of attitudes they consider these best dealt with by integration into skills learning. They argue that without the necessary behavioral skills learners' interactions do not improve despite positive attitudes (Kurtz & Silverman, 1998). However, unexamined attitudes, biases and personal stress can interfere with patient care, and hence educational courses that specifically address these are recommended by some educators (Novack, Epstein, & Paulsen, 1999).

Attitudes are addressed in the formal curriculum of ethics, moral philosophy, law, sociology, psychology, communication skills and community-oriented education programs. However, the informal curriculum is an everyday occurrence. Much of that which is learned, especially in the way of attitudes, is imbibed and copied. Hence, formal teaching around skills and attitudes may be either supported or undermined in the daily educational, practice and clinical environment (Pfeiffer et al., 1998). It is here that social influence and important, respected role models exert considerable effect (Sears et al., 1991). Discussion would seem to be especially important where there is dissonance in espoused professional attitudes and those behaviors observed in practice, or where there is conflict between what different teachers are saying, valuing or expecting of students. The tension that such contradictions in practice and teaching create could usefully be explored in the learning context so that options, choices and appropriate strategies are discussed.

Assessment of attitudes presents particular challenges. Whilst the cognitive aspects regarding ethics and law are amenable to written exams, the underlying affective aspects of patient-centeredness/problem orientation or doctor-centered/disease orientation are commonly inferred from observing behavior (de Monchy et al., 1988). This is explored more fully in the section on assessment instruments.

CRITERIA FOR ASSESSMENT METHODS

Any method should meet the criteria of reliability and validity but must also be feasible if it is to be accepted.

Reliability

Reliability of an assessment is its ability to show stability and consistency over varying conditions of measurement (e.g. different observers, physicians, patients). Inter-rater reliability, the degree of agreement between observers of the same interview, is the most commonly used test of any assessment. Generalizability analysis identifies sources of unreliability such as ambiguous items, undertrained observers, halo effects by biased observers and observers having difficulty with certain items (Thorndike, 1982).

Research has shown that intercase reliability, the generalizability of results for the same physician across different cases or types of patients, is an important limiting factor in the measurement of medical interviewing skills (Van Thiel et al., 1991). The gold standard for a test is cited as Cronbach's alpha of 0.8.

Estimates range from 4 to 25 with 12 to 15 being the consensus for the number of test interviews needed to provide such a reliability. This is a very wide range. The number of cases needed to reach reliability is less when fewer criteria are used in the assessment instrument. Hence the range may reflect differences in assessment design.

Swanson and Norcini (1989) have estimated that 8 hours of testing time or approximately 24 20-minute stations are needed to reliably assess the domains of information gathering and communication skills. With an Objective Structured Clinical Examination designed to cover a wider range of clinical skills, and hence where variance from content area and skill domain is introduced, the estimated test time to achieve a reliability of 0.8 was 10 hours or 30 20-minute stations (Gruppen et al., 1997). Van der Vleuten and Swanson (1990) arrive at a figure of between 3 and 4 hours with 8-10 cases, 20 minutes in length. More recent studies using global ratings are reaching good reliability (0.83) with 2-hour Objective Structured Clinical Examinations using 10 cases (Tann et al., 1997).

Characteristics of the marking schemes that may contribute to poorer rater reliability have been investigated. Items requiring a qualitative grading in contrast to the simple documentation of the presence or absence of an action result in poorer agreement. It would also seem that shorter and more global rating scales have greater reliability than more detailed and lengthy checklists (Van der Vleuten et al., 1991; Van Thiel et al., 1992).

To what extent the need for a wide range of test cases is a reflection of the test's measurement of content in clinical history taking skills, rather than process skills, is unknown. It may be that we still cannot say how many stations or how much testing time is needed to assess communication and interpersonal skills because we do not have instruments that measure only these, without being confounded by clinical content and clinical knowledge issues. However, some believe it is not possible to separate communication from clinical context and that the two dimensions are interdependent (Colliver et al., 1999).

Examiner reliability

Inter-rater reliability is thought to improve with training of observers and simple, unambiguous, behaviorally specific items for scoring (Ovadia et al., 1982).

Taking an individual station overall checklist score correlations have been shown to vary between 0.02 and 0.76 between raters and within rater from 0.06 to 0.80 (Tamblyn et al., 1991a). Training has been most effective in improving the accuracy of non-medical raters and remarkably ineffective in improving physician rater agreements (Van der Vleuten et al., 1989). Selection, it is thought, may be more cost effective than training, whilst calibrating raters in advance and statistically adjusting scores on a *post hoc* basis for systematic rating error is another proposal (Newble et al., 1980).

Standardized patient reliability

Boon and Stewart (1998) in their review article identified two assessment scales which had been designed specifically for use by a standardized patient who is trained to assess students in real-time using Likert scales (Cohen et al., 1996; Schnabl et al., 1995; Kopelow et al., 1995). A variety of other scales exist which have also been used by standardized patients. In this situation the standardized patient both plays the patient role and fills out the rating on the candidate. A significant association was found between the accuracy of case presentation and within rater reliability (Tamblyn et al., 1991). The reliability of standardized patients with accuracy scores of 80% or lower was 0.14 compared to 0.68 for those with 100% accuracy in case presentation. Hence simulated patients who are more accurate in the presentation of the case will likely be more reliable raters. This finding held true irrespective of which test site or trainer was involved in training the standardized patients. In another study standardised patient accuracy was found to be good to very good and consistent even over an examination that lasted as long as 15 days (Vu et al., 1992). Petrusa et al. (1994) found that ratings done by trained standardized patients demonstrated very high reliability on the two scales of socioemotional and communication behaviors (0.93 and 0.95 respectively), indicating a consistent measure of these attributes for students across a 20 case clinical performance examination. Gender bias effects have been investigated by Colliver et al. (1993). Except for women examinees' higher performance in personal manner, men and women performed equally well on interpersonal and communication skills and did so regardless of the gender of the standardized patient.

Stillman (1993) has expressed the need for caution over use of standardized patients in high stakes exams despite the finding that, with careful selection and training, standardized patients can achieve acceptable levels of accuracy and reliability (Tamblyn et al., 1991b; Smee, 1994). Physician raters are believed to be more credible in high stakes exams or in an exam where there is a high failure rate (Colliver & Williams, 1993).

Validity

Valid instruments are those which achieve the intended standard of measure. Content validity is the degree to which the measure samples and represents the domain of the subject in question. Another criterion is whether the test is appropriate to the program's educational objectives and the proficiency levels to be obtained for the target group (e.g. undergraduates, residents).

Predictive validity relates to the instrument's ability to show or predict an increase in competency. Convergent/divergent validity is the ability to measure particular competencies (in this case communication and interviewing skills) and not other competencies (e.g. medical knowledge). This is of particular importance since content knowledge of the task has been shown to affect skills (Hodges et al., 1994, 1996).

Construct validity is achieved when the instrument measures only those theoretical dimensions of interviewing skills that cause changes in outcome such as patient satisfaction, compliance, recalled information or subsequent health behavior. Deriving items from the literature on communication and outcome addresses the issue on construct validity in design, but ideally should be tested for correlation with outcomes after the assessment (e.g. patient satisfaction, increased insight, feeling of involvement, health outcome).

The literature reveals a general lack of validity testing for assessment instruments of communication and interpersonal skills. Most testing that has been done relates to reliability (Boon & Stewart, 1998).

Feasibility

Strategies for maximizing reliability and validity whilst attending to practicality and costs are needed. There needs to be a reasonable test length and scoring time; simple and trainable criteria and definitions for observers; time and labor requirements to minimize costs; and user friendly documentation. The figures for length of exam, needed to reach reliability, vary enormously between studies although the more recent use of global ratings with good reliability and reduced test length is heartening.

ASSESSMENT GUIDES, INSTRUMENTS AND METHOD

Generic doctor-patient interaction skills

There are in existence a considerable number of assessment instruments containing criteria that relate to the underlying model of teaching and learning which the various authors have developed and which are informed by the evidence on behaviors affecting outcome. They vary in the degree of detailed items or globalization and the domains incorporated. Each has its own strengths and weaknesses in regard to the explicit underlying model of medical interviewing, observable categories of skills, inter-rater and inter-case reliability, validity, practicality and usefulness of instrument for feedback (Kraan et al., 1995).

Boon and Stewart (1998) have published a comprehensive review article of all those assessment instruments for patient-doctor communication which had either been published in the literature or were known to experts in the field and were obtainable from these sources. They used 1986-1996 as the time frame and identified a total of 44, of which 16 had been used primarily for educational purposes (teaching, feedback and assessment). The educational instruments are shown in the Appendix. Seven had been used in only one published study and only nine had ever been validated, mostly with patient satisfaction or level of training of examinees. They are generic frameworks for effective patient-doctor communication applicable in many different medical contexts and usually cover varying combinations of communication, interpersonal and history-taking skills. The reviewers subjected them to meta-analysis and collated information covering a brief description, number of items, reliability (inter-rater, intra-rater, reliability, test-retest and internal consistency), validity (convergent, divergent and construct, predictive and face), current use and other specific features.

There was considerable overlap with many items in these instruments, indicating similarities in the conceptual basis of measurement. Such similarities would tend to support the criteria of face/construct validity of these instruments. However, they noted that very little research had been undertaken on reliability and validity of these instruments with the exception of inter-rater reliability. Those most fully tested were the Arizona Clinical Interview Rating Scale and the Maastricht History Taking and Advice Checklist which have good internal consistency with Cronbach alpha values of 0.80-0.85. The former (16 items) lends itself to real-time assessment as well as analysis of videotapes. The latter (68 items) uses videotape analysis with extensive training of observers.

The instruments varied in their method of measurement. Some include qualitative judgements with rating scales such as Likert, allowing observers to rate how well an individual performs a specific behavior or task (Arizona Clinical Interview Rating Scale, Daily Rating Form of Student Clinical Performance, Brown University Interpersonal Skills Evaluation, Campbell et al.'s Assessment of Trainees, Hopkins Interpersonal Skills Assessment, Pendleton's Consultation

Map/Rating Scale). Others used checklists which code for the presence or absence of an activity (Lovett, SEGUE, MAAS).

Practical applications varied and whilst some were primarily used for assessment in real time (Arizona, Calgary-Cambridge, Daily Rating Form of Student Clinical Performance, Interpersonal and Communication Skills Checklist, Interpersonal Skills Rating Form, SEGUE), others were designed and used with video or audio recordings of simulated or real patient encounters which were subsequently graded (Brown University Interpersonal Skill Evaluation, Campbell et al.'s Assessment of Trainees, Hopkins Interpersonal Skills Assessment, MAAS, Pendleton's Consultation Map/Rating Scale, TALK).

Some instruments have been used for assessment of medical students whilst others were designed for use with physicians in continuing medical education (Schnabl et al., 1995; Kurtz et al., 1998; Pendleton et al., 1984; Makoul, 1995; Van Thiel et al., 1992). Low inter-case reliability has been identified as a problem with all the instruments to date with perhaps the exception of the revised MAAS. Van Thiel and colleagues (1992) have produced a simplified MAAS-Global scoring list which includes 12 concrete interview behaviors for communication and interpersonal skills and four for medical performance. Items are case-independent and global, but anchored with detailed criteria. A seven-point Likert scale is used for scoring. Between 8 and 12 cases (with two or one raters respectively) in 2–2½ hours were needed to achieve generalizability coefficients of 0.8 in general practice test settings, using videotape analysis of standardized patient encounters. They found that reliability improves if assessment was restricted to basic interviewing skills. Reports of validity and reliability using the revised MAAS with doctors in general practice settings are encouraging (Ram et al., 1999).

Specific instruments

Whilst the generic schemes include behaviors fundamental to any consultation, some modifications may be necessary in particular circumstances. In interviewing a patient with mania, for example, Hodges (1994) points out that a candidate would be rated on his/her ability to abandon open-ended questions and firmly direct the interview, a technique which would be inconsiderate and inappropriate with, for example, a depressed patient.

Issue specific guides have been designed for clinical situations in which particular skills may also be required. For example there are guides for breaking bad news (Miller et al., 1999), bereavement and palliative care (Argent et al., 1994; Maguire & Faulkner, 1988), revealing hidden depression (Gask et al., 1988), prevention and motivation (Sanson-Fisher et al., 1991), addressing gender and cultural issues (Chugh et al., 1993). Miller et al. (1999) tested their rating scale, specifically designed for assessing breaking bad news, on simulated encounters and found a high internal consistency (Cronbach's alpha 0.93).

Empathy has been singled out for separate assessment in various models, guides and instruments (Evans et al., 1993; Suchman et al., 1997). Suchman's team observed that patients seldom verbalize their emotions directly and spontaneously, tending to offer clues instead. Learners need to actively and consciously use empathy. Their ability to recognize hidden emotions, invite exploration, acknowledge these emotions so that the patient feels understood, avoid using potential empathic opportunity terminators (i.e. cutting patients off as a result of the clinician's preoccupation with diagnosis and problem solving), allow time and avoid premature empathy are all contained in his model. This model is used in training and formative feedback rather than as a graded assessment instrument. There is a lack of instruments reported in the literature that specifically assess empathy, especially non-verbal behaviors (Boon & Stewart, 1998).

Attitudinal assessments

Assessments of patient-doctor communication which focus on the quality of the interpersonal interaction, in contrast to those which assess technical performance, are needed (Roter & Hall, 1989; Wasserman & Inui, 1983). This relationship domain combines both attitudinal and skills aspects of the patient-doctor interaction and is characterized by patient-centered, problem-oriented in contrast to doctor-centered, disease-oriented behavior.

Attitudes are usually measured using questionnaires and attitude scales with Likert type ratings. A number of such questionnaires have been developed to assess and compare the attitudes of different groups of students and practitioners toward the patient-centered, problem-oriented as opposed to the doctor-centered, disease-oriented end of the scale (De Monchy et al., 1988; Grol et al., 1990; Price et al., 1998).

There is some evidence that attitudes correlate with physicians' actual behaviors in consultations. Using a self-report questionnaire with a Likert scale on beliefs about psychosocial aspects of care, those physicians with positive attitudes used more empathy and reassurance, fewer closed questions and provided relatively more psychosocial and less biomedical information than their colleagues (Levinson & Roter, 1995). Patients were more active in these consultations as evidenced by expressing opinions and asking questions. Hence, this type of questionnaire assessment could be helpful in identifying students' attitudinal orientation and potential behavior. Other authors have used measures of moral development and values preferences primarily for evaluation purposes, although these instruments do have potential for assessment (Rezler et al., 1992). Whilst knowledge (cognitive component) of moral, ethical and legal principles may be assessed in written examinations, ethical sensitivity has also been measured (Consensus Statement, 1998; Herbert et al., 1992).

There have been numerous written assessment methods developed to test cognitive components of ethical competence such as ability to discuss concepts, identifying and weighing value-laden aspects of decision making, defining the relevance of principles to a case and arriving at a defensible clinical opinion. There is, however, also debate about humanistic qualities such as compassion, empathy and respect for patients which reflect a student's moral character, and whether, how and when these should be assessed (Goldie, 2000). These elements belong to the non-cognitive factors of ethical competence (Miles et al., 1989; Smith et al., 1994; Wooliscroft et al., 1994; Singer et al., 1993).

Objective Structured Clinical Examinations and simulated surgeries have been used to assess behavioral aspects of attitudes. Singer and colleagues (1993) found reliability of only 0.28 in a four station Objective Structured Clinical Examination designed to test clinical ethics in final-year medical students. To achieve the gold standard of 0.8 would require 41 stations, i.e. almost seven hours of testing. Whilst it has value in formative assessment, Singer advocates additional more reliable methods for assessing ethics (Singer et al., 1996).

Assessment of attitudes has recently been undertaken in the United Kingdom as part of the General Medical Council's performance procedure (Jolly, 1998). Using the simulated surgery assessment format, examples of attitudinal items included acceptance of the patient's perspective on the problem, exploration of the patient's concerns and validation of the patient's anxieties. Practice observations of doctors performing real clinical tasks is another method used to investigate doctors whose performance has been questioned (General Medical Council, 1996). Whilst results from these methods are favorable, the importance of trying to detect attitude problems during undergraduate training has been stressed. It is suggested from pilot studies that many of the problems with doctors' attitudes that come before professional standards and complaints committees probably date back some time (Jolly, 1998). Regular peer/collegiate assessment might have detected problems and ways of collating data in medical schools should be found.

Behaviors such as those cited above are commonly incorporated in Objective Structured Clinical Examination stations and in doctor-patient assessment instruments. However, the less detailed, more subjective and informal assessments of communication and attitude which occur in end of firm clerkship or programme gradings, may be particularly valuable data from real life settings. They provide opportunities to identify any problems, explore the cause and help deal with the student's situation. The major problem again is that of reliability and students frequently complain of the unfairness of these gradings. Nevertheless, attempts have been made to provide clearer and explicit behavioral descriptors for attitudes in daily clinical practice (Bienenstock et al., 1994). Triangulation offers a means whereby data that are acquired from different sources and found to be consistent can corroborate validity and reliability.

Attitude questionnaires have a place in evaluating the outcome of educational programs by assessing changes in students' attitudes at different points during the course. Many studies have revealed that students' psychosocial orientation is high at the outset of their course, declines in the middle years and may increase toward the end as they realize that they will soon be facing the realities of caring for patients themselves (Powell et al., 1987). This may reflect a change of focus in learning needs in the middle years as students are intent on understanding biomedical content and it has implications for when students' attitudes might best be assessed (Kraan et al., 1990). It also demonstrates the power of the social environment to undermine or sustain appropriate professional attitudes (Pfeiffer et al., 1998).

We interpret attitudes from observing a person's behavior. When we see behavior we disapprove of we may assume negative attitudes or indeed the opposite if we see behavior we deem appropriate. The relationship to behavior is, however, not always linear and the effect of situational variables is important in understanding both attitudes and behavior. Moreover, even with positive attitudes, students or doctors may lack skills to achieve effective interactions with patients. Hence, caution is needed since there may be a number of explanations for observed behavior including; emotions (e.g. fear leading to defensiveness), lack of skills, lack of knowledge, a mixture of attitudes (good and bad), competing pressures and the effect of social context, environment and power relations.

Discussion of the affective and cognitive components of attitudes (underlying feelings, thoughts and knowledge) is important in learning sessions that incorporate immediate feedback. At present summative assessment of attitudes confines itself to the knowledge base of ethical principles and reasoning in written examinations and to observed behaviors in Objective Structured Clinical Examination stations. The need for a combination of methods in assessment of students has been made (Case, 1997).

Use of assessment instruments to evaluate the effect of training

Assessment instruments for communication skills, interpersonal skills and attitudes should be able to detect changes and improvements in an individual as a result of training. Boon and Stewart (1998) highlighted the relative lack of longitudinal studies which investigate the development and maintenance of patient-practitioner relationships. Similarly, there is a lack of well-designed intervention studies on how educational strategies influence behaviors and ultimately patient outcomes.

Hulsman and colleagues (1999), in a review of 14 postgraduate training studies, found only three with a good pre and post test and control design, hence conclusions from the rest must be treated with caution. Those with behavioral observations nearly all reported some training effects whilst the areas which improved most were interpersonal and affective rather than information giving behaviors (Levinson & Roter, 1993; Baile et al., 1997; Maguire et al., 1978, 1986; Bowman et al., 1992). The assessment instruments used were mostly designed as study-specific rating scales and only in four studies were previously published rating scales used. The use of so many different instruments makes it difficult to compare the results of studies. It has been suggested that researchers, clinicians and educationalists work together with existing instruments and adapt or modify them in the light of research on validity and reliability (Boon & Stewart, 1998).

Test methods

The assessment instruments described above may be used in a variety of test methods. Methodologies and rating schemes may vary according to the target group, ranging from undergraduate students at different stages of their clinical course to postgraduate clinicians in workplace settings undertaking accreditation and reaccreditation assessments. Some are specifically designed for practicing doctors such as general practitioners (Cox & Mulholland, 1993) or for use as audit tools in hospital settings (Morris et al., 1995). In many cases the target group for the methods used is not specified.

Jolly and Grant (1997) provide a comprehensive guide to assessment methods. Those that particularly relate to assessment of non-cognitive factors include the following:

- Objective Structured Clinical Examination
- Simulated Surgeries
- Video Assessment – real or simulated patients
- Audio-taped Assessments
- Record of Practice – Critical Incident Audit
- Self Assessment
- Peer Assessment & Audit
- Patient Assessments.

Objective Structured Clinical Examination

Objective Structured Clinical Examinations are now a common assessment method for clinical competencies and an important tool for undergraduate and postgraduate training. They are a major component of the licensing exams of the College of Family Physicians of Canada and the Medical Council of Canada (Reznick et al., 1993a). They use either trained real patients or a person trained to act as a patient to maintain standardization. This is the commonest method of testing clinical communication, interpersonal and history taking skills. Each station is marked according to a predetermined list of objectives for demonstrating competence in the particular skill under test. The examiner does not use his or her subjective opinion and each student is exposed to the same test set and criteria. Reliability on marking some of the Yes/No items has been reported to be high whilst it is less so for items requiring qualitative evaluation of a performance item (Kraan et al., 1995).

Frequently the checklists used combine history content either general (e.g. asked about factors that triggered the complaint) or specific (e.g. asked about associated visual disturbances); communication skills (e.g. used comprehensible language, summarized, gave information in small amounts at a time); and interpersonal skills (e.g. sets the proper pace during the interview, puts the patient at ease, reflects emotions properly).

Good agreement can be achieved between raters scoring the same station even with minimal training. There is, however, generally poor agreement between a candidate's performance at different stations; hence it is estimated that between 15 and 20 cases are required to reach high levels of reliability for a score of candidates' skills (Van der Vleuten & Swanson, 1990). This method of testing is valid in that it matches student learning and objectives and encourages practice of key skills.

Despite the relatively widespread use of Objective Structured Clinical Examinations in a number of countries, there is considerable variation in design according to purpose, construction, choice of content, checklists or rating scales, pass/fail decisions, integration of skills and station length (Van der Vleuten et al., 1994).

In practice many rating scales designed and used in Objective Structured Clinical Examinations are probably simplified short scales with global items. An example given by Jolly and Grant (1997, p. 97) shows a five point rating scale with eight items including introduction, puts patient at ease, checks patient knowledge, clarity of explanation/avoiding jargon, checks understanding, sensitivity/empathy, details next step and invites questions. These short scales are commonly used schemes for Objective Structured Clinical Examination stations when marking is done in real time and can be done by either a trained simulated patient or faculty. Such simplified schemes are in contrast to the detailed published assessment instruments and are modified to fit the station length, complexity and feasibility. They will be based on the guides used in training but modified according to the task that the candidate is expected to perform.

Examiner briefing and training is important to ensure that behaviors within global categories have been specified and defined.

Objective Structured Clinical Examinations may be used for formative or summative assessment. Large scale standardized patient-based Objective Structured Clinical Examinations have been held in Quebec since 1990 as part of licensing exams. These are 26 stations in length with cases varying from 7 to 20 minutes duration. Since 1995 the number of longer cases has increased because of the introduction and integration of assessment of doctor-patient communication and organizational skills within all cases (as distinct from separate communication stations). Doctor-patient communication constitutes 8-10% of the marks (Grand'Maison et al., 1997). The cost of running an Objective Structured Clinical Examination is high. In Canada in 1993 the per-student cost was estimated to be between $496 and $870 depending on the accounting model used (Reznick et al., 1993b). However, the importance of the fundamental clinical skills being assessed, and the unique capability of the Objective Structured Clinical Examination method to do so, are arguments for its value.

Simulated surgeries

These involve replication of a clinical scenario in a realistic clinical setting using standardized patients. They are currently used mainly in general practice and have been used by the General Medical Council in the United Kingdom, but could also be used in hospital settings (General Medical Council, 1996).

Video assessment

All of the above may be videotaped for rating of encounters at a later time. However, video assessment has been developed as a particular method. Predominantly reported in relation to postgraduate assessment, recordings are made of real or simulated patient encounters in everyday practice and reviewed later to assess performance. Observer effect is minimized and allows for assessment of real clinical performance in contrast to competence in examination settings (Rethans, 1990). Indeed, a particular concern with Objective Structured Clinical Examinations is whether competence in an exam is a reliable measure of performance in the workplace. Validity in real life settings will be high. Sampling and reviewing a broad enough range of consultations will increase its reliability. In some instances the trainee records as many as 50 consecutive patients to prevent biased selection (Jolly & Grant, 1997). Obtaining ethical consent from patients presents perhaps the main difficulty in ensuring a broad range of test set. It is also a time consuming process. Formative assessment in undergraduate learning commonly makes use of videotaping and review.

Another technique uses video to assess perceptual skills. Individuals watch videotaped consultations and are assessed on their ability to understand the emotion communicated by another through verbal or non-verbal means, such as facial expression, body movements and voice tone (Rosenthal et al., 1979). This particular method is assessing the candidates' perceptual skills rather than their interactional process skills. These are thought to be importantly linked although evidence is not available.

Audio-assessment

This has similar usage to videotaped assessments but lacks data on body language. It has been used specifically in telephone consultation assessment (Kosower et al., 1996). Both video and audiotapes have the advantage of a permanent record which permits easy analysis and where necessary (or desirable) re-analysis. Videotaping of Objective Structured Clinical Examinations has been advocated as this can help to avoid or resolve appeal problems in certifying examinations (Heaton & Kurtz, 1992; Martin et al., 1998).

Record of practice

Using an audit of critical incidents, one study has been described in which nurses were asked to report poor or exceptional performance amongst medical students (Newble, 1983). Whilst having the advantage of a real life setting and potentially adding to its validity, Newble raises doubts over validity, reliability and feasibility. Reliability is thought to be low owing to a large number of assessors and contexts. The technique has not been widely used, suggesting low feasibility (Jolly & Grant, 1997). It could however be argued that concerns about an individual's performance documented by a wide range of people and in different settings could alert teachers to problems. Triangulation is a method which seeks to identify evidence from different sources to corroborate findings. End of firm or clerkship gradings on communication, interpersonal skills and attitudes are not regarded as reliable. However, as previously mentioned, attitudinal problems seen in practicing doctors might have been detected earlier if information had been gathered and reviewed (Jolly, 1998).

Self-assessment

Developing learners' abilities to self assess is desirable. This approach clearly fits in with the learning process, formative assessment with feedback and the development of lifelong learning skills of reflection and self-assessment (Novack, Epstein, & Paulsen, 1999). Video has been used widely in general practice vocational training in the United Kingdom where trainees record and review their performance as part of their training (Hays, 1990; Cox & Mulholland, 1993). The Measure of Patient-Centred Care assesses a physician's perception of his or her care of the last 10 patients seen (Maheux et al., 1997). It uses a Likert scale and has been tested for reliability and validity. It has an internal consistency (Cronbach's alpha) of 0.8 and construct validity has been demonstrated (with level of training). Self-audit questionnaires have been found to be valuable by physicians who have used them (Morris et al., 1995).

In one study 3rd year students' overall self-assessments correlated 0.46 with those of the independent observer, a finding which is higher than typically reported in studies of the validity of self-assessment (Farnill et al., 1997). The students' mean rating of their performance was, however, lower than that of the observer.

Martin et al. (1998) used videotaped benchmarks to improve self-assessment ability of 50 family practice residents in Canada. Following a 10-minute videotaped interview with a difficult communication problem the doctor in question and two experts evaluated the doctor's communication skills. The doctor then watched four performances of the same clinical situation. These ranged from poor to good but the doctor was not told which was which. The doctor evaluated each of these and then re-evaluated his or her own performance. The first correlation between the doctor and experts' evaluations was moderate (r = 0.38) but increased significantly after viewing the other videotapes (r = 0.52). Interestingly, *post hoc* analysis showed that neither the initial nor post-benchmark self-assessment ability was related to the ability to accurately evaluate the benchmarks in a manner consistent with the experts. It would seem that providing a set of benchmarks improves trainees' ability to self evaluate even though this is not strongly linked to the ability to assess others doing the same task, or to an explicit identification of the qualities of the benchmark. Observational, perceptive and analytical skills have been found to improve with training. Students who had received training were better able to identify helpful and unhelpful interviewing behaviors when observing taped consultations than a control group who had not received training (Kendrik & Freeling, 1993).

Peer assessment and audit

Rating forms have been developed for peer assessment and audit. An example is the Physician Assessment Rating Form used by the Royal Australasian College of Physicians in its Maintenance of Professional Standards Programme (Jolly & Grant, 1997, pp. 115-116). Extensively tested it has been reported to have satisfactory validity and reliability. Fifteen ratings on the physician's interpersonal skills and attitudes are obtained from members of the multidisciplinary team.

Peer and self-assessment carry less weight than that by trained observers but are of considerable value in formative assessment and in audit programs. The ability to self assess and request feedback is essential for becoming a life-long learner throughout clinical practice (Hays, 1990).

Patient assessment

A number of questionnaires have been designed for patients to assess the doctor's performance (Henbest & Stewart, 1990). Interviewing of patients requires extensive manpower and large numbers of patients are needed with adjustments for differences in patient populations in order to compare scores among residents (Tamblyn et al., 1994; Henkin et al., 1990). In one study an average of 12.2 satisfaction ratings were collected on a large sample (91) of medical residents and clinical clerks. This provided a reliability of 0.56 (intraclass correlation) for patients' satisfaction scores of residents. 15% were found to have a substantially greater proportion of poor and fair ratings than average. Valuable information was gained on residents' ability to establish a satisfactory patient-physician relationship. However, the numbers of ratings required may limit its feasibility as a way of assessing residents (McLeod et al., 1994).

Another study with intervention and control design gathered data from 5885 patient-completed questionnaires for 68 GP registrars. Ratings were significantly higher for GPs who had participated in the communication skills teaching (Greco et al., 1998).

Standardized patients

Use and role

The standardized patient has been a major influence on both the learning of explicit skills in the doctor-patient relationship and in assessing these competencies. Originally described by Barrows in 1964, these generally healthy people are trained to play a patient with a particular set of symptoms and history (and in some cases physical signs) realistically and reliably (Barrows & Abrahamson, 1964). They provide a means of developing more uniform and controlled instruction and evaluation of basic clinical skills including clinical communication skills in core or key conditions and situations.

In North America these programs are highly developed such that in many cases experienced patient simulators have become trainers themselves and are called patient instructors. They train other simulators, teach medical students communication, interpersonal skills and in some instances clinical method of examination and history taking skills. They also grade students on their performance and give feedback. Additionally, some may have a major part in organization and administration of Objective Structured Clinical Examinations. Stillman (1993) in a review published in 1993 of experiences working with standardized patients for over 20 years reflects in detail on the process and concludes by cautioning that further research must be done before standardized patients can be used as assessors for high-stakes certifying and licensing examinations.

In the United States and Canada in 1994, 80% of medical schools were using standardized patients for training and evaluation (Anderson et al., 1994). It is evident from surveys conducted at that time that they were used most in teaching breast and pelvic examination and for the male genital urinary examination. There is evidence of their increasing use in the area of interviewing skills and medical history taking. The recommendations to include standardised patient based stations in graduation examinations has triggered the establishment of consortia in North America to share expertise, resources, skills and research opportunities (Morrison & Barrows, 1994).

In Europe simulated patients are used in a variety of ways although research data on the overall situation are not available. It would appear, however, that their role is more in relation to learning, feedback, formative assessment and as standardized patients in examinations and less in respect of grading students or training other standardized patients. The more confined role that standardized patients play in Europe may be to do with resources, philosophy or both. One of the debates that exists is whether training standardized patients to rate students' history taking and examination skills (content) alters their situation to such an extent that they are no longer able to stay in the role of "naïve but intelligent" patient.

Selection

Recruitment of local lay people, actors and patients has been used. Smee (1993) cautions that health professionals as patients, and even as trainers, may have difficulty in adopting the patient's perspective and find it harder to simulate a patient's level of naivety in response to medical jargon and the nature of the medical problem. On the other hand standardized patients when trained are more experienced with regard to medical interviewing than a real patient or student. They may be exposed to hundreds of medical interviews and trained to become focused in their evaluation of the students' interpersonal skills. Pololi (1995) defines characteristics needed, including absence of negative or punitive attitudes toward physicians, physical stamina, good memory, ability to express emotions verbally and flexibility of time schedules.

Training and costs

The time required to train standardized patients ranges between one hour and fifteen hours depending on the task, with an average of four hours reported to train a standardized patient in one case for an Objective Structured Clinical Examination (Stillman, 1993; Smee, 1994). Costs are likely to vary across institutions and depend on whether professional actors, lay people or volunteers are involved. It would appear to be easier to arrange standardized patient training than to get faculty examiners along to training sessions. A number of studies have now shown that simulated patients who are trained and standardized provide reliable assessment (Tamblyn et al., 1991a, 1991b). Within training and formative assessment their feedback would appear to be particularly valued (Pololi, 1995).

RESEARCH ON ITEMIZED CHECKLISTS AND GLOBAL RATINGS

In the past items such as "ability to relate to the patient" or "manner" with either a checklist or Likert scale were used to assess communication abilities. These early global ratings, although simple and quick, were too vague and difficult for examiners and learners to interpret or learn from. Progress from research into the components of effective patient-doctor encounters resulted in extremely detailed instruments with many specific items, e.g. MAAS (Kraan et al., 1989), and the Cambridge-Calgary Guide (Kurtz et al., 1998). Support for the level of detail came from the argument that learners need this degree of specificity so as to be clear about the explicit expectations in their medical interviewing and to know that these behaviors will be assessed in a summative situation.

Detailed checklists with many items of specific behavior have helped make transparent to students and assessors what skills are expected. In Boon and Stewart's review of educational assessment instruments, the number of items ranged from 68 in the Maastricht History Taking and Advice Checklist (Kraan et al., 1989) to 6 in the Daily Rating for Student Clinical Performance (White et al., 1991). Very detailed checklists are also said by some authors to ensure an objectivity and help to reduce error from examiner unreliability.

There has, however, been a move in recent years back toward using more global ratings for assessment. The assumption that checklists are more objective and hence better than rating scales with respect to psychometric properties as reliability has been challenged by recent studies (Van der Vleuten et al., 1991; Norman et al., 1991). These authors refer to checklists as being "objectified" rather than objective, and conclude that not only do they not provide more reliable scores but also they may be trivializing the content being measured. Research now indicates that global communication checklists and detailed communication checklists are highly correlated; thus, it is probably unnecessary to employ the time-consuming detailed versions. Although globalizing results in more examiner variation, this hardly influences total test reliability since, with different examiners at different stations, examiner error at individual stages averages out across stations (Van der Vleuten et al., 1994).

More recently Cohen et al. (1996) compared checklist and rating scores using the Interpersonal and Communication Skills Checklist. This 26-item checklist has five sections (eliciting information, non-verbal behavior, patient education, professional manner and patient satisfaction). At the end of each section the standardized patient was asked to provide a global rating of the component indicated by the items in that section. Correlations between the checklist scores and ratings for the five components ranged from 0.6 to 0.8. The inter-case reliability of the checklists and ratings ranged from 0.33 to 0.55 and 0.39 and 0.52, respectively over the five components. Indeed, there were somewhat higher reliabilities for subjective ratings than for the "objectified" checklist. The authors state that the pattern of results lends further support to the claim that *"objectified"* measures, like checklists, *"do not inherently provide more reliable sources"* (p. 89).

Amiel and Lunenfield (1994) found that the total global rating mean score was significantly higher than checklist mean scores and was possibly reflecting qualities not assessed by the checklist. With this particular design the standardized patients went through the process of using the detailed checklist items before giving a global rating for the section. Detailed checklists may still be important at some point for examiner and student training so that expected behaviors are specified (Cohen et al., 1997). It would seem, however, that use of global ratings alone, without the associated use of a detailed checklist, can still provide good reliability with both standardized patient and physician raters (Tann et al., 1997). Moreover, detailed checklists do not allow for the fact that there is usually no single correct approach to a problem and they present examiners with difficulties of how to reward for helpful behaviors which are not on the checklist.

Intuitively the problem with global ratings is that they begin to move toward subjective assessment and risk greater unreliability. The research, however, now suggests greater reliability when adding global scores in history taking stations. The importance of employing experienced and trained examiners is highlighted together with the special importance that interpersonal skills may be afforded in this approach to assessment (Amiel & Lunenfeld, 1994).

Moreover, in the Netherlands there is a clear shift away from detailed prescriptive lists which were encouraging inappropriate student learning (Van der Vleuten et al., 1991, 1994). They had potentially negative effects on study behavior and led to triviality of content being measured. Concern was expressed that students learnt and applied checklists without a more integrated approach to interacting with patients. Furthermore it is difficult to infer from such detail whether the student demonstrates a level of competency. The "gestalt" of the interaction is not apparent and the higher components of clinical competence tend to be overlooked (Cox, 1990).

Other problems with itemized lists in the Objective Structured Clinical Examination format tests is that standardized patients are instructed not to divulge information which the student is expected to obtain until the student explicitly asks for the information (Smee, 1993, 1994). This may run contrary to the whole emphasis in the instructional model of patient-centered interviewing where students are encouraged to use open questions and facilitative behavior to let patients unfurl their story. By doing so, students learn to obtain considerable information in the context of the patient's narrative. However, if the assessment instrument and the corresponding standardized patient behavior direct the candidate toward closed questioning style, then there is a conflict in the learning objectives and the assessment method.

More global items such as empathic and listening abilities, skills at giving explanations, involving patients and use of language provide the opportunity to rate proficiency more meaningfully. The debate over the use of global or very detailed assessment instruments appears to be moving away from the latter for both educational and psychometric reasons.

CAN AND SHOULD COMMUNICATION SKILLS BE ASSESSED SEPARATELY FROM CLINICAL CONTENT?

Are there general aspects of the doctor-patient relationship that can be evaluated in any encounter independent of the type of clinical problem?

Most Objective Structured Clinical Examinations have not contained stations that focus predominantly on communication skills. Typically clinicians when asked to create stations will produce content laden scoring systems that are factually based. Students are required to address content area as a primary goal (e.g. take a history, perform a physical examination, obtain informed consent) whilst communication and interpersonal skills (rapport, empathy, interviewing technique, control of emotions) are secondary. This is also likely to be a reflection of the emphasis on content in the clinical teaching and learning setting. Rarely have stations been created to specifically test communication skills as a primary objective.

Some studies have shown that performance in communication skills stations is not well correlated with performance in other communication stations. Much of the research on performance-based assessments has shown only moderate inter-station reliability (Vu & Barrows, 1994). This applies even when cases are drawn from the same speciality, when the same diagnosis is portrayed with different complaints or when the same complaint, due to different diagnoses, is presented to the students. The authors suggest that, whilst test development may need to be improved, another explanation could be that performance or competence is specific to content and not a generalizable measure. The troubling conclusion to this is that it would be necessary to test students' communication skills on each type of clinical problem, rather than a few "representable" observations (Vu & Barrows, 1994).

It has been pointed out that in many Objective Structured Clinical Examination stations the communication skills component is an add-on to history taking stations which test clinical content. Hodges and colleagues (1994) proposed the need for communication skills stations where the clinical content is an add-on. They postulated that by increasing the difficulty of the communication skills challenge in a station there may be greater variance in students' scores and improved generalizability. Six stations were created each with two versions; a straightforward, easy one where the patient did not display strong emotions or reaction and a complicated one where, with the same clinical problem, the standardized patient demonstrated difficult emotions (fear, anxiety, confusion, depression, anger and sadness). Each student had three easy and three complicated stations. Increasing the station's difficulty in terms of handling more challenging emotional content, resulted in only slightly greater variance between candidates as seen by a trend toward a larger standard deviation. They found that "communication skills" are highly bound to content. The most effective communication checklists appeared to be those that sought very specific behaviors deemed necessary for each specific clinical problem. Increased knowledge of the content "improves" a candidate's apparent communication skills. Conversely poor communication skills may impede the gathering of content even when the candidate possesses adequate knowledge about the problem. The authors think the search for a set of generalizable communication skills will remain elusive and that assessors should define and assess skills that are complementary to specific clinical problems. Colliver et al. (1999) recently reported on the relationship between clinical competence and communication skills in standardized patient assessment. These are two dimensions of the clinical encounter. For each station (15 examinations) simple Pearson's correlations were computed. To overcome halo effect they also computed corrected cross-half and corrected cross-case correlations. Simple correlations were around 0.5 whilst the others were 0.65 to 0.7. He concludes that the moderate relationship is not due to a flaw in the measurement of clinical competence, as has been suggested, but a natural consequence of the clinical encounter, in which there exists an interdependence of these two dimensions. It would appear from the research evidence to date that clinical content and communication in relation to it are such closely linked dimensions that the two cannot be separated. As yet there does not seem to have been any research where students are told the clinical condition in advance and allowed to prepare their knowledge on this topic, such that it would be their communication and interpersonal skills in the encounter alone that were being tested. It has not been possible to test for communication and interpersonal skills independently from the clinical case content.

The approach taken by certification exam designers has been to increase the length of Objective Structured Clinical Examination stations to include doctor-patient assessment in each of the patient-based stations and hence integrate them to account for 8-10% of marks, rather than assess them separately (Grand'Maison et al., 1997).

STANDARD SETTING AND PASS/FAIL DECISIONS

Summative examinations require decisions on pass/fail or borderline scores. It is a complex process and there is currently a lack of a standard available for medical interviewing to decide on such cut off points. The method most commonly used in setting a standard on individual stations is the Angoff method (Angoff, 1971).

A two-stage method has been described using Angoff standard-setting procedure first and followed by a revision of the standard after the exam has taken place. This is in the light of structured discussions of the Objective Structured Clinical Examination scores of real students (Morrison et al., 1996).

Another method is that in use since 1994/5 by the Medical Council of Canada on its large-scale multicenter Objective Structured Clinical Examination for postgraduate physicians (Dauphinee et al., 1997). Physician examiners make global judgments at each station to identify candidates with borderline performances. The scores on those stations where candidates' performances are judged to be borderline are added for each station and an initial passing score is obtained for all stations and then the exam as a whole. The latter score is then adjusted upward one standard error of measurement for the final passing score. The authors state this is not suitable for small scale Objective Structured Clinical Examinations of 100-150 as the numbers of observations are not large enough to dilute any differences in performance from one year to another. This technique requires expert standard setters like physicians rather than trained simulated patients.

Some institutions use a group norm-referencing method. Hence when a student's score is lower than one standard deviation below the mean of the group, the score is considered insufficient (Kraan et al., 1995). Other groups have made decisions to set a pass mark, i.e. criterion referencing. For example Schnabl used the literature to identify 13 items and apply a 7 point Likert scale (Schnabl et al., 1995). They used an average of 5 for each item as a standard for acceptable minimal performance.

Kopelow et al. (1994) set a pass mark of 71% for interpersonal skills, arguing that below a threshold the simulated patient was not making a strong enough positive comment about the student's interpersonal skills for that student to pass. Standard setting is a complex process. Clearly if the standard is set too high too many candidates will fail although they may be competent.

Whilst consensus is an important part of the process the difference between what people say they should do and what they do in practice may be quite different. Hence, problems arise in not only defining the methods of assessing the performance quality of doctors, but even more in defining the level of acceptable care. In other words, there are difficulties in deciding what is "competence", what is "good" and what is "bad". The danger of a panel of experts setting a standard is that it runs the risk of being an "armchair" standard and not one that has a basis in actual practice. Even when consensus groups decide on standards, or when physicians were asked to construct for themselves standards of care for use in everyday clinical practice, they failed to meet their own standards in many instances (Norman et al., 1985).

Rethans and colleagues (1991a) used the framework devised by a consensus group for common cases in primary care which specified essential actions, intermediate actions and superfluous actions for a variety of presenting problems. Although this is measuring technical clinical skills rather than communication or interpersonal skills the findings are of interest. In actual practice the doctors' performance met only 56% of the actions which they had considered to be essential. Coles (1998) refers to the gap between theory (good practice that is theoretically defined and is the ideal) and personal theory (how people translate the ideal into standards of good everyday practice for themselves) and the gap between personal theory and practice (what they actually do). The fact that doctors perform below predetermined standards, even when agreed by them, does not prove they are incompetent. It should at least be tested against the hypothesis that standards for actual care are still not realistic (Rethans et al., 1991b).

The consensus working group pointed out that standard setting is based on expert judgments of students' performances, but that there was a need for outcome (predictive validity) studies, to relate to behaviors captured in the testing of standardized patient interactions to actual patient outcomes. Standard setting remains a difficult issue for every type of assessment including non-cognitive factors.

CONTEXT OF ASSESSMENT – SIMULATED OR WORKPLACE ASSESSMENTS

How important is the context of assessment of non-cognitive factors? Case (1997) draws attention to the three inferences made in assessment. Evaluation aims to make a decision good, bad or indifferent about a candidate's performance in a test. Generalization entails being sure that the results of this test reflect performance in the universe and is dependent on sampling. Extrapolation, the third inference, involves the assumption that the performance in an artificial test setting will be the same on a daily basis in real life contexts. Increasing standardization of tests and extending sampling improves evaluation and generalization judgments but the former reduces the ability to extrapolate. Conversely, tests in real life settings are difficult to standardize and control for sampling.

Rethans (1990) distinguishes competence and performance: two different concepts in the assessment of quality of medical care. Performance relates to "what a doctor does in his day to day practice" whilst competence is "what a doctor is capable of doing". Most authors use the terms interchangeably without drawing these important distinctions. Intuitively passing exams should tell us about future performance of doctors, i.e. they should have predictive validity, but as Rethans pointed out, no evidence existed to validate this assumption.

Doctors have also pointed out the inhibitive effect of observed stations in clinical exams and the possibility of this affecting their behavior. Hence, the intrusive nature of the test, anxiety created and distortion of behavior may be an issue in the reliable assessment of competence and performance. To control for patient variation, one approach being used to assess performance is to send simulated patients to the clinic unannounced and for the simulator to assess the clinician's performance. Clinicians know that simulators will be coming so consent has been gained, but do not know when or who they are (Burri et al., 1976; Norman et al., 1985; Rethans et al., 1991b). This methodology was acceptable to the doctors in question (Rethans & Van Boven, 1987; Rethans et al., 1991a).

Some research has shown that students and clinicians cannot distinguish simulated from real patients in history taking and that there is no difference in their interviewing behavior between the two (Sanson-Fisher & Poole, 1980; Colliver & Williams, 1993; Rethans & Van Boven, 1987; Rethans et al., 1991c). Other studies, however, have suggested that this might not always be the case and care needs to be taken to ensure standardized patients have carefully constructed cover stories and are sufficiently well matched to and briefed about the local area of the practice (Brown et al., 1998).

Videotaped consultations with real patients and the application of rating scales to provide feedback to general practitioners has been used in training for a number of years (Pendleton et al., 1984; Hays, 1990). More recently the General Practice training schemes in the United Kingdom have devised an approach for reviewing a number of videotaped real consultations which span different clinical situations (Royal College of General Practitioners, 1996). There continues to be debate about feasibility, cost, reliability and validity, particularly in relation to global versus detailed skills and competencies with as yet very little research data available on these issues (Campbell et al., 1995; Campbell & Murray, 1996). General practitioners have reported greater satisfaction with analysis of their videotaped real consultations which they deemed as natural and more recognizable as their normal working practice style (Ram et al., 1999). Acceptable levels of reliability were reached after 2½ hours of observation, of 12 consultations with a single observer. Validity was high and costs and feasibility were acceptable compared to assessment in simulated standardized settings.

Some studies have been carried out in Canada with residents in ambulatory settings and using patient satisfaction as the outcome variable. Valuable information was gained on residents' ability to establish a satisfactory patient-physician relationship. However the large numbers of ratings required may limit its feasibility as a way of assessing residents (McLeod et al., 1994). Interestingly, patient satisfaction ratings were found to have a strong correlation with faculty ratings of resident humanism. There was no association between residents' self-ratings and those by faculty and patients. The two sources, patient and faculty, provide triangulation of data and support for the findings. The authors suggest that the ambulatory care setting offers a useful context for assessment of non-cognitive behavioral features of resident performance.

Audit tools for communication have been piloted. In one such project consultants reviewed their own communication skills and compared their self-assessment with the feedback from their patients (Morris et al., 1995). It was seen as a useful process by the consultants and patients although design, methodological features and small numbers did not allow any further conclusions.

The incorporation of communication skills in both audit and appraisal are an inevitable result of both the high proportion of patient complaints that relate to communication and attitude, and of the increasingly recognized importance of these domains of professional practice (Audit Commission, 1993).

CONCLUDING COMMENTS

The development of reliable and valid assessments of communication skills, interpersonal skills and attitude poses considerable difficulties for the traditional methods of closed systems research. There are a number of variables operating, including the "patient", the examiner, the clinical content, the clinical task, and the context as confounding variables to any underlying communication and interpersonal relationship. The ability of the assessment schedule to reliably measure these non-cognitive factors and then to make a judgment about what constitutes competence and incompetence is no small challenge.

The literature points to an emerging consensus of those elements in the doctor-patient interaction which should be assessed. There are many assessment instruments designed to match instructional models in different institutions. The absence of assessments of non-verbal behaviors in the interaction between patients and physicians has been noted. Attitudes in all their complexity can be explored in learning settings that provide immediate feedback but it should be recognized that summative assessments based only on observed behaviors are not necessarily measuring attitude.

There are a number of instruments covering communication, interpersonal and history taking skills, with considerable similarities as well as variation. Some have undergone psychometric testing, mostly interrater reliability, but few have been tested for internal consistency or for validity. The call for research, using stored and new data banks of videotaped consultations, to improve the instruments and their application is perhaps long overdue. Educators should be encouraged to review existing instruments and collaborate over research instead of re-inventing the wheel.

There is debate about the merits of detailed checklists versus global ratings and a move toward the latter for summative assessments. The former are useful for specifying behaviors in learning and feedback contexts, whilst global instruments would seem to fulfill the requirements of reliability and validity and provide easier, more practical and feasible methods.

Research evidence available points to the conclusion that reliable assessment of an individual's communication skills and interpersonal skills using any one method is problematic. Knowledge of clinical content is a confounding variable and the range and length of test-set needed to provide the statistical gold standard have been unrealistic for many institutions. Recent studies are indicating shorter test times with more reliable global assessment instruments. Well-designed longitudinal studies are needed to establish the validity of these measures in terms of patient outcomes.

Simulated patients trained and selected for accuracy in portraying cases reliably and authentically would seem to be as reliable in assessments of students as faculty. Whilst cost may well point to the advantages of using standardized patients rather than faculty, the latter provide greater credibility and confidence in rating for high stakes exams. Standardized patients are particularly valued in formative assessment and can be realistically used in workplace setting assessments. Selection of simulated patients and examiners for their accuracy and reliability would appear to be a more cost-effective means of developing valid and reliable assessment methods than training alone.

Communication and interpersonal skills, whilst separated in focused learning and training feedback contexts, are currently integrated with the clinical content and history taking skills in summative assessments. Testing to date has not identified generalizable communication and interpersonal skills that are independent of clinical content. There would appear to be no research on whether it is possible to assess communication and interactional skills independent of clinical problems if students are given the clinical content in advance. This would seem worthy of research.

Any summative judgment made of a student's competence or incompetence has to be defensible. As Marinker (1997) notes: *"Reliability is about competitive fairness to students. Validity is about responsible justice to their future patients"* (p. 295). Both are important and no one method of assessment is likely to meet all requirements. Learning and assessment are integral to each other, we must ensure students are learning what we want them to and take care not to let reliability override that which is truly important.

Despite the difficulties, assessment of non-cognitive factors is possible and, given their central importance to clinical practice, every effort should be made to include these both formatively as students learn and in certification and recertification examinations. Further research will enable educators to build upon the advances already made.

REFERENCES

Amiel, G. E., & Lunenfeld, E. (1994). Increasing reliability of an Objective Structured Clinical Examination by further assessing performance with a global scale. In A. I. Rothman & R. Cohen (Eds.), *Proceedings of the Sixth Ottawa Conference on Medical Education* (pp. 273-274). Toronto, Ontario: University of Toronto.

Anderson, M. B., Stillman, P. L., & Wang, Y. (1994). Growing use of standardised patients in teaching and evaluation in medical education. *Teaching & Learning in Medicine, 6,* 15-22.

Angoff, W. H. (1971). Scales, norms and equivalent scores. In R. L. Thorndike (Ed.), *Educational Measurement* (pp. 508-600). Washington, DC: American Council of Education.

Argent, J., Faulkner, A., Jones, A., & O'Keefe, C. (1994). Communication skills in palliative care: development and modification of a rating scale. *Medical Education, 28*(6), 559-565.

Audit Commission (1993). *What seems to be the matter; communication between hospitals and patients.* National Health Service Report No.12. London: HMSO.

Baile, W. F., Lenzi, R., Kudelka, A. P., Maguire, P., Novack, D., Goldstein, M., Myers, E. G., & Bast, R. C. Jr. (1997). Improving physician-patient communication in cancer care: outcome of a workshop for oncologists. *Journal of Cancer Education, 12*(3), 166-173.

Bales, R. F., & Hare, A. P. (1965). Diagnostic use of the interaction profile. *Journal of Social Psychology, 67,* 239-258.

Balint, M. (1972). *The doctor, his patient and the illness*, 2nd ed. New York: International Universities Press.

Barlett, E., Grayson, M., & Barker, R. (1984). The effects of physician communication skills on patient satisfaction, recall and adherence. *Journal of Chronic Disease, 37,* 755-764.

Barrows, H. S., & Abrahamson, S. (1964). The programmed patient: A technique for appraising student performance in clinical neurology. *Journal of Medical Education, 39,* 802-805.

Ben-Sira, Z. (1980). The function of the professional's affective behaviour in client satisfaction: A revised approach to social interaction theory. *Journal of Health and Social Behaviour, 21,* 170.

Bienenstock, A., Keane, D. R., Cohen, M., Eaman, S., Hollenberg, R., Cavanagh, P., & Watson, S. (1994) Defining and evaluating professional behaviour in the clinical encounter. In A. I. Rothman & R. Cohen (Eds.), *Proceedings of the Sixth Ottawa Conference on Medical Education* (pp. 174-177). Toronto, Ontario: University of Toronto.

Bird, J., & Cohen-Cole, S. A. (1990). The three-function model of the medical interview: an educational device. In M. Hale (Ed.), *Models of consultation-liaison-psychiatry* (pp. 65-88). Basel, Switzerland: S Karger AG.

Bird, J., Hall, A., Maguire, P., & Heavy, A. (1993). Workshops for consultants on the teaching of clinical communication skills. *Medical Education, 27,* 181-185.

Bloom, S. (1983). *The doctor and his patient: a sociological interpretation.* New York Russel Sage.

Boon, H., & Stewart, M. (1998). Patient-physician communication assessment instruments: 1986 to 1996 in review. *Patient Education and Counselling, 35,* 161-176.

Bowman, F. M., Goldberg, D. P., Millar, T., Gask, L., & McGrath, G. (1992). Improving the skills of established general practitioners: the long-term benefits of group teaching. *Medical Education, 26*(1), 63-68.

Brown, J. A., Abelson, J., Woodward, C. A., Hutchison, B., & Norman, G. (1998). Fielding standardized patients in primary care settings: lessons from a study using unannounced standardized patients to assess preventive care practices. *International Journal for Quality in Health Care, 10*(3), 199-206.

Burchand, K. W., & Rowland-Morin, P. A. (1990). A new method of assessing the interpersonal skills of surgeons. *Academic Medicine, 65,* 274.

Burri, A., McCaughan, K., & Barrows, H. (1976). The feasibility of using simulated patient as a means to evaluate clinical competence in a community. *Proceedings of the Annual Conference of Research in Medical Education, 15,* 295.

Byrne, J. M., & Long, B. E. L. (1976). *Doctors talking to patients.* London: HMSO.

Campbell, L. M., & Murray, T. S. (1996). Summative assessment of vocational trainees: results of a 3-year study. *British Journal of General Practice, 46,* 411-414.

Campbell, L. M., Howie, J. G. R., & Murray, T. S. (1995). Use of videotaped consultations in summative assessment of trainees in general practice. *British Journal of General Practice, 45,* 137-141.

Carkuff, R. R. (1969). The prediction of the effects of teacher-counselor education: the development of communication and discrimination selection indexes. *Counselor Education Supervision, 8,* 265-272.

Case, S. (1997). Assessment truths that we hold as self-evident and their implications. In A. J. J. A. Scherpbier, C. P. M. Van der Vleuten, J. J. Rethans, & A. F. W. Van der Steeg (Eds.), *Advances in medical education* (pp. 2-6). Dordrecht: Kluwer Academic Publishers.

Chugh, U., Dillman, E., Kurtz, S. M., Lockyer, J., & Parboosingh, J. (1993). Multicultural issues in the medical curriculum: implications for Canadian physicians. *Medical Teacher, 15,* 83-91.

Cohen, D. S., Colliver, J. A., Marcy, M. S., Fried, E. D., & Schwartz, M. H. (1996). Psychometric properties of a standardised-patient checklist and rating-scale used to assess interpersonal and communication skills. *Academic Medicine, 71,* Suppl 1, 87-89.

Cohen, D. S., Colliver, J. A., Robbs, R. S., & Schwartz, M. H. (1997). A large-scale study of the reliabilities of checklist scores and ratings of components of interpersonal and communication skills evaluated on a standardised patient examination. In A. J. J. A. Scherpbier, C. P. M. Van der Vleuten, J. J. Rethans, & A. F. W. Van der Steeg (Eds.), *Advances in medical education* (pp. 424-426). Dordrecht: Kluwer Academic Publishers.

Coles C. (1998). Education in the OP clinic: purposes, content and methods. In J. W. R. Peyton (Ed.), *Teaching and learning in medical practice* (pp. 182-184). Manticore Europe Ltd.

Colliver, J. A., & Williams, R. G. (1993). Proceedings of the AAMC's Consensus Conference on the Use of Standardised Patients in the Teaching and Evaluation of Clinical Skills. Section 2, Technical Issues: Test Applications. *Academic Medicine, 68*(6), 454-463.

Colliver, J. A., Swartz, M. H., Robbs, R. S., & Cohen, D. S. (1999). Relationship between clinical competence and interpersonal and communication skills in standardized-patient assessment. *Academic Medicine, 74*(3), 271-274.

Colliver, J. A., Vu, N. V., Marcy, M. L., Travis, T. A., & Robbs, R. S. (1993). Effects of examinee gender, standardized-patient gender, and their interaction on standardized patients' ratings of examinees' interpersonal and communication skills. *Academic Medicine, 68*(2), 153-157.

Consensus Statement (1998). Teaching medical ethics and law within medical education: a model for the United Kingdom core curriculum. *Journal of Medical Ethics, 24,* 188-192.

Cox, J., & Mulholland, H. (1993). An instrument for the assessment of videotapes of general practitioners' performance. *British Medical Journal, 306,* 1043-1046.

Cox, K. (1990). No Oscar for Objective Structured Clinical Examination. *Medical Education, 24*(6), 540-545.

Dauphinee, W. D., Blackmore, D. E., Smee, S. M., Rothman, A. I., & Reznick, R. K. (1997). Optimizing the input of physician examiners in setting standards for a large scale Objective Structured Clinical Examination: Experience with Part II of the qualifying examination of the Medical Council of Canada. In A. J. J. A. Scherpbier, C. P. M. Van der Vleuten, J. J. Rethans, & A. F. W. Van der Steeg (Eds.), *Advances in medical education* (pp. 656-658). Dordrecht: Kluwer Academic Publishers.

Davis, H., & Fallowfield, L. (1991). *Counselling and communication in health care* (pp. 3-60). Chichester: John Wiley & Sons.

De Monchy, C., Richardson, R., Brown, R. A., & Harden, R. M. (1988). Measuring attitudes of doctors: the doctor-patient (DP) rating. *Medical Education, 22,* 231-239.

DiMatteo, M. R., Hays, R. D., & Prince, L. M. (1986). Relationship of physicians' nonverbal communication skill to patient satisfaction, appointment non-compliance and physician workload. *Health Psychology, 5,* 581-594.

DiMatteo, M. R., Taranta, A., Friedman, H. S., & Prince, L. M. (1980). Predicting patient satisfaction from physicians' nonverbal communication skills. *Medical Care, 18,* 376-387.

Engel, G. L. (1977). The need for a new medical model: a challenge for biomedicine. *Science, 196*(4286), 129-136.

Evans, B. J., Stanley, R. O., & Burrows, G. D. (1993). Measuring medical students' empathy skills. *British Journal of Medical Psychology, 66*(Pt 2), 121-133.

Farnill, D., Hayes, S. C., & Todisco, J. (1997). Interviewing skills: self evaluation by medical students. *Medical Education, 31,* 122-127.

Gask, L., Goldberg, D., Lesser, A. L., & Millar, T. (1988). Improving the psychiatric skills of general practice trainees: an evaluation of a group training course. *Medical Education, 22,* 132-138.

General Medical Council (1998). *Duties of a doctor.* G.M.C., London. www.gmc-uk.org

General Medical Council (1993). *Tomorrow's doctors: recommendations on undergraduate medical education.* G.M.C., London.

General Medical Council (1996). *Performance procedures – a summary of current proposals.* G.M.C., London.

Goldie, J. (2000). Review of ethics curricula in undergraduate medical education. *Medical Education, 342,* 108-119.

Grand'Maison, P., Brailovsky, C. A., & Lescop, J. (1997). The Quebec Licensing Objective Structured Clinical Examination: modifications and improvements over 6 years of experience. In A. J. J. A. Scherpbier, C. P. M. Van der Vleuten, J. J. Rethans, & A. F. W. Van der Steeg (Eds.), *Advances in medical education* (pp. 437-440). Dordrecht: Kluwer Academic Publishers.

Grayson, M., Nugent, C., & Oken, S. L. (1977). A systematic and comprehensive approach to teaching and evaluating interpersonal skills. *Journal of Medical Education, 52*(11), 906-913.

Greco, M., Francis, W., Buckley, J., Brownlea, A., & McGovern, J. (1998). Real-patient evaluation of communication skills teaching for GP registrars. *Family Practitioner, 15*(1), 51-57.

Grol, R., de Maeseneer, J., Whitfield, M., & Mokkink, H. (1990). Disease-centred versus patient-centred attitudes: comparison of general practitioners in Belgium, Britain and The Netherlands. *Family Practice, 7,* 100-103.

Gruppen, L. D., Davis, W. K., Fitzgerald, J. T., & McQuillan, M. A. (1997). Reliability, number of stations, and examination length in an Objective Structured Clinical Examination. In A. J. J. A. Scherpbier, C. P. M. Van der Vleuten, J. J. Rethans, & A. F. W. Van der Steeg (Eds.), *Advances in medical education* (pp. 441-442). Dordrecht: Kluwer Academic Publishers.

Hays, R. B. (1990). Assessment of general practice consultations: content validity of a rating scale. *Medical Education, 24,* 110-116.

Heaton, C. J., & Kurtz, S. M. (1992). Videotape recall: learning and assessment in certifying exams. In I. R. Hart & R. Hardin. (Eds.), *International Conference Proceedings: Developments in Assessing Clinical Competence* (pp. 541-547). Montreal: Heal Publications.

Henbest, R. J., & Stewart, M. A. (1990). Patient-centredness in the consultation. 2: Does it really make a difference? *Family Practice, 7*(1), 28-33.

Henkin, Y., Friedman, M., Bouskila, D., Drora, K., & Glick, S. (1990). The use of patients as student evaluators. *Medical Teacher, 12*(3/4), 278-289.

Herbert, P. C., Meslin, E. M., Dunn, E. V., Byrne, N., & Reid, S. R. (1992). Measuring the ethical sensitivity of medical students: A study at the University of Toronto. *Journal of Medical Ethics, 18,* 142-147.

Hodges, B., Turnbull, J., Cohen, R., Bienenstock, A., & Norman, G. (1996). Evaluating communication skills in the objective structured clinical examination: reliability and generalizability. *Medical Education, 30,* 38-43.

Hodges, B., Turnbull, J., Cohen, R., Bienenstock, D., & Norman, G. (1994). Assessment of communication skills with complex cases using Objective Structured Clinical Examination format. In A. I. Rothman & R. Cohen (Eds.), *Proceedings of the Sixth Ottawa Conference on Medical Education* (pp. 269-272). Toronto, Ontario: University of Toronto.

Hulsman, R. L., Ros, W. J. G., Winnubst, J. A. M., & Bensing, J. M. (1999). Teaching clinically experienced physicians communication skills. A review of evaluation studies. *Medical Education, 33*(9), 655-668.

Hundert, E. M., Douglas-Steele, D., & Bickel, J. (1996). Context in medical education: the informal ethics curriculum. *Medical Education, 30,* 353-364.

Jolly, B. (1998). Assessment of attitudes in professional competence – lessons from the new 'GMC Performance Procedures'. Paper presented at Conference on 'Core Clinical Competence: Meeting the Assessment Challenge'. Leeds, 2 April.

Jolly, B., & Grant, J. (1997). *The good assessment guide.* Joint Centre for Education in Medicine, 33 Millman St, London WC1N 3EJ, U.K.

Kendrik, T., & Freeling, P. (1993). A communication skills course for preclinical students: evaluation of general practice based teaching using group methods. *Medical Education, 27*(3), 211-217.

Koppelow, M., Schnabl, G., Chochinov, A. Beazley, G., Gill, E., Leslie, W., Macpherson, J., Moroz, S., Morris, M., & Parker, J. (1994). Criterion referenced standard setting for a standardized patient examination. In A. I. Rothman & R. Cohen (Eds.), *Proceedings of the Sixth Ottawa Conference on Medical Education* (pp. 105-107). Toronto, Ontario: University of Toronto.

Koppelow, M. L., Schnabl, G. K., Hassard, T. H., Tamblyn, R. M., Klass, D. J., Beazley, G., & Hechter (1995). Assessing practising physicians in two settings using standardised patients. *Academic Medicine, 67* (Suppl 10), S19-21.

Korsch, B. M. (1989). The past and the future of research in doctor-patient relations. In M. Stewart & D. Roter (Eds.), *Communicating with medical patients* (pp. 246-251). Newbury Park, CA: Sage.

Korsch, B. M., & Negrete, V. F. (1972). Doctor-patient communication. *Scientific American, 227*, 66-74.

Kosower, E., Inkelis, S., Seidel, J., & Berman, N. (1996). Evaluating telephone T.A.L.K. *Journal of Biocommunication, 23*(1), 27-32.

Kraan, H. F., Crijnen, A. A., de Vries, M. W., Zuidweg, J., Imbos, T., & Van der Vleuten, C. P. (1990). To what extent are medical interviewing skills teachable? *Medical Teacher, 12*(3-4), 315-328.

Kraan, H. F., Crijnen, A. A. M., Van der Vleuten, C. P. M., & Imbos, T. (1995). Evaluating instruments for medical interviewing skills. In M. Lipkin, S. M. Putnam, & A. Lazare (Eds.), *The medical interview; clinical care, education & research* (pp. 460-472). New York: Springer-Verlag.

Kraan, H. F., Crijnen, A. A. M., Zuidweg, J., Van der Vleuten, C. P. M., & Imbos, T. (1989). Evaluating undergraduate training – a checklist for medical interviewing skills. In M. Stewart & D. Roter (Eds.), *Communicating with medical patients* (pp. 167-177). Newbury Park, CA: Sage.

Kurtz, S. M., Silverman, J. D., & Draper, J. (1998). *Teaching and learning communication skills in medicine,* Appendix 2 (pp. 225-232). The two-guide format of the Calgary-Cambridge Observation Guide. Abingdon: Radcliffe Medical Press.

Levenstein, J. H., Brown, J. B., Weston, W. W., Stewart, M., McCracken, E. C., & McWhinney, I. (1989). Patient-centred clinical interviewing. In M. Stewart & D. Roter (Eds.), *Communicating with medical patients* (pp. 107-120). Newbury Park, CA: Sage.

Levinson, W., & Roter, D. L. (1993). The effects of two continuing medical education programs on communication skills of practising primary care physicians. *Journal of General Internal Medicine, 8*(6), 318-324.

Levinson, W., & Roter, D. (1995). Physicians' psychosocial beliefs correlate with their patient communication skills. *Journal of General Internal Medicine, 10*(7), 375-379.

Levinson, W., Roter, D. L., Mullooly, J. P., Dull, V. T., & Frankel, R. M. (1997). Physician-patient communication. The relationship with malpractice claims amongst primary care physicians and surgeons. *Journal of the American Medical Association, 277*(7), 553-559.

Ley, P. (1988). *Communication with patients: improving satisfaction and compliance.* London: Croom Helm.

Lovett, L. M., Cox, A., & Abou-Saleh, M. (1990). Teaching psychiatric interview skills to medical students. *Medical Education, 24,* 243.

McLeod, P. J., Tamblyn, R., Benaroya, S., & Snell, L. (1994). Faculty ratings of resident humanism predict patient satisfaction ratings in ambulatory medical clinics. *Journal of General Internal Medicine, 9*(6), 321-326.

Maguire, P., & Faulkner, A. (1988). Communicate with cancer patients: 1. Handling bad news and difficult questions. *British Medical Journal, 297*(6653), 907-909.

Maguire, P., Fairbairn, S., & Fletcher, C. (1986). Consultation skills of young doctors: benefits of feedback training in interviewing as students persist. *British Medical Journal, 292,* 1573-1576.

Maguire, G. P., Roe, P., Goldberg, D. P., Jones, S., Hyde, C., & O'Dowd, T. (1978). The value of feedback in teaching interviewing skills to medical students. *Psychological Medicine, 8,* 695-704.

Maheux, B., Beaudoin, C., Jean, P., Des Marchais, J., Côte, L., Tiraoui, A. M., & Charbonneau, A.. (1997). Development and validation of a measure of patient-centred care in medical practice. In A. I. Rothman & R. Cohen (Eds.), *Proceedings of the Sixth Ottawa Conference on Medical Education* (pp. 186-190). Toronto, Ontario: University of Toronto.

Makoul, G. (1995). SEGUE: a framework for teaching and evaluating communication in medical encounters. *Division 1 of the American Educatorial Research Association.* San Francisco.

Marinker, M. (1997). Myth, paradox and the hidden curriculum. *Medical Education, 31*(4), 293-298.

Martin, D., Regehr, G., Hodges, B., & McNaughton, N. (1998). Using videotaped benchmarks to improve the self-assessment ability of family practice residents. *Academic Medicine, 73*(11), 1201-1206.

Marvel, M. K., Doherty, W. J., & Weiner, E. (1998). Medical interviewing by exemplary family physicians. *Journal of Family Practice, 47*(5), 343-348.

Miles, S. H., Lane, L. W., Bickel, J., Walker, R. M., & Casse, C. K. (1989). Medical ethics education: coming of age. *Academic Medicine, 64,* 705-714.

Miller, S. J., Hope, T., & Talbot, D. C. (1999). The development of a structured rating schedule (the BAS) to assess skills in breaking bad news. *British Journal of Cancer, 80*(5-6), 792-800.

Morris, P., Freire, D., Batstone, G., & Patel, H. (1995). *The satisfactory consultation: development of a communication audit tool.* The College of Health, St Margaret's House, 21 Old Ford Rd, London E2 9PL.

Morrison, H., McNally, H., Wylie, C., McFaul, P., & Thompson, W. (1996). The passing score in the Objective Structured Clinical Examination. *Medical Education, 30*(5), 345-348.

Morrison, L. J., & Barrows, H. S. (1994). Developing consortia for clinical practice examinations: The Macy project. *Teaching and Learning in Medicine, 6*(1), 23-27.

Newble, D. I. (1983). The critical incident technique: a new approach to the assessment of clinical performance. *Medical Education, 17,* 401-403.

Newble, D., & Wakeford, R. (1994). Primary certification in the United Kingdom and Australasia. In D. Newble, B. Jolly, & R. Wakeford (Eds.), *The certification and recertification of doctors* (pp. 13-18). Cambridge: Cambridge University Press.

Newble, D. I., Hoare, J., & Sheldrake, P. F. (1980). The selection and training of examiners for clinical examinations. *Medical Education, 14,* 345-349.

Norman, G. R., Neufeld, V. R., Walsh, A., Woodward, C. A., & McConvey, G. A. (1985). Measuring physicians' performances by using simulated patients. *Medical Education, 60,* 925-934.

Norman, G. R., Van der Vleuten, C. P. M., & De Graaf, E. (1991). Pitfalls in the pursuit of objectivity: issues of validity, efficiency, and acceptability. *Medical Education, 25,* 119-126.

Novack, D. H., Epstein, R. M., & Paulsen, R. H. (1999). Toward creating physician-healers: fostering medical students' self-awareness, personal growth and well-being. *Academic Medicine, 74*(5), 16-20.

Ovadia, A. B., Yager, J., & Heinrich, R. L. (1982). Assessment of medical interview skills. In J. Yager (Ed.), *Teaching psychiatry and behavioural science* (pp. 485-500). Toronto: Grune & Stratton.

Parsons, T. (1951). *The social system.* Glencoe IL: Free Press.

Pendleton, D., Schofield, T., Tate, P., & Havelock, P. (1984). *The consultation: an approach to learning and teaching.* Oxford, England: Oxford University Press.

Petrusa, E. R., Camp, M. G., Harward, D. H., Richards, B. F., Smith, III A. C., Willis, S. E., & Bolton, C. A. (1994). Measuring the doctor-patient relationship and communication in a clinical performance exam. In A. I. Rothman & R. Cohen (Eds.), *Proceedings of the Sixth Ottawa Conference on Medical Education* (pp. 259-261). Toronto, Ontario: University of Toronto.

Pfeiffer, C., Madray, H., Ardolino, A., & Willms, J. (1998). The rise and fall of students' skills in obtaining a medical history. *Medical Education, 32,* 283-288.

Pololi, L. (1995). Standardised patients: as we evaluate, so shall we reap. *Lancet, 345,* 966-968.

Powell, A., Boakes, J., & Slater, P. (1987). What motivates medical students: how they see themselves and their profession. *Medical Education, 21*(3), 176-182.

Price, J., Price, D., Williams, G., & Hoffenberg, R. (1998). Changes in medical students' attitudes as they progress through the medical course. *Journal of Medical Ethics, 24,* 110-117.

Ram, P., Grol, R., Rethans, J. J., Schouten, B., Van der Vleuten, C., & Kester, A. (1999). Assessment of general practitioners by video observation of communicative and medical performance in daily practice: issues of validity, reliability and feasibility. *Medical Education, 33,* 447-454.

Rethans, J. J. (1990). Competence and performance: two different concepts in the assessment of quality of medical care. *Family Practice, 7,* 168-174.

Rethans, J. J., & Van Boven, C. P. A. (1987). Simulated patients in general practice: a different look at the consultation. *British Medical Journal, 294,* 809-812.

Rethans, J. J., Sturmans, F., Drop, R., & Van der Vleuten, C. (1991a). Assessment of the performance of general practitioners by the use of standardized (simulated) patients. *British Journal of General Practice, 41,* 97-99.

Rethans, J. J., Sturmans, F., Drop, R., Van der Vleuten, C. P. M., & Hobus, P. (1991b). Does competence of general practitioners predict their performance? Comparison between examination setting and actual practice. *British Medical Journal, 303,* 1377-1380.

Rethans, J. J., Drop, R., Sturmans, F., & Van der Vleuten, C. P. M. (1991c). A method for introducing standardised (simulated) patients into general practice consultations. *British Journal of General Practice, 41,* 94-96.

Rezler, A. G., Schwartz, R. L., Obenshain, S. S., Gibson, J. M., & Bennahum, D. A. (1992). Assessment of ethical decisions and values. *Medical Education, 26,* 7-16.

Reznick, R. K., Blackmore, D., Cohen, R., Baumler, J., Rothman, A., Snode, S., Chalmers, A., Poldre, P. Birthwhistte, R., & Walsh, P. (1993a). An objective clinical examination for the licentiate of the Medical Council of Canada; from research to reality. *Academic Medicine, 68*(10), S4-6.

Reznick, R. K., Smee, S., Baumber, J. S., Cohen, R., Rothman, A., Blackmore, D., & Berard, M. (1993b) Guidelines for estimating the real cost of an objective structured clinical examination. *Academic Medicine, 68*(7), 513-517.

Rosenthal, R., Hall, J. A., DiMatteo, M. R., Rogers, P. L., & Archer, D. (1979). *Sensitivity to nonverbal communication: the PONS test.* Baltimore: Johns Hopkins University Press.

Roter, D. (1989). Which facets of communication have strong effects on outcome? A Meta-analysis. In M. Stewart & D. Roter (Eds.), *Communication with medical patients* (pp. 183-196). Newbury Park, CA: Sage.

Roter, D. L., & Hall, J. A. (1989). Studies of doctor-patient interaction. *Annual Review of Public Health, 10,* 163-180.

Royal College of General Practitioners Membership Examination (1996). *Assessment of consulting skills workbook.* London: RCGP.

Saltini, A., Cappellari, D., Cellerino, P., Del Piccolo, L., & Zimmermann, C. (1998). An instrument for evaluating the medical interview in general practice: VR-MICS/D (Verona-Medical Interview Classification System/Doctor). *Epidemiologia e Psychiatra Sociale, 7*(3), 210-223.

Sanson-Fisher, R., & Cockburn, J. (1997). Effective teaching of communication skills for medical practice: selecting an appropriate clinical context. *Medical Education, 31*(1), 52-57.

Sanson-Fisher, R., & Poole, A. D. (1980). Simulated patients and the assessment of medical students' interpersonal skills. *Medical Education, 14,* 249-253.

Sanson-Fisher, R. W., Redman, S., Walsh, R., Mitchell, K., Reid, A. L., & Perkins, J. J. (1991). Training medical practitioners in information transfer skills: the new challenge. *Medical Education, 25,* 322-323.

Schnabl, G. K., Hassard, T. H., & Kopelow, M. L. (1991). The assessment of interpersonal skills using standardized patients. *Academic Medicine, 66*(9 Suppl), S34-36.

Sears, D. O., Peplau, L. A., & Taylor, S. E. (1991). *Social psychology,* 7th ed. 'Social Cognition and Attitudes, Ch 5 & 6. NJ: Prentice Hall.

Silverman, J., Kurtz, S., & Draper, J. (1998). *Skills for communicating with patients.* Abingdon: Radcliffe Medical Press.

Simpson, M., Buckman, R., Stewart, M., Maguire, P., Lipkin, M., Novack, D., & Till, J. (1991). Doctor-patient communication: the Toronto consensus statement. *British Medical Journal, 303,* 1385-1387.

Singer, P., Cohen, R., Robb, A., & Rothman, A. (1993). The ethics Objective Structured Clinical Examination. *Journal of General Internal Medicine, 8,* 23-28.

Singer, P. A., Robb, A., Cohen, R., Norman, G., & Turnbull, J. (1996). Performance-based assessment of clinical ethics using an objective structured clinical examination. *Academic Medicine, 71*(5), 495-498.

Smee, S. M. (1993). Standardised patients: a trainer's perspective. *Annals of Community-Oriented Education, 6,* 273-281.

Smee, S. M. (1994). Training standardised patients for different types of Objective Structured Clinical Examination stations. In A. I. Rothman, & R. Cohen (Eds.), *Proceedings of the Sixth Ottawa Conference* (pp. 336-342). Toronto, Ontario: University of Toronto.

Smith, S. R., Balint, A., Krause, K. C., Moore-West, M., & Viles, P. H. (1994). Performance-based assessment of moral reasoning and ethical judgement among medical students. *Academic Medicine, 69,* 381-386.

Stewart, M., & Roter, D. (Eds.) (1989) *Communicating with medical patients.* Newbury Park, CA: Sage.

Stewart, M., Brown, J. B., Boon, H., Galajda, J., Meredith, L., & Sangster M. (1999). Evidence on patient-doctor communication. *Cancer Prevention & Control, 3*(1), 25-30.

Stillman, P. L. (1993). Technical issues: logistics of AAMC (Review). *Academic Medicine, 68*(6), 464-468.

Stillman, P. L., Brown, D. R., Redfield, D. L., & Sabers, D. L. (1977). Construct validation of the Arizona Clinical Interview Rating Scale. *Educational Psychological Measurement, 37*(4), 1031-1038.

Suchman, A. L., Markakis, K., Beckman, H. B., & Frankel, R. (1997). A model of empathic communication in the medical interview. *Journal of the American Medical Association, 277*(8), 678-682.

Swanson, D. B., & Norcini, J. J. (1989). Factors influencing the reproducibility of tests using standardised patients. *Teaching and Learning in Medicine, 1,* 158-166.

Tamblyn, R. M., Klass, D. J., Schnabl, G. K., & Kopelow, M. L. (1991a). Sources of unreliability and bias in standardised-patient rating. *Teaching and Learning in Medicine, 3*(2), 74-85.

Tamblyn, R. M., Klass, D. J., Schnabl, G. K., & Kopelow, M. L. (1991b). The accuracy of standardised patient presentations. *Medical Education, 25,* 100-109.

Tamblyn, R., Benaroya, S., Snell, L., McLeod, P., Schnarch, B., & Abrahamowicz, M. (1994). The feasibility and value of using patient satisfaction ratings to evaluate internal medicine residents. *Journal of General Internal Medicine, 9*(3), 146-152.

Tann, M., Amiel, G. E., Bitterman, A., Ber, R., & Cohen, R. (1997). Analysis of the use of global ratings by standardised patients and physicians. In A. J. J. A. Scherpbier, C. P. M. Van der Vleuten, J. J. Rethans, & A. F. W. Van der Steeg (Eds.), *Advances in medical education* (pp. 191-192). Dordrecht: Kluwer Academic Publishers.

Thorndike, R. L. (1982). *Applied psychometrics.* Boston, MA: Houghton-Mifflin.

Tuckett, D., Boulton, M., Olson, C., & Williams, A. (1985). *Meetings between experts: an approach to sharing ideas in medical consultations.* London and New York: Tavistock Publications.

Van der Vleuten, C. P. M., & Swanson, D. B. (1990). Assessment of clinical skills with standardised patients: state of the art. *Teaching and Learning in Medicine, 2,* 58-76.

Van der Vleuten, C. P. M., Norman, G. R., & De Graaf, E. (1991). Pitfalls in the pursuit of objectivity: issues of reliability. *Medical Education, 25,* 110-118.

Van der Vleuten, C. P. M., Scherpbier, A. J. J. A., & Van Luijk, S. J. (1994). Use of Objective Structured Clinical Examinations in the Netherlands. In A. I. Rothman & R. Cohen (Eds.), *Proceedings of the Sixth Ottawa Conference* (pp. 320-321). Toronto, Ontario: University of Toronto.

Van der Vleuten, C. P. M., Van Luyk, S. J., Van Ballegooijen, A. M. J., & Swanson, D. B. (1989). Training & experience of examiners. *Medical Education, 3,* 290-296.

Van Thiel, J., Kraan, H. F., & Van der Vleuten, C. P. M. (1991). Reliability and feasibility of measuring medical interviewing skills: the revised Maastricht History-Taking and Advice Checklist. *Medical Education, 25*(3), 224-229.

Van Thiel, J., Van der Vleuten, C. P. M., & Kraan, H. (1992). Assessment of medical interviewing skills: generalizability of scores using successive MAAS-versions. In R. M. Harden, I. R. Hart, & H. Mulholland (Eds.), *Approaches to the assessment of clinical competence* (pp. 526-540). Dundee: Centre for Medical Education.

Vu, N. V., & Barrows, H. S. (1994). Use of standardised patients in clinical assessments: recent developments and measurement findings. *Educational Researcher, 23*(3), 23-30.

Vu, N. V., Marcy, M. M., Colliver, J. A., Verhulst, S. J., Travis, T. A., & Barrows, H. S. (1992). Standardized (simulated) patients' accuracy in recording clinical performance check-list items. *Medical Education, 26*(2), 99-104.

Wasserman, R. C., & Inui, T. S. (1983). Systematic analysis of clinician-patient interactions: a critique of recent approaches with suggestions for future research. *Medical Care, 21*(3), 279-293.

White, D. G., Tiberius, R., Talbot, Y., Schiralli, V., & Ricket, M. (1991). Improving feedback for medical students in a family medicine clerkship. *Canadian Family Physician, 37,* 64-70.

Wooliscroft, J. O., Howell, J. D., Patel, B. P., & Swanson, D. B. (1994). Resident-patient interactions: the humanistic qualities of internal medicine residents assessed by patients, attending physicians, program supervisors and nurses. *Academic Medicine, 69,* 216-224.

APPENDIX A. EDUCATIONAL COMMUNICATION ASSESSMENT TOOLS

	Assessment	Description	No. of items	Reliability	Validity	Current use	Special notes
1	Arizona Clinical Interview Rating (ACIR); Stillman et al., 1977	Assessment of interviewing skill in the following areas: organization, skills timeline, transitional statements, questioning, documentation, rapport; 5-point scale	16 specific	Inter-rater = 0.52-0.87; intra-rater = 0.85-0.90; internal consistency = 0.80 (Cronbach's alpha)	Construct validity (level of training) demonstrated; no correlation with BUISE	Teaching and assessing medical students (in practice settings)	External assessment of videotaped or real-time interviews
2	Brown University Interpersonal Skill Evaluation (BUISE); Burchard et al., 1990	Assessment of physicians' interpersonal skills in following categories: rapport, clinical skills or procedures, feedback, closing; 7-point scale	37	Inter-rater = 0.91	None reported; no correlation with ACIR	Ditto	External assessment of videotaped interview
3	Calgary-Cambridge Referenced Observation Guides: 1. Interviewing the Patient; 2. Explanation and Planning with the Patient; Kurtz et al., 1998	Practical teaching tool which delineates and structures skills which aid in doctor-patient communication; descriptive feedback	1. 37 2. Varies	Testing ongoing	Testing ongoing	Ditto	External assessment of real-time interviews

	Assessment	Description	No. of items	Reliability	Validity	Current use	Special notes
4	Campbell et al.'s Assessment of Trainees, 1995, 1996	Assessment of videotaped interactions to determine the competence of general practice trainees: presence of error scored present/absent; other tasks scored on 6-point scale	7	Inter-rater = 0.2–0.5 "high" level of agreement with overall decision pass or refer for more training	None reported	Assessing medical students in general practice settings	External assessment of 204h videotaped interviews
5	Daily Rating Form of Student Clinical Performance; White et al., 1991	Daily evaluation form for rating clinical clerks: each skill rated as fail, pass, excellent, n/a (1-12 scale)	6	None reported	Construct validity (level of training) demonstrated	Teaching and assessing medical students on a daily basis	External assessment by supervisor
6	Hopkin's Interpersonal Skills Assessment; Grayson et al., 1977; Bartlett et al., 1984	Assessment of MD's interpersonal skills in 4 categories: sensitivity; interchange of information; organization; and environmental factors	14	Inter-rater = 0.52 intra-rater = 0.77	None reported	Teaching and assessing medical students (in practice settings)	External assessment videotaped interview
7	Interpersonal and Communication Skills Checklist; Cohen et al., 1996	Standardized patients assess students' skills during a 20-min "case" (six cases have been developed): Likert scale	17	Inter-case = 0.65	Convergent validity (correlated with a non-validated rating scale)	Assessing medical students	Standardized patients to assess students in real-time

	Assessment	Description	No. of items	Reliability	Validity	Current use	Special notes
8	Interpersonal Skills Rating Form; Schnabl et al., 1995; Kopelow et al., 1995	Standardized patients assess their perceptions of the interviewer; Likert scale	13	Reliability coefficients ranged from 0.68 to 0.85	None reported	Assessing medical students and physicians	Trained standardized patients to assess students in real-time
9	Lovett et al.'s Techniques of Interviewing Peer-assessment Form	Peer-assessment of interviewing skills; yes/no response to specific behaviors; global assessment ranked on a 4-point scale from strongly agree to strongly disagree	22	None reported	None reported	Assessment of interviews with psychiatric patients in workshops	Peer-observation of interviews and peer assessment
10	Maastricht History Taking and Advice Checklist (MAAS); Kraan et al., 1989	Assessment of specific skills; first 3 subscales scored present/absent; last 2 subscales scored: yes/indifferent/no	68	Percentage agreement between observers = 0.70-0.90; inter-rater (individual scales) 0.00-0.98	Convergent and divergent (comparison with medical knowledge global expert and self ratings)	Teaching and assessing medical students (in practice settings)	External assessment of videotaped interview; observers require extensive training

Assessment	Description	No. of items	Reliability	Validity	Current use	Special notes
11 Measure of Patient-Centered Care; Maheux et al., 1997	Assessment of physician's perception of his/her care of the last 10 patients seen; self-report; Likert scale	14	Internal consistency = 0.85 (Cronbach's alpha)	Construct validity (level of training) demonstrated	Assessing medical students (in practice settings)	Self report; no external observer necessary
12 Patient Evaluation Questionnaire; Henkin et al., 1990	Assessment of patients' perception of medical students' behavior during interactions	15	None reported	None demonstrated; no correlation with tutors' evaluations	Ditto	Extensive manpower to interview patients
13 Pendleton's Consultation Map Rating Scale 1984/	Consultation map provides a method for describing a consultation. Consultation scale is designed to evaluate a consultation; visual analogue scale	Map = 11; Scale = 14	None reported	None reported	Teaching and assessing medical students/ trainees in practice settings	External assessment of videotaped interviews

	Assessment	Description	No. of items	Reliability	Validity	Current use	Special notes
14	SEGUE Framework; Makoul, 1995	Assessment of specific communication tasks; nominal (i.e. yes/no) scale	Short = 25 Long = 31	Inter-rater = 0.88 intra-rater = 0.98	Convergent validity (correlated with patient satisfaction)	Teaching and assessing medical students and residents in general medical practice	Can be used for videotaped, audio-taped or real-time encounters; includes section for comments
15	Standard Index of Communication (SIC)/Standard Index of Discrimination (SID)/Levels of Response Scale (LRS); Carkuff, 1969	SIC is a video-tape of stimuli used to elicit helper responses rated on the LRS (9-point scale). SID is a videotape of 4 sample responses to each of the stimuli in the SIC, which the participant is asked to rank on the LRS	SIC:16 SID:64 LRS:1 (9-point scale)	Inter-rater = 0.89 Rate-rerate = 0.93-0.95	None reported	Teaching and assessing medical students (in practice settings)	External assessment of responses
16	Telephone Assessment of T.A.L.K.; Kosower et al., 1996	Assessment of interpersonal communication skills of physicians on the telephone; Likert scale	22	Inter-rater identified as "good"	Face validity (evaluated by expert panel)	Teaching and assessing medical students (in pediatric settings)	Has been modified for assessing inter-personal communication in medical interviewing

Note. Reprinted from: Patient Education and Counseling, 35, Boon H. and Stewart M., Patient-physician communication assessment instruments: 1986 to 1996 in review, 161-176. Copyright 1998, with permission from Elsevier Science.

23 The Use of Computers in Assessment

BRIAN E. CLAUSER
National Board of Medical Examiners, Philadelphia

LAMBERT W.T. SCHUWIRTH
University of Maastricht

SUMMARY

Computers have had a pervasive impact on contemporary life, an impact that has been felt strongly in educational assessment. Interestingly, although the potential advantages of computerized testing have been studied and discussed for more than two decades, it is only within the last few years that computers have begun to have a large-scale practical impact on assessment. This chapter will examine the role of computers in medical education assessment. The chapter is broadly divided into three sections. The first examines the use computers as a platform for the delivery of standard testing formats (e.g., multiple-choice items). In this application, the computer eliminates costs associated with printing test materials, allows for enhancements such as audio and video, and may allow for increased flexibility in scheduling and administration. The computer also facilitates the implementation of various types of adaptive testing. Computer-adaptive testing (CAT) is a means of improving the efficiency of testing by targeting the test to the individual examinee. Most computer-adaptive testing procedures are based on item response theory (IRT). A brief (and relatively non-mathematical) description of IRT will be presented followed by a discussion of the logic and potential of CAT. This section will end with a description of some recent innovations related to computerized testing, including alternative item selection and test construction methodologies and procedures for automated test assembly.

The second section of this chapter will focus on computer simulations for use in assessment. As with other aspects of computer-based testing, discussion, planning and research date back decades but results from large-scale implementation are only now becoming available. This section begins with an historical perspective, describing the precursor of the computer simulation, the paper-and-pencil based patient management problem. Two examples of currently available simulations are described. A significant question with the use of computerized patient management simulations is, "How should the performance be scored"? A conceptual framework

International Handbook of Research in Medical Education, 757–792.
G.R. Norman, C.P.M. Van der Vleuten, D.I. Newble (eds.)
© 2002 *Dordrecht: Kluwer Academic Publishers. Printed in Great Britain.*

for considering scoring approaches is described and recent published results are summarized. Validity and reliability issues are discussed for assessments based on computerized simulations.

The third section of this chapter briefly describes what may be the future of computers in assessment. Research in the areas of natural language processing and virtual reality provide a basis for sensible speculation about the potential for the use of technology in future assessment. Recommendations are made to temper enthusiasm so that technology may be a means to improved assessment rather than an end in itself.

INTRODUCTION

This chapter examines the role of computers in medical education assessment from three perspectives. The first section considers the use of computers as a platform for the delivery of standard testing formats. In this application, the computer may eliminate costs associated with printing test materials, allows for enhancement of the stimulus materials, and provides increased flexibility in scheduling and administration. The computer also facilitates the implementation of various types of computer-adaptive testing. The second section focuses on computer simulations for use in assessment, including a detailed description of two simulation formats that are currently in use. A significant question with the use of computerized patient management simulations is, "How should the performance be scored?". A conceptual framework for considering scoring approaches is presented. The third section describes what may be the future of computers in assessment. Research in the areas of natural language processing and virtual reality are presented as a basis for speculation about the use of technology in future assessment. Recommendations are made to temper enthusiasm so that technology may be seen as a means to improved assessment rather than an end in itself.

COMPUTER DELIVERY OF STANDARD TEST FORMATS

Logistical advantages and disadvantages of computer administration

The use of computers for test administration offers both theoretical and practical advantages. Practically speaking, paper administration of an examination requires printing test books. This simple requirement has numerous implications. In medical evaluation, it is often appropriate to have high-quality color photographs included in the stimulus materials. However, color printing remains a significant expense; so much so that testing programs may be forced to limit or eliminate the use of this sort of stimulus. With computer delivery, presenting colored stimulus materials requires only that the photograph be digitized. Eliminating the printing costs may practically remove restrictions on the use of color pictures which are only one type of stimulus material that the computer facilitates. Although audio and video have been used in certification tests, presentation has been problematic. As with color, the computer makes presentation of this type of material relatively convenient, assuming that the required hardware and software are available.

In addition to the costs and practical limitations in terms of the nature of stimulus materials, printed test booklets may create a substantial logistical challenge. For large-scale high-stakes testing, a significant problem is created in the distribution of the booklets. To ensure security, booklets must be printed, shipped, and stored at the administration site, under secure conditions. The loss of a single copy of the test (for even a brief period) calls into question the security of the examination. In the common circumstance that test materials are to be reused, the problem does not end with the test administration. Security must continue after administration while test materials are collected and shipped back to the test administrator. Again, if even a single copy is missing, the security of the test material may be compromised.

By contrast, when the test is administered on computer, encryption procedures can be used to ensure that the test material is only available during the period that the authorized examinee is viewing the item on the screen. Systems involving separate passwords given to the test administrator and the examinee can be implemented to ensure that the material is only decrypted under authorized conditions. Scoring can be completed on-line or an electronic file can be returned to be scored. In either case, there is no need for further transportation of the secure test materials and the encrypted files can simply be deleted when testing is complete.

Computerization also has the potential to offer flexibility in test administration. For large-scale assessments, tests are typically administered on a relatively small number of dates annually. Administrative efficiency and printing costs dictate this restriction. By contrast, when examinations are administered via computer-testing, centers can be established and test forms can be administered at the examinee's convenience. This flexibility may also appear highly advantageous in small-scale (intramural) testing contexts. Testing on demand makes it convenient to establish educational programs in which students work at their own rate, demonstrating mastery at each level before moving to the subsequent unit.

This section has described some of the "promise" of computer-based testing from a practical and logistical perspective. Before moving on to examine the additional theoretical advantages of computerization, a few comments on the practical limitations are warranted. Clearly computerization eliminates printing costs. However, it does introduce other administration expenses. The evaluator must either establish the required computer center(s) or pay for administration at commercial centers. In general the cost of computer administration will exceed the cost of paper administration for large-scale testing (when economy of scale makes printing more efficient). In smaller-scale administrations, where the cost of high-quality printing may be much higher per examinee, this relationship may shift.

Although certain aspects of administration may become more convenient because of computerization, issues arise which may not have an analogue in paper administration. For example, when color pictures are part of the test material, it is possible to print the pictures so that each test booklet will contain an accurate and uniform representation. By contrast, the image on a computer screen may vary from machine to machine, depending on specifics of the hardware and software, and also on monitor adjustments. Similar issues may arise when audio or video are included in the stimulus materials. Even when the test is entirely text based, the specifics of the computer equipment may lead to concerns about the standardization of administration (e.g., the size and quality of the monitor may influence the readability of the material).

Another issue that arises in computerization of assessment is the possible impact of examinee computer experience. When examinees differ in terms of how often they use computers, issues of comfort and familiarity may become a concern. In some circumstances there may be examinees who experience anxiety when using a computer. Although there is empirical evidence suggesting that computer experience may have a negligible impact on outcomes, the issue requires consideration when planning a computerized assessment.

As described previously, computerization may dramatically reduce the vulnerability of a testing program to certain types of security breaches. If test booklets are not printed, there is no need for concern that a booklet may be taken, copied, and distributed before or after the administration. If the test is administered as a single simultaneous sitting for all examinees, this may create the optimal security conditions. However, if computerization means moving from occasional administrations to ongoing availability, it will most likely be necessary to reuse items from day to day. This creates the possibility that examinees may memorize or otherwise carry away specifics about the items. Organized efforts to collect information may lead to subsequent examinees having information about large numbers of items. Varying test forms administered and constructing substantial numbers of forms from a pool containing a large number of items may effectively minimize the advantage that any individual is likely to gain from information gathered by other examinees. The drawback is that item writing is typically expensive and writing the items required to produce numerous forms with minimal overlap will be costly.

Finally, the convenience of scheduling may prove to be a limited advantage. No doubt some examinees will find a single scheduled test date inconvenient. Illness or other personal conflicts my be problematic. But the other side of the convenience of examinee scheduling may be that when all (or most) examinees wish to test during a brief period, the available computer facilities may be insufficient to accommodate them. There are likely to be circumstances in which the guarantee of test availability during some critical period is more attractive than the convenience on self-scheduling without that guarantee.

Theoretical advantages of computerized testing

For more than two decades, researchers have examined the potential advantages associated with computer-adaptive testing (CAT). The logic behind CAT is that each item response provides information about the examinee; however, the amount of information provided varies. The information provided by an item is maximized when the difficulty of the item is well matched to the proficiency of the examinee (i.e., when the probability of the examinee responding correctly is about 0.5). The mathematical definition of information and the logic behind this relationship are complex but it is intuitively apparent that if a highly proficient examinee is presented with a very easy item and answers correctly, the evaluator has learned little. By contrast, if the highly proficient examinee responds correctly (or incorrectly) to a very difficult item, this response provides some basis for raising or lowering the estimation of that examinee's proficiency. CAT allows the evaluator to select a set of test items that is optimally targeted to the examinee's proficiency. In effect, this approach selects a set of items that minimize measurement error in the vicinity of the individual examinee's estimated proficiency.

Item response theory

Classical test theory provides a variety of extremely useful tools for evaluating the performance of tests and test items. One limitation of this framework is that the resulting conclusions about test and item performance must be interpreted in the context of the specific sample of examinees whose responses were evaluated. Similarly, inferences about examinees must be interpreted in the context of the sample of items which they completed. For example, to describe the difficulty of a test item (scored as 0 or 1) in the classical test theory framework, an index would be calculated representing the proportion of examinees scoring 1 on the item. This index, referred to as the p-value, is informative, but it may vary dramatically if the item is re-administered to a more (or less) competent sample of examinees. Similarly, a description of examinee proficiency is likely to take the form of a percent correct or number correct score. This value will also vary if the examinee is retested with a sample of more (or less) difficult items.

In contrast to classical test theory, IRT provides a means of estimating item difficulty which is theoretically invariant with regard to the sample of examinees that responded to the item. Similarly, it provides an estimate of examinee proficiency which is invariant to the sample of items used to measure the examinee. Practically, it is this invariance which makes proficiency estimates based on computer-adaptive testing possible. This means that a potentially unique set of items can be administered to each examinee to optimize the information available about that examinee's proficiency.

In the typical conceptualization of CAT, an examinee is presented with a small number of items. Based on the responses to those items an estimate is made of the examinee's proficiency. The next item is then selected to provide maximum information at that proficiency level. After the examinee responds, the examinee's proficiency is estimated again, and based on the revised estimate an item is selected to provide maximum information. This process of sequential and iterative testing and proficiency estimation continues until the criterion for ending the test is met. By optimally selecting the items in this sequential manner, it may be possible to substantially increase the information available about an examinee's proficiency relative to that provided by a fixed administration.

As with the potential logistical advantages of computerized testing, the advantages arising from the use of CAT require careful consideration and evaluation. The discussion that follows is a brief summary. (See Hambleton & Swaminathan, 1985; Hambleton, Swaminathan, & Rogers, 1991; for a more complete description of IRT and Wainer et al., 1990, for a more detailed description of computerized adaptive testing.) Even in summary form, it is necessary to have some sense of IRT. The discussion, therefore, begins with a description of item response theory. It then considers some of the specifics of CAT implementation. The discussion concludes with a description of some of the more recent innovations in computerized test delivery.

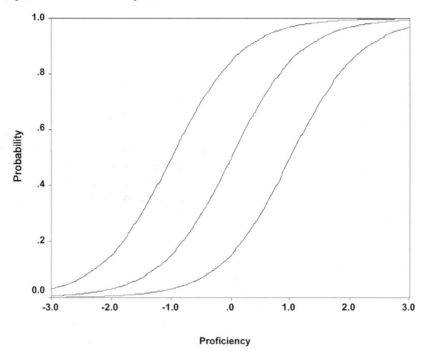

Figure 1. Item characteristic curve for the one-parameter logistic IRT model

Most currently used IRT models apply a logistic function to describe the relationship between an examinee's proficiency and the probability that that examinee will respond correctly to a given test item. The most common models are shown in the appendix, although a mathematical understanding of the models is not required to follow the present discussion. In this framework, examinee proficiency and item difficulty are placed on the same scale. Using the simplest of the models, the one-parameter model, item difficulty is represented by a horizontal shift in the logistic curve along the scale. The logistic curve represents the probability of a correct response to the item as a function of examinee proficiency. Figure 1 presents three of these curves for items of varying difficulty. (Again, the item difficulty scale and the examinee proficiency scales are identical.) In this model, the item which provides the most information about an examinee's proficiency is the one with the curve that has its point of inflection closest to the examinee's proficiency; the best guess as to the examinee's actual proficiency is the current estimate. The curves demonstrate two important features of the one-parameter model. First, for examinees of low proficiency, the probability of a correct response is approximately zero. This aspect of the model may be problematic when it is applied to multiple-choice items where even random guessing leads to a proportion correct in excess of zero. The other important feature of this model is that the curves have the same shape. In IRT terminology, this requires that all items have equal discrimination. This requirement is similar to the condition that the item to total test score (point-biserial) correlation is the same for all items.

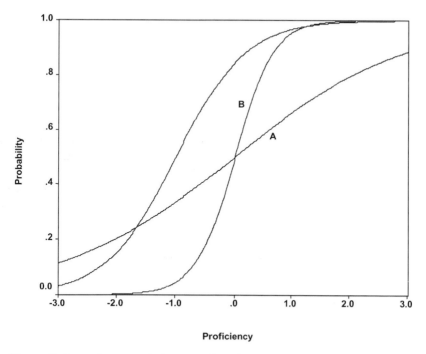

Figure 2. Item characteristic curve for the two-parameter logistic IRT model

The remaining two commonly used IRT models are appropriate for use in conditions in which these two aspects of the one-parameter model may make it inappropriate. In the two-parameter logistic model, items differ not only in difficulty, but in discrimination. In this model, discrimination is represented by the slope of the logistic curve. Figure 2 provides examples of items that differ in both discrimination and difficulty. Again, without focusing on the mathematics, it should be intuitive that the steeper curve, the one in which the probability of a correct response between examinees with greater and lesser proficiency. This distinction is significant in the CAT context because items which are more discriminating, when properly targeted in terms of difficulty, are more informative. Conceptually this is again intuitive in that it reduces to the idea that an item which correlates more highly with the proficiency of interest provides more information about examinee proficiency than does an equivalent item with a lower correlation. In this case, the optimal item may no longer be the one with a difficulty most closely targeted to the examinee's proficiency, but instead it will be the item that optimally combines targeting of difficulty with high discrimination.

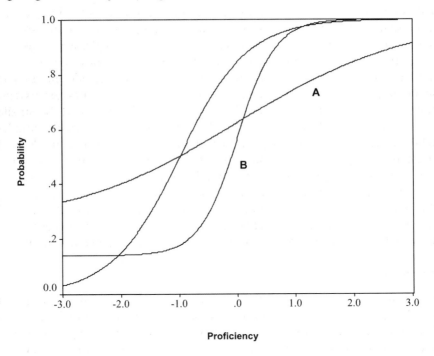

Figure 3. Item characteristic curve for the three-parameter logistic T model

The most complex of the three common IRT models is the three-parameter logistic model. In this model, as with the two-parameter logistic model, the response function may vary both in position on the scale (reflecting differences in item difficulty) and in slope (reflecting differences in discrimination). The three-parameter model is adapted to additionally allow for the possibility that an examinee with extremely low proficiency will have a non-zero probability of a correct response to the item. Figure 3 provides examples of curves representing items using a three-parameter model.

Even this brief explanation of IRT should provide a sense of the usefulness of these models. When the data fit the model, the estimated parameters are invariant with respect to the sample used (although in practice, efficient estimation will be dependent on the sampling design).

The models provide a means of selecting items that will be optimal in terms of the information they provide about an examinee's proficiency. The invariance property means that the required item parameters can be estimated based on one group of examinees and applied to another group or to an individual examinee. Since the parameters describe items and not tests, the examinee's ability can subsequently be estimated based on any selected set of items.

This is clearly a powerful theory. The price of that power is that the parameter estimation requires strong assumptions. It is assumed that the proficiency being measured is unidimensional and that the individual item responses are independent (after conditioning on that proficiency). Beyond that, the choice of the specific model can be based on the fit of the data to that model. For example, when guessing is not a significant issue and all items are of approximately equal discrimination, the one-parameter model may be the best option. When these requirements are not met, the more complex models may be preferred. When the data reasonably approximate the requirements of the one-parameter model, it has the advantage that the smaller number of parameters allow for reasonable estimation with smaller samples. Acceptable parameter estimates may be obtained in the one-parameter model with approximately 200 examinee responses on each item. By contrast, the three-parameter model may require 500 to 1000 examinees per item.

Taken together, the sample-size requirements and the required assumptions may limit the applicability of these models. Clearly, small-scale (e.g., intramural) examination programs may be unable to meet the sample requirements. The unidimensionality and independence assumptions provide additional limitations.

Computer adaptive testing

The conceptual basis for CAT is that item selection should occur in a manner that provides the greatest possible information about examinee proficiency. IRT procedures often use some form of maximum likelihood estimation. This means that, as soon as the examinee has answered at least one item correctly and at least one item incorrectly, it is possible to estimate that examinee's proficiency. After making the estimate, the next item will be selected to provide the greatest information at that proficiency level. This process continues until a specified number of items has been administered. With this approach, the number of items is fixed, as with most paper-and-pencil testing, but to the extent that the items in a fixed form are less than an optimal selection from the set of all items available in the pool, CAT allows examinee proficiency to be estimated more efficiently. This means that the standard error of measurement is likely to be reduced for some (or all) examinees. With this approach, the precision of testing will vary across examinees because the available items will allow for more optimal testing of some examinees than others.

Completion of a fixed number of items is only one basis for terminating a CAT administration for an examinee. With each item administered, the available information about an examinee's proficiency increases. This information is an inverse function of the precision with which the examinee's proficiency can be estimated. A second rule for stopping a CAT administration is that the test is terminated when the examinee's proficiency has been estimated with a specified level of precision. With this approach the CAT will typically stop after different numbers of items for different examinees. Although the test length will differ across examinees, the precision of measurement will be similar for each examinee.

When a test is administered to classify examinees (e.g., certification testing) rather than to estimate examinee proficiency, it may be that the measurement precision of primary interest is the classification accuracy of the resulting test scores. In this circumstance, a stopping rule can be established to end the test when the probability that the examinee is mis-classified reaches some predetermined level (Kingsbury & Weiss, 1983). A variation of this strategy (Spray & Reckase, 1996) uses Wald's sequential probability ratio test (Wald, 1947). This approach provides a basis for structuring the stopping rule to reflect the fact that the cost associated with incorrectly failing an examinee whose true proficiency is above the standard (due to measurement error) may be different than the cost associated with incorrectly passing an examinee whose true proficiency is below the standard.

The basic CAT framework is based on the idea that, after each proficiency estimation, item selection is designed to optimize information about examinee proficiency. This abstract model leads to two potential problems in practical testing situations. First, tests are typically built to meet content specifications. If items are chosen to optimize information, the content specifications may be seriously violated. A second issue is that, in high-stakes testing, security concerns dictate that test forms taken by examinees on different days have minimal overlap. This minimal overlap will occur when all items in the pool are used at a similar (hopefully low) rate. In the typical CAT scenario, certain items will appear optimal for many examinees while other items may rarely be selected.

The same general logic applies to the resolution of both of these problems; item selection must not be based solely on the potential contribution of the item in terms of information. One simple (and possibly simplistic) answer to the first problem would be to sequentially select items from each content category in the table of specifications so that the selected item provided maximum information from those available within the specified category. This approach results in satisfying the requirements of the content specifications. Similarly, the security issues related to over-use of certain items can be resolved by limiting the number of times any item can be administered. This can be accomplished either by removing the item from use after a specified number of exposures or by developing a more complex algorithm that selects an item based on both its potential information contribution and the frequency of previous use. It is obvious that these constraints on item selection will reduce the precision of tests developed from a practically limited item pool. Much of the recent psychometric research done to support computerized testing has focused on these problems. The next section describes some of the strategies that have been developed during recent years.

Approaches to item selection

The general approach to exposure control in which items become unavailable (or less available) as testing continues over an administration period leads to a problem. Examinees completing the examination on day one of administration will in general be presented with a better test than those completing the test later in the administration. As the item pool is depleted through repeated selection of the most informative items, it is inevitable that an optimal test produced from a depleted pool will be inferior to one from the same pool before depletion. Two very promising approaches to this dilemma have been developed based on the availability of automated test assembly software. This software does exactly what the name implies, it constructs tests to meet pre-specified constraints while maximizing certain statistical characteristics of the test. Unlike CAT item selection software, this system constructs complete tests or subtests. The types of constraints that can be accommodated are: upper and lower bounds for the number of items that must appear from specified content categories; balances on secondary factors such as age or gender of patients described in items; specification of individual items that must or cannot appear on the same test form; and item overlap between forms. Taking these factors into consideration, the software will use the items in an available pool to construct a specified number of forms of the test maximizing the measurement precision on each form. One approach that takes advantage of this technology is computer adaptive sequential testing (CAST). With CAST, a branching strategy is used to deliver blocks of items. (See Luecht and Nungester, 1998, for a more complete description of CAST). At the end of each block, the examinee's proficiency is estimated and predetermined branching rules are used to identify the most appropriate next block for that examinee. Figure 4 provides a diagram showing the possible pathways through a simple CAST administration.

In this example, all examinees complete a module of medium difficulty. At the end of this module, examinees are classified into one of three levels of proficiency. The most proficient examinees are then administered a relatively difficult module, less proficient examinees are administered a module of medium difficulty, and the least proficient examinees are administered a relatively easy module. At the conclusion of this module, examinee proficiency is again estimated and examinees are again assigned the module that provides the most information at their proficiency level. Using IRT item parameters, it is possible to produce scores on a common scale for all examinees, regardless of the relative difficulty of the modules completed.

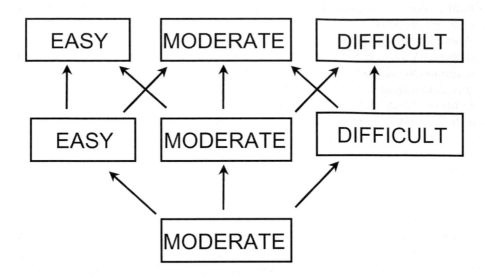

Figure 4. Pathway diagram for a simple CAST administration

The CAST approach has some important practical advantages. Because all alternative modules can be created from a pool simultaneously, prior to administration, it is possible to constrain the automated test assembly software to limit item overlap. Additionally, because the alternate modules are created at the same time, rather than with the CAT approach where the forms are created sequentially as examinees test, the software can be constrained to create forms with similar measurement characteristics. This approach also gives considerable flexibility in terms of meeting overall test content constraints. Content balancing can occur within each module or it can be structured so that any choice of a single module from each level results in satisfying the content specifications. Finally, because the modules are constructed in advance, test development committees or other groups or individuals responsible for the test can review sample forms or all forms of the test in advance in order to be sure that the various forms are acceptable.

Van der Linden has recently proposed an alternative procedure, also based on the potential to use computer software to simultaneously construct multiple forms of a test that meet required content and statistical constraints. Rather than selecting a single item after each iteration of proficiency estimation, the computer constructs an entire test form ensuring that all content constraints can be met. The most informative item is then selected from the previously unadministered items in this "shadow test". Following administration of the item, the examinee's ability is re-estimated and the process is repeated with a new test form (that includes all items previously administered to the examinee) being constructed to meet all constraints. The advantage in measurement efficiency associated with item selection based on the item's potential information contribution is therefore maintained and when the administration is complete the content constraints have necessarily been met (Van der Linden, in press).

Another recently developed strategy for CAT administration was suggested by Chang and Ying (1998). This approach stratifies items for selection based on the discrimination parameter. The procedure takes advantage of the fact, evident from Figure 2, that when a highly discriminating item is poorly targeted for an examinee, in terms of difficulty, the available information may actually be lower than that of a less discriminating item targeted in the same way. An item with low discrimination (e.g., item A in Figure 2) will have a gentle slope across a wide range of the score scale. By contrast, a highly discriminating item will have a very steep slope across a narrow part of the score scale and a relatively flat slope outside of that range (e.g., item B in Figure 2). By stratifying item selection on the discrimination parameter, items with relatively low discrimination can be selected early in the CAT administration when there is little information about the examinee's proficiency. As testing continues and the precision of proficiency estimation increases, more highly-discriminating items can be accurately targeted to examinee proficiency. The main advantage of this approach is that it makes efficient use of low discriminating items which might otherwise not be selected in a CAT administration. This reduces the disparity in item selection rate across low and high discriminating items and reduces or eliminates the need for more artificial controls on item selection required to control overlap of items across forms.

A final comment is warranted on the potential utility of CAT and other procedures involving strategies for optimal item selection. The theoretical usefulness of these procedures over random item selection is obvious. Early research suggested that it might be possible to maintain a set level of measurement precision while reducing test lengths by one-third or more, but evaluators considering the use of these methodologies should consider the specifics of the situation. For example, if a paper-and-pencil test is to be used to make classification decisions based on a single cut-score and the current forms are constructed to optimize measurement precision in the vicinity of the cut-score, sophisticated item selection procedures may offer relatively little improvement in measurement efficiency. Similarly, even when the intention of the assessment is to precisely estimate examinee proficiency rather than to classify the examinee, the usefulness of these procedures for optimal item selection will be limited by the size and quality of the item pool and the extent of the constraints created by the need to construct test forms to meet content and security specifications. Finally, there may be situations in which political pressures limit the use of these approaches. For example, it may be possible to reliably classify some examinees as proficient (or non-proficient) after they have completed as few as 50 to 75 items. From a measurement perspective, this would seem to be a highly efficient and clearly desirable situation. However, if the test is being administered to make a high-stakes decision (such as medical licensure) it may be politically unacceptable to allow (or deny) a candidate a license to practice medicine based on responses to only 50 test items.

Limitations of IRT and CAT

Rapid increase in the availability of computer technology and intensive research on the practical problems of computerized testing make this approach increasingly attractive. As more experience is gained with computer delivery of assessments in medical education, the ease with which evaluators can confidently move to this modality will increase. Regardless of the extent of these improvements, it is unlikely that IRT based computerized adaptive testing will be an appropriate choice for all evaluation programs. Beyond the need for computer hardware and software, several limitations will remain. These may be particularly problematic for small evaluation programs. First, IRT models require reasonably large samples of examinee responses for item parameter estimation; 100 to 1000 responses per item, depending on the model. Second, as this section makes clear, considerable psychometric expertise is required to make decisions about which IRT models and which item selection procedures are most appropriate for the specific context. For small programs, such as intramural assessment at an individual medical school or certification testing in highly specialized areas, this may make application of this technology impractical. This does not eliminate the possibility of computer administration, only the use of IRT based administration procedures.

COMPUTER SIMULATIONS

Simulations as an item format

The bedside examination and other oral examination formats have been a mainstay of the evaluation of medical students for generations. However, as the use of multiple-choice items became widespread in the 1950s and 1960s, the efficiency and reliability of these traditional evaluation formats was called into question. Organizations, such as the National Board of Medical Examiners, made heroic efforts to standardize bedside evaluation in order to improve the reliability but ultimately found that satisfactory reliability could not be obtained (Hubbard & Levit, 1985). The resulting decision to drop the bedside evaluation from the National Board's licensure examination was followed by similar steps on the part of many other large-scale licensure and certification agencies. At the National Board of Medical Examiners and elsewhere this decision motivated a major interest in development of alternative formats that might be used to examine a candidate's ability to integrate information and make decisions. In 1968, the National Board made a commitment to develop a computer simulation to evaluate physicians' patient management skills.

The decision to drop the use of the bedside examination by the National Board of Medical Examiners also led to increased interest in paper-and-pencil based simulations referred to as patient management problems or PMPs (Berner, Hamilton, & Best, 1974). With this format, the examinee was provided with initial information about a patient and then given choices regarding the tests or examinations that should be ordered. After making a selection, the examinee would be given access to the resulting information. A variety of approaches were available for accessing the information; the examinee may be given a special pen that could be used to make a latent image visible or a special ink or other covering might be removed with an eraser. Although PMPs were administered on paper, the motivation for the use of PMPs was the same as that for computerized simulations. The perceived measurement importance of this format is reflected in the fact that by 1985 PMPs represented a significant part of the National Board of Medical Examiners' Part III examination. Nonetheless, evaluators were beginning to have concerns about the format and several problems were identified.

Typically, detailed scoring keys for PMPs were developed by expert panels. Experts were asked to score and weight all the possible decisions an examinee could make when working through a PMP. It was found that, although experts could readily agree on the final solution for a case, they were much less likely to reach consensus about the optimal route an examinee should take to reach that solution. Differences of opinion frequently existed about the scoring and weighting of individual actions (Swanson, Norcini, & Grosso, 1987).

In addition to difficulties in developing scoring keys, it was found that when experts were examined using PMPs their scores were often lower than those of so-called "intermediates" (physicians who recently graduated from medical schools) or even final year medical students (Schmidt, Boshuizen, & Hobus, 1988). This unexpected finding challenged the construct validity of these scores.

Perhaps the most problematic limitation of PMP scores was their low reliability. Inter-case correlations tended to be low, meaning that the score an examinee received on one case tended to be a poor predictor for that examinee's performance on other cases (Elstein, Shulmann, & Sprafka, 1978; Swanson et al., 1987). Evidence that problem-solving ability is considerably more context (or domain) specific than originally assumed had serious consequences for the conceptual assumptions about the nature of the proficiency PMPs were intended to evaluate. Medical evaluators originally tended to assume that problem-solving ability was a stable and generic trait (i.e. once a person had become a successful problem solver, (s)he would be able to solve any given problem within the same broad domain). The implication of these results for examinations based on complex PMP formats is the same as those for examinations involving other forms of complex performance assessment; in order to obtain scores that are adequately generalizable very lengthy tests may be required (Swanson, 1987).

A final limitation with the PMP resulted from the fact that the format provided cueing. Because the examinee chose from a list of options at each point in the test process, it was possible for the examinee to look ahead in the booklet and make decisions about the most appropriate choices at the beginning of the case in light of the options that would be available at subsequent stages. As long as the format was delivered in a printed booklet, this cueing represented a potentially serious problem. The obvious solution to the problem was computerized test delivery. With this format examinees could not gain access to information about subsequent stages of the examination until they had completed the earlier steps. Acting on this potential led to computerized PMPs, one of the first forms of computer-based simulation for medical evaluation.

These limitations led most testing organizations to the decision to abandon the use of PMPs. Interest in replacing PMPs, along with the belief that computers would allow for collection of even richer assessment information, resulted in considerable interest in computer simulations of the patient-care environment. Numerous systems have been developed. Most have been limited to the application of intramural assessment, but some projects have been targeted at licensure or certification assessment. This chapter will describe two examples representing different testing contexts, different levels of complexity and, to some extent, different test construction philosophies.

Computerized case-based testing (CCT)

CCT was developed at the University of Maastricht in the Netherlands as a response to the problems encountered with PMPs. The system is used to assess students during their clerkship years. The intended purpose of CCT is to assess the competence of medical students in applying their knowledge to solve patient problems. The test material is based on the so-called "key-feature" approach (Bordage, 1987).

A central server at the University contains the test material, allowing authorized individuals to draw or select tests from the item bank. Separate banks have been developed for testing within specified disciplines. The test administered to a given examinee is created by randomly selecting cases within the constraints of a pre-specified blueprint (Schuwirth, Van der Vleuten, De Kock, Peperkamp, & Donkers, 1996). The system can be accessed from a limited number of locations (affiliated hospitals) during a specified time frame. Although use of CCT is currently limited to the medical faculties of the University of Maastricht and the University of Amsterdam, dissemination to other medical faculties is planned.

The case presentations in CCT are brief. Considerable effort is made to produce descriptions that are authentic but succinct. Unlike the format typically used in PMPs, in which patient information is provided sequentially, with CCT the entire case is presented at once. In this presentation relevant signs, symptoms, and findings are given including the necessary contextual information. Multimedia are used when relevant, but these applications are restricted to circumstances in which interpretation of visual or auditory stimuli is central to the measurement objective of the case. Figure 5 provides an example of the item interface.

Each case description is followed by one to five questions, and questions are aimed at essential decisions (i.e. those key-decisions that decide whether a case would be managed successfully or not). Routine decisions or general medical knowledge questions are avoided (Schuwirth et al., 1999). A number of question formats are used with the content typically dictating format. The choice of constructed response versus fixed format is based on the number of realistic alternatives facing the physician in practice. For example, examinees are likely to be requested to select lab tests from a list while questions asking for a differential diagnosis may be open-ended.

Although software for evaluating natural language is currently in use in high-stakes testing, these applications are highly specialized and at present require resources well beyond those likely to be available to any but the largest testing organizations (Burstein et al., 1998). In CCT, open-ended questions use the so-called "long menu format" (Schuwirth, Van der Vleuten, & Donkers, 1995). These items consist of a list of possible answers (totaling over 9000 alternatives) out of which the examinee has to "select" the correct answer. Rather than scanning all alternatives, the examinee generates the answer by making free-text entry and the program identifies matches to the list. This question format closely approximates a true open-ended question format (Schuwirth, Van der Vleuten, Stoffers, & Peperkamp, 1996).

When using these short cases, some loss of fidelity is inevitable. Therefore, considerable time and energy is devoted to ensuring that the stimulus materials are realistic. All cases are based on actual patients, and are written by the physician who actually provided the consultation.

These initial case descriptions are thoroughly reviewed and edited by an expert panel. Each case is then presented to an independent panel of experts for review of the answer key. A case is only used if consensus regarding the correct answers can be reached among the experts. A typical CCT test contains about 60 cases. Again, for each examinee, a separate test is drawn from the item bank by randomly selecting items within the constraints of a discipline-specific blueprint. Within each discipline the item bank contains at least 1200 to 1500 cases. These large banks are important both because they allow for appropriate sampling within the discipline and because they discourage examinees from viewing memorization of test material as an effective test preparation strategy.

Examinees have a fixed time limit for completing the test; testing time per case is not limited. Examinees are allowed to use textbooks for reference. This use of reference material is both consistent with conditions in practice and carries the additional advantage that it reminds case developers to avoid simplistic factual questions.

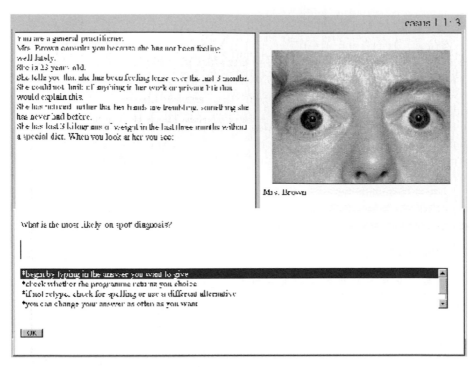

Figure 5. CCS interface showing sample problem

Scores for CCT are produced by summing correct responses. This approach is consistent with the philosophy used for case development, with each case being associated with a small number of questions and all questions focusing on central aspects of the specific management challenge. Students receive their results immediately after taking the test.

The approach used in CCT was aimed at avoiding the problems of the long PMPs. By using short cases and limited numbers of questions many different cases can be presented per test, thus sampling the domain more adequately. Obviously, this represents a compromise. Shortening and focusing the cases allows for superior sampling but it necessarily represents an abstraction of the problem solving challenge that physicians face in practice. It therefore somewhat reduces the authenticity of the task. CCT also changes the focus of the assessment from the problem solving process to the outcome.

Research on CCT has assessed the quality and appropriateness of case content, score reliability, and the relationship between CCT and other item formats (Schuwirth, 1998). A large-scale study is currently underway to assess the consequential validity (Messick, 1989) of CCT by examining its influence on student learning behavior. Specifics are referenced in the following sections describing validity issues.

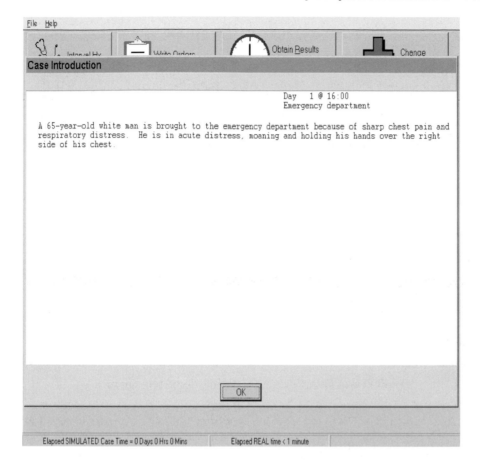

File   Help

Obtain Results

Chance

Case Introduction

Day   1 @ 16:00
Emergency department

A 65-year-old white man is brought to the emergency department because of sharp chest pain and respiratory distress. He is in acute distress, moaning and holding his hands over the right side of his chest.

OK

Elapsed SIMULATED Case Time = 0 Days 0 Hrs 0 Mins   Elapsed REAL time < 1 minute

Figure 6. CCS interface showing sample opening scenario
Primum® Computer-Based Case Simulation, copyright © 1988-2001 by the National
Board of Medical Examiners®. Reprinted by permission. All rights reserved.

Primum® computer-based case simulations

This system has been under development by the NBME since the 1960s. From the outset, the intention has been to include the format in the assessment sequence for physician licensure in the United States. Primum provides a largely unprompted simulation of the patient-care environment. The examinee is presented with a brief opening scenario describing the patient's presentation. Figure 6 provides an example of the screen presenting the opening scenario. The examinee then reviews history and physical-examination information. The challenge is to collect diagnostic information and provide appropriate treatment. Tests, consultations, treatments, and procedures are ordered by using a standard keyboard to make free-text entries on an order sheet. The system recognizes over 12,500 terms, abbreviations, acronyms, brand and generic names, representing nearly 2500 unique actions. Figure 7 shows the order screen.

In addition to making entries on the order screen, the examinee is responsible for making decisions about the patient's location and for advancing the case through simulated time. The clock and location icons at the top of the screen in Figure 6 give the examinee control over these aspects of the case.

The Primum simulation is dynamic in that the patient's condition changes over time as a function of both the underlying problem and the actions taken by the examinee. If an examinee orders vital signs or diagnostic tests, the results will reflect the conditions at that time. The simulation is also realistic in that test results only become available after an appropriate passage of simulated time. Similarly, medications take effect only after a realistic period of simulated time.

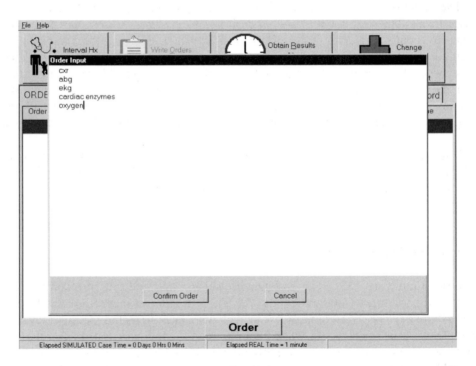

Figure 7. CCS interface showing order screen
Primum® Computer-Based Case Simulation, copyright © 1988-2001 by the National Board of Medical Examiners®. Reprinted by permission. All rights reserved.

Primum produces a complex and realistic simulation of the patient-care environment, but it has been designed to test only specified aspects of patient management, and so the simulation is not complete. For example, the examinee is not asked to interpret x-rays. If an x-ray is ordered, the findings are presented in written form. The decision to limit the simulation in this way was based on the view that if assessment of the examinee's ability to interpret x-rays is of interest, it can be more efficiently accomplished by presenting sets of x-rays in the more traditional fixed-response format.

Similarly, the simulation is not designed to assess the examinee's ability to take a history or perform a physical examination. Another aspect of patient care explicitly excluded from the evaluation is the need to make decisions about optimal dosage for medications. The examinees must indicate whether the medication is to be given one time only or on an ongoing basis, they must also indicate the route of administration, and they must take responsibility for terminating ongoing medications at the appropriate time, but information about the specific dosage is not requested and examinees are instructed to assume that the dosage delivered is optimal.

The duration of the case (in simulated time) is programmed based on the assessment objective that the case is designed to evaluate. Cases may last from hours to months. All cases end uniformly, with a note thanking the examinee for taking care of the patient. Cases end after some pre-specified period of simulated time, when the examinee has fulfilled all of the assessment objectives, or when, owing to inappropriate care, the patient's condition has deteriorated to the point that continued management would call upon proficiencies that were not part of the original assessment objective for the case. Each case is also limited in terms of real time.

When an examinee finishes managing a case, Primum retains a complete record of the actions ordered by the examinee along with the simulated time at which the action was ordered. Scoring is accomplished through a computerized review of this record.

Scoring simulations

Several limitations of paper-and-pencil patient management problems were described previously. The problem of potential prompting associated with allowing the examinees access to options associated with later branches before they had completed earlier steps is eliminated with computer administration. Unfortunately, moving to computer does little to resolve issues related to scoring. One lesson from the PMP experience is clear: an assessment task is only useful if it can be used to produce meaningful scores. With this in mind, it is not surprising that considerable effort has gone into refining and evaluating scores produced for computer simulations.

The first step in developing a scoring system is to make a decision about what is to be measured. It is tempting to develop the most complex and realistic simulation possible assuming that realism must support valid inference. This approach turns scoring into a *post hoc* activity. A more sensible approach is to construct the simulation and the scoring system simultaneously to support the specific inferences of interest. With this approach, the nature of the proficiency being measured rather than the limitations of the simulation will drive scoring decisions.

The use of this approach is apparent in the previous description of CCT. The focus on "key features" and on the outcome rather than the process of decision making is clearly reflected in the construction of CCT test materials. In the case of Primum, the concern was to evaluate the process of examinee decision making in the context of patient management. This focus resulted in development of a more complex simulation allowing for evaluation not only of actions ordered by the examinee but of the sequence and timing of those orders. Nonetheless, as described previously, there was no effort made to develop a complete simulation of the environment. For example, the need to interpret imaging studies was not part of the design of this simulation. Although a potentially important skill, this was not considered to be a part of the proficiency that Primum was intended to assess.

Once the proficiencies of interest are carefully identified, the question of scoring moves from which aspects of the performance are to be quantified to how this quantification is to be achieved. In some circumstances, both in medicine and in other professions, it is possible to evaluate a performance using a completely objective standard. An early version of the National Board of Medical Examiners' certification examination required (among other things) that the candidate suture a section of animal intestine. The intestine was then attached to a water source exerting a fixed pressure and observed to see if the suture leaked (Hubbard & Levit, 1985). In areas where complex skills are evaluated, absolute standards are the exception. Scoring performance assessments has more commonly relied on expert judgment. This is clearly the norm for oral examinations. Even computer simulations, taking advantage of up-to-the-minute technology to present the stimulus, may be scored by having experts review the record of examinee performance. However, particularly when simulations are used for large-scale assessment, the problems of using expert judges may be extremely limiting. The use of judges invariably leads to error. Even with careful training, different judges may evaluate the same performances differently or make errors due to fatigue or inattention. The number of hours of experts' time required to rate the performances of the thousands of examinees assessed annually in many testing programs may also make this approach highly impractical.

The potential advantage of creating a scoring system that allows the computer to replace these experts has justified a considerable research effort. Again, one sensible strategy is that represented by CCT. By avoiding the sequencing of examinee responses so that earlier responses do not alter the context in which later responses are made, a system that simply matches the examinee response to the key is workable. For more complex simulations, particularly those that involve sequencing through the simulation of time, this approach is likely to be unworkable. In the case where there is no single correct answer, the simplest approach is to create a key specifying desirable and undesirable actions that an examinee might order and following the approach used with PMPs, credit the appropriate actions ordered and debit the non-indicated and risky actions. This approach is likely to produce a score that correlates moderately with expert ratings of the performance. Unfortunately, it is clear that experts will often apply a more complex judgment policy and the simplicity of this system may result in reduced validity. This sort of approach is also likely to lead to the problems described earlier in the scoring of PMPs (resulting in a system that favors thoroughness over efficiency). What is needed is an algorithm that more accurately imitates the judgment policies used by experts. Two general approaches have been attempted for automated scoring of computer-based performance assessments (see Clauser [in press] for a discussion of the use of these methodologies in a variety of non-medical assessments). Both of these methods have been evaluated as part of the National Board of Medical Examiners' research on computer-based case simulations.

The first approach, which will be referred to as "rule-based" scoring, requires that experts articulate the policies that they use in rating performances. These decision rules are then reduced to logical arguments that can be represented as computer code. The process typically begins by assigning scores to general levels of performance. For example, a score of "1" may indicate that the examinee showed no evidence of understanding the problem presented by the patient; a score of "3" may require that the examinee took appropriate steps to arrive at the correct diagnosis; a score of "5" may require that the examinee ordered actions that would have led to the correct diagnosis and that the examinee provided at least minimally effective treatment; and so on. The next step requires that the experts articulate the specific actions required to achieve these general levels of performance. For example, the diagnosis may require that the examinee order one of three alternative imaging studies plus at least one of two alternative lab studies. Sequencing and timing factors may also come into play at this stage (e.g., to receive credit for a bacterial culture, it may be necessary to order it prior to the initiation of antibiotic; under some circumstances, higher scores may be achieved if the correct treatment is initiated sooner instead of later). The resulting code may be quite complex because it must account for all alternative patterns of action that may lead to the same level of performance. (The interested reader is referred to Clauser et al. (1997) and Clauser, Margolis, Clyman, and Ross (1997) for a more detailed description of this approach and specific examples of the code used for scoring.) Empirical evaluation of this approach has produced encouraging results. These rule-based scores have been shown to have moderate to high correlations to expert ratings of the same performances.

The second approach to computerized scoring also represents an effort to capture the policies used by experts in rating transaction lists. This approach uses a regression-based procedure to differentially weight varying types of actions ordered by examinees. With this approach, a key which specifies all actions considered potentially beneficial or indicated for management of the case is developed by a committee of experts. These actions are then categorized into levels of importance.

Actions which are not considered indicated for management of the case are similarly categorized into levels based on associated risk and degree of intrusiveness. A regression equation can then be developed for the case with expert ratings of examinee performance acting as the dependent measure and counts of actions ordered by the examinee in each of the beneficial and risky categories acting as the independent measures. Additional independent measures may be included which represent timing or other relevant features of the performance. In effect, the examinee's rating is being predicted based on these easily computed variables. These regressions are typically developed using large samples of examinees, with the dependent measure produced by averaging ratings from several experts. The regression weights are then used to weight actions ordered by future examinees to produce scores. As with the rule-based scores, the logic behind the algorithm can be complex because it is possible for the defined actions to include specification about timing and sequencing. As with the rule-based approach, evaluation of scores produced with this regression-based procedure has been encouraging.

Other potential scoring strategies remain to be examined. For example, one possible scoring methodology for patient management simulations has been applied to the scoring of computerized architectural problems. The idea is that the computer simulates the real life conditions and then evaluates the outcome. For example, the architect may be asked to develop a plan for grading the ground around a building. The computer can then simulate the conditions of a heavy rain and determine whether water would run off or inappropriately pool (Bejar, 1995). A similar approach is also used in evaluating pilots in flight simulators. When sufficiently complete models are available to describe human response to treatments, this sort of approach may be useful.

Validity issues

Much of the reported research on Primum has focused on scoring the simulation. Specific attention has been given to the relationship between scores produced by the system and expert ratings of the same performance. This focus is typical of research on computerized scoring procedures in other assessment contexts as well (Braun, Bennett, Frye, & Soloway, 1990; Bejar, 1995; Bennett & Sebrechts, 1996; Kaplan & Bennett, 1994; Page & Petersen, 1995; Sebrechts, Bennett, & Rock, 1991). When an automated scoring system is to be used to replace expert raters, it is reasonable that consistency between the two approaches would be a focus of attention. It should be emphasized that this is only one part of the overall validity question. Evaluators appear to have some awareness of the complexity of validating paper-and-pencil tests. Even when practice is inconsistent with principles, the importance of this validation process is acknowledged. By contrast, with computer simulations and with performance assessments in general there seems to be a view that the realism of the stimulus materials provides an end-run on the problem of validation. This is a naive view, limited in two important ways. First, the evaluation is a sample of examinee behavior and that sample is influenced by the specifics of the conditions of sampling. Variability across those conditions is inevitable and this variability impacts the stability of the resulting measurement. Issues related to this variability will be discussed in a subsequent section, but it is important to keep in mind that in general the more elaborately realistic the evaluation setting the greater the impact on precision of measurement. The second limitation is that, except in the most trivial situations, placing an examinee in a realistic setting does nothing to ensure valid measurement. A realistic setting may provide a context for measuring a variety of relevant proficiencies. It also provides a context for measuring a variety of irrelevant proficiencies. There is no insurance as to which will result. As noted previously, valid measurement will require careful definition of the proficiency of interest. The simulation should be constructed to elicit evidence about this proficiency and the scoring system should be constructed to quantify that evidence in a way that supports the intended inferences about examinees. In some cases it will be possible to base the construction of the simulation and the scoring system on empirical evidence about the proficiency of interest. More typically, both of these construction projects will be driven primarily by expert opinion, and it will be appropriate to collect evidence after the fact to support the validity argument. Evidence to show that the scores are related to other measures of the same proficiency provides a useful line of argument. If a simulation is designed to evaluate patient management, it would be expected that students early in their training will score less well than those at a more advanced level and that practicing physicians with demonstrable competence will score better yet. Scores on other tests of medical proficiency would also be expected to correlate with those from the simulation, even if the simulation is intended to measure aspects of proficiency not captured in other formats.

Several studies related to CCT illustrate these issues. Efforts were made to examine (1) the relationship between CCT scores and the level of medical training completed by the examinee, and (2) the relationship between CCT scores and performance on other tests of medical proficiency. Additionally, efforts were made to more directly gain understanding of the nature of the proficiency assessed by CCT and how that differed from the proficiency assessed by more traditional fixed-format questions. The relationship between the level of examinee training and test scores was examined by comparing performance on equated tests administered before and after a clerkship. The examinees showed large score increases after training. Although additional studies are needed, this result would seem to provide evidence that CCT measures some aspect of what was taught in the clerkship. Comparison of CCT scores with scores from other knowledge-based tests produced surprisingly low disattenuated correlations (between 0.15 and 0.30). Unfortunately, the data did not provide a basis for determining the extent to which these low correlations reflected differences in the content sampling as opposed to differences in the proficiency measured by these alternate formats.

Striking differences between CCT items and traditional knowledge-based test items were found by analyzing think-aloud protocols. These differences were consistent with expectations. It was found that decisions that are presented within an authentic and meaningful context require the examinee to read and process the case information and to relate this to the knowledge in his/her knowledge base to reach decisions. With test items that focus on superficial factual knowledge, less information processing may be required (Schuwirth, Verheggen, Van der Vleuten, Boshuizen, & Dinant, 2001).

Of course neither these findings nor the previously reported correlational results provide insight into the extent to which the proficiency assessed by CCT differs from that assessed by more sophisticated fixed format items. Well-trained item writers learn to produce items that require the application of knowledge rather than recall of isolated facts (Case & Swanson, 1998). In fact, the fixed format items currently used in medical licensure assessment in the United States are in concept strikingly similar to CCT cases (FSMB & NBME, 1998).

With simulations, there should also be concern that scores may reflect irrelevant sources of variance. In spite of the complexity of interpretation, this line of reasoning is important. With complex assessment formats it will be essential to consider both those arguments that support the relationship between test scores and the construct the test is intended to assess and those arguments which suggest different interpretations.

Studies relating test scores to the construct of interest have been given priority in this presentation because they are more likely to be ignored in practice, regardless of the assessment format. A second essential basis for arguments about the validity of inferences based on test scores is the content representation in the assessment. There are typically two aspects to this argument. The first will be based on the expertise of the content specialists who develop the test specifications. In some contexts, expert opinion will be the only criterion available, or practically possible, and expert opinion is only as good as the experts. The second aspect of the content argument will be based on empirical evidence.

Again to provide an example from CCT, an extensive survey of examinees and experts provided evidence that the content of the cases (and the associated questions) closely matches the challenges presented by practice. In general, experts judged the case presentations to be authentic and the decisions addressed in the questions to be realistic, although there was not complete agreement for all cases. (The specific characteristics of the cases in which no consensus could be reached are under study.) Consensus about the value of CCT was even higher in the examinee groups. Examinees agreed almost invariably that the tasks set by CCT were similar to those set to them in real practice. Clearly, results of this sort, which are based solely on opinion, are limited (Ericsson & Simon, 1993; Nisbett & Wilson, 1977). None the less, they provide encouraging initial evidence regarding the validity of inferences made based on CCT scores.

The most likely form of this empirical evidence supporting test content will be analysis of tasks and responsibilities of the practitioner. This may be collected through surveys or through direct observation. This does not imply that the content of a simulation-based assessment must directly match an empirically-based content model of practice. It may be that the assessment is designed to focus on some subset of the tasks within the purview of the practitioner. In this case, inferences drawn from scores must be similarly limited.

Precision of measurement

It is a truism of psychometric theory that the upper bound for validity is a function of reliability. Although more current views may argue against summarizing validity in terms of a simple correlation coefficient (Cronbach, 1971; Messick, 1989), it is incontestible that an assessment that is unstable across implementations cannot provide a basis for making generalizable inferences about examinees. It may be appealing to believe that an examinee called upon to perform relevant tasks in a highly realistic setting under the observation of competent experts is being validly evaluated. The problem is that the evaluation is a report on the examinee's performance on specific tasks, on a specific occasion, under the observation of specific experts applying a specific scoring procedure, and the interpretation of the score will almost always be intended to refer to a proficiency that generalizes across at least some of these conditions. When an assessment based on a simulation presents challenges in terms of separate patient-based cases, the interpretation of the score is usually intended to generalize across similar cases of which those on the assessment are considered a sample. When experts score a performance it is not typically the opinion of *those* experts that is of interest, but the opinion of experts overall. The specific individuals involved might again be seen as a sample from a pool of eligible experts. Additionally, although these experts score the performance on a single occasion, it is not their view on that occasion that is of interest. If their decisions vary across hours of the day or days of the week, randomly or systematically, this variability interferes with the potential to make valid inferences about examinee proficiency.

Each of these factors has the potential to introduce error into the scores produced by a simulation. The actual impact of these conditions of measurement will depend on the specifics of the test and on the intended interpretation of the scores. For example, for most performance assessments the variability of examinee response across tasks is substantial. When the set of tasks used on a test is considered a sample, this instability represents a significant source of error. As with other forms of performance assessment, this is a significant problem in assessment based on simulations. This result has been clearly observed in research on the National Board of Medical Examiners' computer simulations (Clauser, Swanson, & Clyman, 1996, 1999). It may be possible to reduce this variability by limiting the range of content represented in the simulation, but this strategy limits the usefulness of the resulting score. Alternatively, the impact of this source of variability can be reduced by increasing the number of cases included in the assessment. Unfortunately, this strategy is limited by the fact that simulations typically take a reasonably extended period to complete. This issue draws attention to an important consideration in constructing simulations. If simplifying the task presented in the simulation can shorten the time required without changing the essential challenge, the reduction in realism that results from simplification can lead to increased reliability and consequently improve validity.

In the context of CCT, the strategy of simplifying case presentation allows for administration of 60 cases in two hours, resulting in reliability estimates for a CCT examination of 0.65 to 0.70. These values are modestly higher than those that would be expected from a two hour examination based on more elaborate simulations but the values remain in the range typically reported for performance assessments. As such, they are likely to be considered an insufficient basis for high-stakes decisions. In the case of CCT, this limitation is ameliorated by the fact that the scores are not used in isolation. Additionally, because the current use of CCT is to make pass/fail classifications rather than focusing on increasing the precision of measurement across the entire score scale, it has been possible to improve the accuracy of decisions by using a sequential administration procedure. Examinees with estimated scores close to the cut-score are not classified based on the initial examination. Instead, these examinees are identified to receive additional cases.

If the simulations are scored by having experts review and rate the performance, another potentially important source of measurement error will come from rater error. Raters may introduce two types of error: errors associated with rater severity, which will tend to be stable across judgments about different tasks and different examinees, and errors related to the specifics of the rater-performance interaction. In the circumstance that some raters are more severe than others, the impact of the resulting measurement error can be limited by having different raters score different tasks. With this approach, each examinee will be judged by multiple raters and the effects of doves and hawks will tend to balance in the total score.

The second type of error may result from a variety of causes. Raters may view the requirements of different tasks differently. Similarly, raters may view specific characteristics of examinees differently. In addition to these systematic differences in rater behavior, error will also result due to rater mistakes. Raters may make clerical mistakes in recording their decisions or they may overlook an aspect of the examinee's performance that they would typically consider important, due to inattention. In general, reducing the impact of this second type of error will require increasing the number of ratings each examinee receives. Generalizability theory provides an appropriate means of evaluating the impact of these various sources of error. The generalizability theory perspective also provides a basis for designing rating procedures that efficiently control these sources of error. Several papers are available that provide a discussion of this application with performance assessments and the framework presented in those papers will be applicable in this context

(Brennan, 1996; Swanson, Clauser, & Case, 1999). Reports of applications specific to computer simulations are also available (Clauser, Clyman, & Swanson, 1999; Clauser, Harik, & Clyman, 2000; Clauser, Swanson, & Clyman, 1996, 1999).

The generalizability framework provides a means of assessing the magnitude of these sources of error and allows the evaluator to design a framework for efficiently using available resources, but there can be no question that the most appropriate starting point for controlling rater error is rater training. Practicing clinicians are expert in the content being assessed. This is a necessary but not sufficient condition for qualification as an expert rater.

It is appealing to believe that computerized scoring procedures for computer simulations eliminate the errors associated with using expert raters. Clearly, the computer algorithm will be implemented uniformly. Clerical errors and lapses in rater attention will be eliminated. But computerization of scoring may not eliminate sources of error resulting from differences in expert perspective. It is unreasonable to assume that two scoring algorithms developed independently for the same task by equally qualified groups of experts would be identical. In most practical circumstances the scoring algorithms will only be developed once for any given task, so it will be impossible to determine the extent to which differences in algorithms developed by different groups of experts will lead to different scores. Clauser et al. (2000) examined this issue and determined that this source of error could be easily controlled in practical implementations settings. It should be noted, however, that the different groups of experts in this study were randomly equivalent and were given careful and identical training. Without such training, it is possible that the resulting scores could vary substantially and systematically due to different views of the proficiency that the test should measure.

In the previous discussion of scoring complex simulations, three general approaches were described; use of expert raters, rule-based systems, regression-based systems. The art and science of scoring computer simulations is still in its infancy, so it is too early to draw final conclusions. Nonetheless, it is of interest to consider the relative reliability of scores produced with these differing approaches. Research from the National Board of Medical Examiners' computer simulation project has compared the generalizability of tests scored with these three methods (Clauser, Clyman, & Swanson, 1999; Clauser, Swanson, & Clyman, 1996, 1999). These initial results indicate that in operational settings the regression-based scoring approaches may be as generalizable as scores produced by expert raters. Specifically, the results showed the regression-based scores to be of equivalent generalizability to scores produced by having two experts rate each performance. It is unlikely that in a large-scale operational setting it would be practical to have each performance rated by more than two experts. By contrast, the rule-based scoring system was less generalizable than either of the other two systems. As part of the process for developing and validating computerized scoring systems for other simulation systems, it will be necessary to repeat these types of studies. There is an important practical consideration in evaluating the results of this type of study; that is the extent to which the high-quality rating which can be produced in small-scale research projects can be maintained in more large-scale operational settings. It may be that the need to recruit less able or less interested experts, or the fatigue that will result from asking experts to increase their rating workload, will make preliminary studies mis-representative of operational outcomes.

Another issue to be considered when comparing the generalizability of alternative scoring systems is the extent to which the procedures are evaluating the same dimension or proficiency. In classical test theory terms, the question is, do the true-scores for the different procedures have a perfect correlation? If the true-score correlation between scores produced by the computerized scoring procedure and those produced from expert ratings is not very close to 1.0, the implication is that the evaluated proficiencies are not identical. In this circumstance, if the generalizability of the computer-generated scores is equal to, or superior to, that of the ratings, there must be some source of scoring-method-specific variance that is captured by the computerized method. For example, it may be possible that a computerized scoring system is sensitive to some aspects of examinee test-taking behavior which are common across tasks. Scoring-method-specific variance is clearly a threat to validity. Two of the cited papers report true-score correlations between ratings and computer generated scores (Clauser, Harik, & Clyman, 2000; Clauser, Swanson, & Clyman, 1999). In general, these results show correlations of approximately 1.0, suggesting that scoring-method-specific variance is not present in these cases. These studies also provided a detailed description of the methods used to estimate the correlations, in the respective appendices.

TECHNOLOGIES FOR THE FUTURE

With the continuing movement toward the use of computers for test delivery and the current interest in expanding assessment beyond fixed-format items, it is likely that interest in computer simulations will continue to grow. The widespread availability of increasingly powerful computer hardware and more and more sophisticated software makes it inevitable that evaluators will be able to make future simulations increasingly complex. The addition of audio and video components and interfaces that allow for more lifelike interaction with the patient and other members of the healthcare team will greatly increase the realism of the simulation.

While it may be inevitable that computer capabilities will increase, it is not inevitable that this will lead to more valid testing. Increasing the sophistication of the testing interface will inevitably increase the complexity of the scoring model required to transform an examinee response into an interpretable score. Each level of increase in complexity of the simulation and scoring models will lead to an exponential increase in the complexity of the validation studies which will be needed to fully understand the implications of the resulting scores. Allowing the availability of computer sophistication to drive assessment practice may lead to face validity for assessments but not to valid inferences about important examinee proficiencies.

The next generation of simulations should be developed based on careful study of the results from this generation. Two questions should guide the creation of the next generation. Firstly, how do current simulation interfaces interfere with an examinee's ability to demonstrate proficiency? And secondly, what proficiencies are we failing to assess with the current formats? The answer to these questions may on occasion be the same as the answer to the question: what does computer technology allow us to do that we could not do before? But there is no reason to assume that this will be the case. The driving force in assessment should be based on what we need to assess and not on what we can assess.

It is axiomatic that in predicting the impact of technological advances short-term progress will be over-estimated and what will be accomplished in the long-term will be under-estimated. Nonetheless, it seems that there is reason to be optimistic about both the short- and long-term future of computerized assessment. As was mentioned at the beginning of this chapter, researchers have been examining the potential of computerized testing for decades, but the last few years have provided something which was previously absent, large-scale experience in computerized testing. This experience has provided a basis for refocusing research on practical problems. This has led to a number of the innovations referred to in this chapter including CAST, a-stratification-based item selection for CAT, and shadow test construction to meet content constraints. If the last few years are any indication, this area will remain one of considerable productivity and continued technical advances leading to practical improvement in assessment practice should be expected.

It is also reasonable to expect considerable short-term improvement in computer-based assessment involving simulations and other more complex item formats. Recent innovations have included significant enhancements in the assessment interface and improvements in scoring (Clyman, Melnick, & Clauser, 1999; Clauser, Margolis, Clyman, & Ross, 1997). With the move to operational use of computer simulations as part of the United States Medical Licensure Examination, results from large-scale high-stakes testing will be available to motivate a new cycle of research and development. Hopefully large-scale testing experience will lead to rapid improvement in the current generation of simulations. In addition to this short-term improvement in computerized simulations, there are two technologies that are under development for application in other contexts that will have obvious potential in medical assessment; virtual reality and natural language processing. Technology to create virtual reality provides visual, auditory and tactile stimuli to simulate the experience of an actual environment. Current forms may be somewhat simplistic, creating something that may appear more like a cartoon world than a real one, but rapid advances are being made. The second of these technologies, natural language processing, is an effort to allow computers to interpret human speech or written language. As these technologies become fully developed, the potential will exist to create a fully interactive simulated patient. Unlike the human standardized patients currently used in medical education and evaluation, with these computer simulated virtual patients it will be possible to simulate an unlimited range of pathological conditions and to allow the physician to implement intrusive evaluations and treatments.

It is difficult for anyone familiar with computer simulations to fail to give at least a passing thought to the potential of virtual reality technologies; the possibility of placing the physician in the operating room or the emergency room, complete with realistic visual, auditory, and tactile stimuli seems obvious. In fact, it seems not only obvious, but inevitable. Without belaboring the point, some caution is warranted. Realism and complexity should be a means (to better assessment) and not an end. This aside, there are at least two good reasons to develop these technologies for assessment. The first is that, as these technologies become more advanced, they may allow the simulation to appear more seamless to the examinee. To the extent that the task presented to the examinee appears more natural, testing artifacts may be reduced.

The second reason for developing these technologies appears far more important. As medicine advances, more and more of what the physician actually does will involve computerized systems. Surgery may increasingly be performed using lasers and other computer-guided tools so that the physician will observe a computer monitor rather than looking directly at the patient. As these changes in medical practice take place, the simulation interface will cease to be an approximation of medical practice. Interacting with the computer interface will actually be an important part of medical practice (Satava & Jones, 1999).

As with virtual reality technologies, natural language processing capabilities are no longer a dream but are still far from being fully developed. Computer programs for recognizing spoken language and for creating spoken language are in common use. The complexity arises from the difficulty of training the computer to "understand" the natural language statements. Even for the relatively simple situation in which the examinee collects medical history information by questioning the simulated patient, the number of different ways that an examinee could ask the same question is almost without limit. And as the complexity of the task increases, the complexity of the language also increases. Consider for example the nuances involved in evaluating patient education or counseling. This complexity is part of the reason that, despite thirty years of research, computerized scoring of essays is still a limited application (Burstein, Kukich, Wolff, & Lu, 1998). Computers are capable of assessing writing skills, but only a relatively simplistic evaluation of content is possible with current programs.

Nonetheless, there is reason for optimism. Both virtual reality and natural language processing technologies have commercial applications well beyond educational assessment, so it is likely that research and development outside of the field of medical education will create innovations far beyond any that could be produced with the resources of a medical school or testing organization. These two technologies are additionally attractive because together they offer the potential to enhance the assessment of both the technical and interpersonal aspects of clinical skill. Although technology is only one part of the work needed to produce assessment, and considerable effort will be required to demonstrate the validity of the resulting scores, these technologies do offer exciting possibilities.

REFERENCES

Bejar I. I. (1995). From adaptive testing to automated scoring of architectural simulations. In E. L. Mancall & P. G. Bashook (Eds.), *Assessing clinical reasoning: The oral examination and alternative methods* (pp. 115-130). Evanston, IL: American Board of Medical Specialities

Bennett, R. E., & Sebrechts, M. M. (1996). The accuracy of expert-system diagnoses of mathematical problem solutions. *Applied Measurement in Education, 9*, 133-150.

Berner, E. S., Hamilton, L. A., & Best, W. R. (1974). A new approach to evaluating problem-solving in medical students. *Journal of Medical Education, 49*, 666-672.

Bordage, G. (1987). An alternative approach to PMP's: the "key-features" concept. In I. R. Hart & R. Harden (Eds.), *Further developments in assessing clinical competence, Proceedings of the second Ottawa conference* (pp. 59-75). Montreal: Can-Heal Publications.

Braun, H. I., Bennett, R. E., Frye, D., & Soloway, E. (1990). Scoring constructed responses using expert systems. *Journal of Educational Measurement, 27*, 93-108.

Brennan, R. L. (1996). Generalizability of performance assessments In G. W. Phillips (Ed.), *Technical issues in large-scale performance assessments.* Washington, DC: National Center for Educational Statistics.

Burstein, J., Kukich, K., Wolff, S., & Lu, C. (1998, April). Computer analysis of essay content for automated score prediction. Paper presented at the meeting of the National Council on Measurement in Education, San Diego.

Case, S. M., & Swanson, D. B. (1998). *Constructing written test questions for the basic and clinical sciences.* Philadelphia, PA: National

Chang, H., & Ying, Z. (1998). A-stratified multistage computerized testing. *Applied Psychological Measurement.*

Clauser, B. E. (in press). Recurrent issues and recent advances in scoring performance assessments. *Applied Psychological Measurement.*

Clauser, B. E., Clyman, S. G., & Swanson, D. B. (1999). Components of rater error in a complex performance assessment. *Journal of Educational Measurement, 36*, 29-45.

Clauser, B. E., Harik, P., & Clyman, S. G. (2000). The generalizability of scores for a performance assessment scored with a computer-automated scoring system. Paper presented at the meeting of the National Council on Measurement in Education, New Orleans.

Clauser, B. E., Margolis, M. J., Clyman, S. G., & Ross, L. P. (1997). Development of automated scoring algorithms for complex performance assessments: A comparison of two approaches. *Journal of Educational Measurement, 34*, 141-161.

Clauser, B. E., Ross, L. P., Clyman, S. G., Rose, K. M., Margolis, M. J., Nungester, R. J., Piemme, T. E., Pinceti, P. S., Chang, L., El-Bayoumi, G., & Malakoff, G. L. (1997). Developing a scoring algorithm to replace expert rating for scoring a complex performance based assessment. *Applied Measurement in Education, 10*, 345-358.

Clauser, B. E., Swanson, D. B., & Clyman, S. G. (1996). The generalizability of scores from a performance assessment of physicians▯ patient management skills *Academic Medicine, 71*(RIME Supplement), S109-S111.

Clauser, B. E., Swanson, D. B., & Clyman, S. G. (1999). A comparison of the generalizability of scores produced by expert raters and automated scoring systems. *Applied Measurement in Education, 12*, 281-299.

Clyman, S. G., Melnick, D. E., & Clauser, B. E. (1999). Computer-based case simulations from medicine: Assessing skills in patient management. In A. Tekian, C. H. McGuire, & W. C. McGahie (Eds.), *Innovative simulations for assessing professional competence* (pp. 29-41). Chicago: University of Illinois, Department of Medical Education.

Cronbach, L. J. (1971). Test validation. In R. L. Thorndike (Ed.), *Educational Measurement*, (2nd ed., pp. 443-507). Washington, DC: American Council on Education.

Elstein, A. S., Shulmann, L. S., & Sprafka, S. A. (1978). *Medical problem-solving: An analysis of clinical reasoning.* Cambridge, MA: Harvard University Press.

Ericsson, K. A., & Simon, H. A. (1993). *Protocol analysis.* Cambridge, MA: Massachusetts Institute of Technology.

Federation of State Medical Boards of the U.S., Inc. (FSMB) and National Board of Medical Examiners (NBME) (1998). *Step 3 general instructions, content description, and sample items.* Philadelphia: FSMB and NBME.

Hambleton, R. K., & Swaminathan, H. (1985). *Item response theory: Principles and applications.* Boston: Kluwer.

Hambleton, R. K., Swaminathan, H., & Rogers, H. J. (1991). *Fundamentals of item response theory.* Newbury Park, CA: Sage.

Hubbard, J. P., & Levit, E. J. (1985). *The national board of medical examiners: The first seventy years.* Philadelphia: National Board of Medical Examiners.

Kaplan, R. M., & Bennett, R. E. (1994). *Using a free-response scoring tool to automatically score the formulating-hypotheses item* (RR 94-08). Princeton, NJ: Educational Testing Service.

Kingsbury, G. G., & Weiss, D. J. (1983). A comparison of IRT-based adaptive mastery testing and sequential mastery testing procedure. In D. J. Weiss (Ed.), *New horizons in testing: Latent trait test theory and computerized adaptive testing* (pp. 257-283). New York: Academic Press.

Luecht, R. M., & Nungester, R. J. (1998). Some practical examples of computer-adaptive sequential testing. *Journal of Educational Measurement, 35,* 229-249.

McCarthy, W. H. (1966). An assessment of the influence of cueing items in objective examinations. *Journal of Medical Education, 41,* 263-266.

Messick, S. (1989). Validity. In R. L. Linn (Ed.), *Educational measurement* (3rd ed., pp. 13-103). New York: American Council on Education.

Nisbett, R. E., & Wilson, T. D. (1977). Telling more than we can know: verbal reports on mental processes. *Psychological Review, 84*(3), 231-259.

Page, E. B., & Petersen, N. S. (1995). The computer moves into essay grading. *Phi Delta Kappan, 76,* 561-565.

Satava, R. M., & Jones, S. B. (1999). The future is now: Virtual reality technologies. In A. Tekian, C. H. McGuire, & W. C. McGahie (Eds.), *Innovative simulations for assessing professional competence* (pp. 29-41). Chicago: University of Illinois, Department of Medical Education.

Schmidt, H. G., Boshuizen, H. P. A., & Hobus, P. P. M. (1988). Transitory stages in the development of medical expertise: The "intermediate effect" in clinical case representation studies. *Proceedings of the 10th Annual Conference of the Cognitive Science Society* (pp. 139-145). Montreal, Canada: Lawrence Erlbaum Associates.

Schuwirth, L. W. T. (1998). *An approach to the assessment of medical problem solving: Computerised case-based testing.* Universiteit Maastricht, Maastricht.

Schuwirth, L. W. T., Blackmore, D. B., Mom, E., Van de Wildenberg, F., Stoffers, H., & Van der Vleuten, C. P. M. (1999). How to write short cases for assessing problem-solving skills. *Medical Teacher, 21*(2), 144-150.

Schuwirth, L. W. T., Van der Vleuten, C. P. M., De Kock, C. A., Peperkamp, A. G. W., & Donkers, H. H. L. M. (1996). Computerized case-based testing: a modern method to assess clinical decision making. *Medical Teacher, 18*(4), 295-300.

Schuwirth, L. W. T., Van der Vleuten, C. P. M., & Donkers, H. H. L. M. (1995). Computerized long-menu questions, an acceptable un-cue-version. In A. I. Rothman & R. Cohen (Eds.), *The sixth Ottawa Conference on Medical Education* (pp. 178-181). Toronto: University of Toronto Bookstore Custom Publishing.

Schuwirth, L. W. T., Van der Vleuten, C. P. M., Stoffers, H. E. J. H., & Peperkamp, A. G. W. (1996). Computerized long-menu questions as an alternative to open-ended questions in computerized assessment. *Medical Education, 30,* 50-55.

Schuwirth, L. W. T., Verheggen, M. M., Van der Vleuten, C. P. M., Boshuizen, H. P. A., & Dinant, G. J. (2001). Do short cases elicit different thinking processes than factual knowledge questions do? *Medical Education, 35,* 348-356.

Sebrechts, M. M., Bennett, R. E., & Rock, D. A. (1991). Agreement between expert-system and human raters on complex constructed-response quantitative items. *Journal of Applied Psychology, 76,* 856-862.

Spray, J. A., & Reckase, M. D. (1996). Comparison of SPRT and sequential Bayes procedures for classifying examinees into two categories using a computerized test. *Journal of Educational and Behavioral Statistics, 21*, 405-414.

Swanson, D. B. (1987). A measurement framework for performance-based tests. In I. Hart & R. Harden (Eds.), *Further developments in assessing clinical competence* (pp. 13 – 45). Montreal: Can-Heal Publications.

Swanson, D. B., Norcini, J. J., & Grosso, L. J. (1987). Assessment of clinical competence: written and computer-based simulations. *Assessment and Evaluation in Higher Education, 12*(3), 220-246.

Swanson, D. B., Clauser, B. E., & Case, S. M. (1999). Clinical skills assessment with standardized patients in high-stakes tests: A framework for thinking about score precision, equating, and security. *Advances in Health Science Education, 4*, 67-106.

Van der Linden, W. J. (in press). Constrained adaptive testing with shadow tests. In W. J. Van der Linden & C. A. W. Glas (Eds.), *Computerized adaptive testing: theory and practice*. Boston: Kluwer.

Wainer, H., Dorans, N. J., Flaugher, R., Green, B. F., Mislevy, R. J., Steinberg, L., & Thissen, D. (1990). *Computerized adaptive testing: A primer*. Hillsdale, NJ: Lawrence Erlbaum Associates.

Wald, A. (1947). *Sequential analysis*. New York: Wiley.

APPENDIX

This appendix presents the three common item response theory models. In the following equations:

$P_i(\theta)$ is the probability that a randomly selected examinee with ability θ will answer item i correctly.

b_i is the difficulty parameter for item i.

a_i is the discrimination parameter for item i.

c_i is the pseudo-guessing parameter for item i. That is, the probability of a correct response on item i for an examinee with extremely low ability.

D is a scaling value of 1.7. This scaling value brings the logistic model into close equivalence with the cumulative normal distribution represented by the normal ogive.

The one-parameter logistic model:

$$P_i(\theta) = \frac{e^{(\theta - b_i)}}{1 + e^{(\theta - b_i)}}$$

The two-parameter logistic model:

$$P_i(\theta) = \frac{e^{Da_i(\theta - b_i)}}{1 + e^{Da_i(\theta - b_i)}}$$

The three-parameter logistic model:

$$P_i(\theta) = c_i + (1 - c_i)\frac{e^{Da_i(\theta - b_i)}}{1 + e^{Da_i(\theta - b_i)}}$$

24 Assessment of Clinical Performance: In-Training Evaluation

JEFF TURNBULL
University of Ottawa

CHRISTINA VAN BARNEVELD
University of Toronto

SUMMARY

Of those evaluation methods currently available for the assessment of clinical competence, in-training evaluation comes closest to measuring true performance. Unfortunately, current methods are neither reliable nor valid, leaving evaluative decisions made on this basis indefensible. The objectives of this chapter are to characterize existing methods of in-training evaluation, and discuss what we know from the literature pertaining to their strengths and weaknesses. Drawing upon evidence from the cognitive and psychometric sciences, new models and methods of in-training evaluation are proposed. The chapter will conclude with a future agenda for research in this domain.

INTRODUCTION

Performance-based evaluation methods are used to assess selected clinical competencies (e.g. patient history and physical examination, communication skills, interpersonal skills) in the medical training context. Performance-based evaluations allow medical trainees to "show" how they perform in a structured context (Miller, 1990). The implication is that the skill or ability that is demonstrated in this setting will be subsequently demonstrated in actual clinical practice.

In general, evaluation methods are "biopsies" of knowledge, skills or attitudes that are believed to describe a defined trait that predicts some future performance. In order to be meaningful, evaluation methods must reflect the objectives that they have been developed to measure. An evaluation tool that measures *"the degree to which the individual can use the knowledge, skills, and judgement associated with a profession to perform effectively in the domain of possible encounter defining the*

International Handbook of Research in Medical Education, 793–810.
G.R. Norman, C.P.M. Van der Vleuten, D.I. Newble (eds.)
© 2002 *Dordrecht: Kluwer Academic Publishers. Printed in Great Britain.*

scope of professional practice" (clinical competency defined by Kane, 1992, p. 166) may vary in appropriateness depending upon the target competency. In this context, appropriateness of the evaluation method depends on the degree to which the tool measures the desired objective (validity), the consistency or reproducibility of scores (reliability) and the ease-of-use of that method in one's own environment (feasibility).

There are a number of clinical evaluation methods that involve learners "showing" their clinical competence in a structured circumstance. Among these are triple-jump examinations; clinical oral examinations; assessments based on standardized patients, such as the objective structured clinical examination; portfolios and logs, and in-training evaluation reports. The in-training evaluation report (sometimes referred to as the clinical evaluation form) attempts to document student or resident performance while in the practice of patient care in a structured environment.

DEFINING IN-TRAINING EVALUATION

We define the ongoing observation, assessment and documentation through the in-training evaluation report of clinical performance in a practice setting as in-training evaluation.

In-training evaluation reports are a performance assessment strategy employed by undergraduate and graduate medical schools to evaluate student progress during training. An in-training evaluation report is a rating form (which may be paper and pencil format, completed electronically via computer or through an interactive voice response system) used by observers to formally document the learner's performance. Typically, the supervising physician observes student performance in a particular department or discipline, one or more times during the training period. Sometimes, other sources of evaluative information are solicited from nurses, other allied health professionals, patients, peers and even the trainee (e.g., Tamblyn et al., 1994; Ramsey et al., 1993; Henkin et al., 1990). While institutions may vary in some of the details (like the number of observers), the purpose of in-training evaluation reports is to provide a summative evaluation of student performance during patient care, and be a source of information for decisions regarding promotion. In-training evaluation reports may also serve a formative function, as a source of feedback to students during the training period.

While other methods of assessment during a clinical rotation have varying degrees of objectivity, they do not measure performance in the setting of day-to-day practice (McManus et al., 1998).

THE SCOPE AND PURPOSE OF IN-TRAINING EVALUATION WITHIN THE CONTEXT OF PERFORMANCE ASSESSMENT

It is accepted wisdom that the farther away medical trainees get from demonstrating abilities in a clinical setting the more difficult it will be to predict whether their test performance truly reflects ability in subsequent clinical practice. While this wisdom has been challenged, it is agreed that the ongoing assessment of clinical competency by supervisors in a practice circumstance is the best method to measure many essential competencies, and is an invaluable evaluation tool. However, it is not the only method that is utilized to assess the knowledge, skills and attitudes comprising clinical competency. It is, however, important to define what these competencies are, to outline the scope and purpose of in-training evaluation.

Historically, one's perception of a good doctor was that of a knowledgeable and technically competent individual. Evaluation strategies were developed to reflect these concepts. Clinical abilities were usually evaluated using an end of rotation performance checklist. Generally, a rotation supervisor, usually remote from the activities of the learner, completed this (if at all) weeks after the end of a rotation. This form of assessment has focused primarily on knowledge and interpersonal abilities and has been subject to ongoing critical scrutiny. Several important initiatives have caused medical teachers to refocus on the specific goals of medical education and how these should be reflected in general and specific objectives, with corresponding evaluation strategies.

As a result of internal and external pressures, the definition of required clinical performance has expanded. Initiatives have forced us to consider additional competencies such as professionalism, communication skills, managerial and advocacy skills, collaboration skills as well as ethical ability, scholarship, compassion, and a population perspective (e.g., Neufeld, 1993; Societal Needs Working Group for the CanMEDS 2000 Project, 1996; Hastings Center Report, 1996; Neufeld et al., 1998; Medical Schools Objective Writing Group, 1999; Maudsley, 1999; Pangaro, 1999).

In addition to these new competencies, the way we think of clinical ability has been redefined. Pangaro (1999) has identified a hierarchy of clinical behaviors that reflect a progressive mastery of the practice of medicine. He has identified a series of roles: reporter (accurately gathering and clearly communicating clinical facts); interpreter (prioritizing among problems identified, offering differential diagnoses and interpreting data); manager (developing management plans tailored to the patient's circumstances and preferences); and educator (going beyond the basics to question and understand and then share knowledge while critically evaluating outcomes).

As well as evaluation methods that truly measure the essential aspects of medical expertise, methods must be developed and implemented that reliably measure these new competencies (Fowell et al., 1999). Our traditional standardized measures of multiple-choice questions, and even objective structured clinical examinations, are unlikely to be able to evaluate some of these complex competencies. In-training evaluation, the ongoing observation, assessment and documentation of performance in the care of patients, if done successfully, has the potential to measure such important domains (not easily measured in other settings) as those listed in Table 1. While this list is by no means complete, the comprehensive evaluation of student or resident performance in the clinical setting must include in-training evaluation, while also supplemented by other more objective measures of competency where indicated. For example, the multiple-choice question is a reliable measure of learner knowledge and the OSCE provides a greater opportunity for the standard assessment of technical skills, yet can either adequately measure professionalism?

Table 1. Competencies best evaluated through in-training evaluation

General Competency	Specific Competency
1. History and physical examination skills	
2. Medical communication skills	- with patients - with colleagues - verbal and written
3. Diagnostic reasoning skills	- problem solving and diagnosis
4. Management skills	- decision-making - cost effective investigation and care - technical skills - preventative skills including counseling
5. Critical appraisal skills (e.b.m.)	- self-assessment - information literacy - critical appraisal
6. Management skills	- practice management - time management - patient care management
7. Continued learning skills	
8. Teaching skills	
9. Advocacy skills	
10. Professional behaviors/attitudes	- "ethics" and "professionalism" to self, patients, colleagues - interpersonal skills
11. Knowledge as it pertains to problem solving	

While the primary purpose of assessment is to provide some overall level of accountability related to the ability of a candidate to practice medicine within a community, there are other important purposes, such as providing meaningful feedback, motivating learning and teaching and assisting in the selection process. Systems developed for the assessment of clinical ability must also reflect these important roles of assessment. In-training evaluation provides the opportunity for ongoing feedback and it highlights what is truly important in the eyes of the student and faculty member.

Ongoing performance assessment has also been suggested as a method of ensuring continued performance competency for practicing physicians as part of the process of continued licensure. As such, the application of the principles of in-training evaluation is not confined to the assessment of students and residents only, but applies to the continuum of practice.

Only recently has attention been paid to the relative merits of the different evaluation strategies as a result of requirements for internal and external accountability (especially those used to make high-stakes decisions). As such, our understanding of the best approach to in-training evaluation must be informed by the existing literature.

LESSONS LEARNED FROM THE LITERATURE

The ongoing assessment of clinical practice performance is done principally through in-training evaluation, and documented through the in-training evaluation report. This section focuses on a summary and analysis of the measurement issues related to in-training evaluation, and identifies the lessons learned from work done to date. We include research on other methods that use raters in the assessment of clinical competency; however, the principal focus of this review is the assessment of ongoing practice performance through in-training evaluation. We believe that this area is where the greatest potential for improvement in the assessment of clinical competence lies.

Reviews of literature on methods used to assess the clinical competence of medical trainees have been completed elsewhere. For example, Neufeld and Norman (1985) describe methods to assess clinical competence and their psychometric properties. Among the methods discussed are direct observation, oral and written examinations, global rating scales, medical record review, patient management problems, computer simulations and methods involving simulated patients. Gray (1996a) provides a primer for resident evaluation describing the strengths and weaknesses of in-training evaluation reports and other methods of evaluating residents. Gray (1996b) has also completed an extensive review of the literature on the roles, strengths and weaknesses of rating scales as evaluation tools. More recently, Holmboe and Hawkins (1998) reviewed the literature from 1966 to 1998 on methods for evaluating the clinical competence of residents, including in-training examinations, medical record audits, clinical evaluation exercises and assessment methods that use SPs. The triple-jump examination and other multi-trait, multi-method approaches have also been described elsewhere (Smith, 1993; Hull et al., 1995). Also, qualitative methods are being explored to enrich and explain interpretations based on in-training evaluations (e.g., Van der Vleuten, 2000). We refer you to these excellent sources for a complete description of the methods to assess clinical competency in medical education.

Reliability

If two "similar" assessment tools were administered to a group of students, it would be unlikely that each person would receive *exactly* the same score on both instruments. Similarly, if two raters observed the same student performance, they may not assign *exactly* the same grade. Each score assigned to a student is subject to errors of measurement (i.e., factors other than clinical competence that influence the student's score). These errors may be random, from a purely chance happening (e.g., disruption in the assessment situation, administration or scoring errors, fluctuations in the individual examinee's state during testing), or they may be systematic errors, consistently affecting an individual's score (e.g., a "hawk" or "dove" rater or the influence of dyslexia on an assessment that involves reading). Both random and systematic errors influence the interpretation of assessment scores. Thus, the extent to which we minimize error variance or "signal noise" while maximizing true variance is an important aspect of any measurement tool. It is desirable to have a consistent (or reproducible) measure of medical trainee clinical performance – i.e., one that reliably differentiates between student performances. Reliability is the ability to detect differences in performance.

The reliability of clinical assessment methods has been investigated in a variety of contexts. Potential sources of measurement error are identified in the literature and include rater stringency or leniency, student characteristics, rater/student interaction, the measurement tool/task, the occasion of observation and the timeliness of the evaluation (i.e., time between observation and documentation). These sources of measurement error are summarized below.

Rater

A predominant criticism of current methods of assessing clinical competency, especially in-training evaluation, is that raters do not consistently distinguish between different levels of student performance. This occurs between raters or for the same rater over different occasions, with reliability coefficients approaching zero (Van der Vleuten & Norman, 1991; Stillman, 1991; McGuire, 1993; Gray, 1996b). Littlefield et al. (1991) found that 27% of raters were lenient or stringent in assigning in-training evaluation scores, when compared to their colleagues, reflecting a large variability in the standards and expectations held for third-year medical students. They attributed these results to raters giving inaccurate ratings, rather than to unique observations that eluded all other raters who evaluated the same student. They also suggest that these rater differences may reflect individual differences in information processing when making the ratings. Fisher et al. (1997) looked at removing the rater effects from medical clerkship evaluations (ITER). They found that raters do not agree in their student ratings, but are consistent in the ordering of the students and so the amount of rater-dependent variability can be estimated and removed from the measures using Rasch calibration. A pilot is currently underway to assess a clerkship evaluation system that is free of rater-dependent variability.

Other work (Speer et al., 1996) suggests that in-training evaluation reliability was acceptable (0.90 with three raters rating all students) when student competency was defined in specific observable behaviors, and when assigning a numeric score was done through an objective group review. McCrae et al. (1995) studied physician ratings as measures of observed student history and physical examination skills, and found that generalizability was 0.85 (pooled across four cases, when three raters rated each case). This was notably higher than the reliability of checklist scores (generalizability of 0.34 across two cases) or database scores (0.59 across four cases).

Some studies have included other sources of evaluative information (i.e., nurses, patients and peers) into the in-training evaluation measurement strategy. Butterfield and Mazzaferri (1991) assessed the reliability of nurse-rater evaluation of the humanistic behaviors of students, obtaining a generalizability (a reliability-like coefficient) greater than 0.90 64% of the time when 10 nurses provided ratings. For patient-raters, 12.2 resident satisfaction ratings were required to obtain a reliability of 0.56 (Tamblyn et al., 1994). Work done by Henkin et al. (1990) reported that patients appeared to be poor discriminators in the evaluation of medical students. For peer-raters, 11 peer ratings per content area were required to obtain a generalizability of 0.70 (Ramsey et al., 1993, 1996). Many of these studies conclude that the number of ratings required to obtain a reliable estimate of student performance may limit the feasibility of using nurse-, peer- or patient-raters to evaluate clinical competence of students and are well above our current norm.

Finally, concerns have been raised pertaining to the ability of raters to discriminate between different content domains when evaluating in-training performance. Reports of high item-total correlations raise concerns that evaluators do not discriminate between the items on an evaluation form. While high internal consistency is desirable when assessing a unidimensional trait, it is less desirable when assessing complex tasks where a multidimensional model may be more appropriate. We will revisit this issue in the next section in a discussion on results on factor analytic work for in-training evaluation.

Student

There are a number of student characteristics that are not a component of the competency being assessed (e.g., first language, tiredness and extroversion) that influence student performance while caring for patients. Work done by Thomas (1993) suggests that variability due to the extroversion of the examinee or other examinee characteristics may influence the results of a clinical oral examination. Unfortunately, it is difficult to isolate all possible factors affecting student performance at a given moment, but it is important to note that they exist and may contribute to errors of measurement of clinical competency.

Rater/student interaction

While not thoroughly researched, the dissonance between faculty roles of "teacher" and 'evaluator' has been mentioned as a potential source of error when attending physicians evaluate their student team members (Turnbull et al., 1998). Ramsey (1993) found moderate correlations (0.08 to 0.03) between the number of patient-related contacts, the number of patients referred between the physician being evaluated and the peer-evaluator, and the peer-ratings that the rater provided. Work done by Eldin (1998) suggests that face-to-face evaluation contexts may yield higher scores than when the rater is not in contact with the student.

Measurement tool/task

Items, administration and scoring of clinical competency assessment measures are potential sources of measurement error. For example, some items on OSCE stations may be more difficult to perform or rate than others (Norcini & Shea, 1992). Foldevi and Svendin (1996) attributed low correlation between three assessments of consultation skills to inter-case (and inter-rater) variability. Concerns of content specificity, i.e., the extent to which the observer can generalize from the observed student's clinical competence to overall competence, may be placed under this heading as well. While usually described as a validity issue, content specificity relates to the reliability of an instrument as well. If performance on one task, problem or case does not necessarily predict performance on other tasks, problems or cases (Schmidt et al., 1990), then our ability to generalize from one performance to overall competence is deflated, because we may be measuring different constructs between occasions.

Occasion

Errors associated with the occasion of observation may be a potential source of measurement error. For example, the performance of a student at the end of the call, rotation or school year may vary from performance at the beginning of these occasions. Factors that relate to learning and experience in patient care, the context of the assessment and other factors may influence the observed clinical competence score. If direct observation of student performance is infrequent, the variability due to occasion may have a large influence on the student's scores.

Time

In some cases, faculty administration officers have reported receiving evaluation forms from faculty up to 2-3 months after the training period (Hunt, 1992). Clearly, this has an impact on the evaluations provided for the student, as evaluators must rely on memory to assess student performance. Research done in cognitive psychology on the accuracy of recall suggests that we may not depend on memory to reliably evaluate student performance (Regher, 1996). When evaluations take place a long time after the event, supervisors tend to "average" their responses and therefore miss the opportunity to document important individual variances. Documentation of the student behavior must take place as close to the time of behavior as possible (preferably immediately).

Other issues that influence the reliability of student in-training evaluation scores are group homogeneity, time limits and number of observations of student performance (Crocker & Algina, 1986). Since reliability depends on variation among individuals on both their true scores and error scores, homogeneity of the group is an important factor. A test may reliably measure competency in a diverse group of students, but the same test may not be as reliable in assessing competency in a more homogeneous group. When in-training evaluation methods are administered to highly competent trainees (as is usually the case in medical training), the differences between student competency levels are small, and this is reflected in a low reliability for the instrument. Note that reliability is a property of the scores on the in-training evaluation *for a particular group of examinees.*

For timed clinical competency assessment methods, the variance in the rates at which the examinees work becomes confounded with their true competence (assuming speed is not a construct being measured). In this case, differences among students are a reflection of both their competency levels and the rates at which they work. This may lead to artificially inflated reliability coefficients, especially when split-half or internal consistency approaches are used to determine reliability.

The number of observations of student performance relates to the reliability coefficient, with multiple observations yielding higher reliability coefficients. This makes intuitive sense, since multiple observations allow the rater to rate a student's competence several times, leading to a more consistent estimate of that student's clinical competence.

Validity

In order to justify interpretations of student clinical competence based on assessment scores, the assessment method must be reliable and valid. A high reliability is necessary but insufficient evidence that the interpretations about a student's clinical competence based on his or her assessment score are accurate. Indeed, a clinical assessment method may consistently measure the wrong thing. While reliability is a measure of the tool itself, validity is a measure of the soundness of inferences based on the results of the test itself (see Messick, 1995 for other conceptions of validity, e.g. consequential validity). Validation of any assessment method is the process by which evidence is collected to support the types of inferences that are to be drawn from the resulting score (Cronbach, 1971).

Content-, criterion-, and construct-related evidence of validity are among the major types of validation information collected (see Moss, 1995 for a discussion of alternative frameworks for the concept of validity). Content-related evidence of validity is related to whether the contents of the in-training evaluation tool (e.g., items, stations, cases) adequately represent a performance domain of specific interest. Criterion-related evidence of validity determines the extent to which the in-training evaluation score predicts scores on a selected criterion that is not directly measured by the assessment but is assumed to be parallel. The criterion may be either a measurement made at the time the test was given or one that will be made at some point in the future (i.e., predictive validity). Construct-related evidence of validity refers to the operational definition of the "unobservable" area being assessed (e.g., empathy), and its relationship with other variables. Crocker and Algina (1986) describe and discuss issues related to these types of validation evidence.

The validity of different methods of assessing clinical competency has been studied. Hull et al. (1995) used a multi-trait multi-method approach to analyze the construct (convergent and divergent) validity of three methods to assess the clinical performance of internal medicine residents: a clinical evaluation form (i.e., in-training evaluation report); an OSCE; and the National Board of Medical Examiners (U.S.A.) Medicine Subject Scores. Results suggested that the ability of these methods to differentiate among traits was low, even when corrected for attenuation. There was a strong method effect among the clinical evaluation form ratings, suggesting a halo effect and/or fuzziness in the definition of the clinical skills and knowledge traits. Hull et al. (1995) concluded that validity is limited by low reliability and that there is a need for additional measures of clinical performance that can differentiate between clinical skills. Pearson et al. (1998) explored the predictive validity of assessment measures at the Newcastle Medical School in Australia on performance ratings during internship (i.e., in-training evaluation). Of five content domains, one (identification, prevention and management of illness) was predictive of later intern performance ratings. They conclude that medical school assessment scores are not highly predictive of intern performance. Restriction of range and sources of variability (field of previous study, self-confidence, motivation, assessing different domains) are discussed as potential sources of concern. Weaver et al. (1993) developed and explored the validity of a questionnaire to assess a resident's humanistic behaviors through patient evaluations. They found that scores correlated significantly with two criterion measures, but there was a lack of agreement between patients and attending physicians. They noted that observations, criteria or standards may vary. Haber and Avins (1994) explored the validity of the American Board of Internal Medicine resident evaluation form to detect differences in clinical competence. They found that the form could detect global differences in competence, but was less useful for providing feedback in specific areas to individual residents.

Factor analytic approaches have been used to determine the latent (unobservable) traits measured by assessments of clinical competence. For example, Foldevi and Svendin (1996) used factor analytic techniques to evaluate the construct validity of their "phase examination", an assessment of consultation and integrative knowledge based on general practice. Their results identify two factors, one representing the solving of a learning task, and the other consultation skill. Similarly, results of work done by Ramsey et al. (1993, 1996) suggest a two-factor model for the evaluation of practicing physician performance by peers. One factor represents cognitive and clinical management, and the other represents humanistic qualities and management of psychosocial aspects of illness. In both these examples, raters distinguish only two constructs or domains of ability, leading one to question either the validity of the instruments, or the validity of using more than a couple of constructs to assess performance.

Other work has found some limited support for the validity of in-training evaluation methods. MacRae et al. (1995) compared checklists and databases with physicians' ratings as measures of student history and physical examination skills. Checklist scores correlated relatively higher than database scores with physician ratings, suggesting validity for their use. Butterfield and Mazzaferri (1991) explored the reliability and validity of an evaluation form for assessing humanistic behavior of internal medicine house-staff. The form was reliable with 5 to 6 nurses-raters and results suggested content- and criterion-related validity.

Other issues related to the collection of validity-related evidence include weighting of items or cases to reflect their importance; quality of the predictor and selected criterions; sample sizes; and restriction of range. Each of these issues influences the validity of the inferences based on these scores (see Crocker and Algina, 1986, for more on these issues).

Overall strengths and weaknesses of existing models of in-training evaluation

In general, evaluation methods used for the assessment of clinical competency suffer principally from the need to increase the reliability of observations by making multiple and objective observations of performance. Unfortunately, these requirements adversely affect the feasibility of the assessment measure. It is clear that no one measure of assessment should be utilized exclusively. Rather, they should be integrated into an overall comprehensive evaluation system. In-training evaluation does have significant potential to measure the essential components of continuous professional performance but its current difficulties, summarized below, have led to serious questions pertaining to its utility.

The strengths of existing models for in-training evaluation are that they are inexpensive and easy to use, although they require some initial developmental resources and some of the raters' time for training and implementation. In-training evaluation models provide an opportunity to evaluate continuous practice performance with the assumption that the skills demonstrated closely approximate those necessary for future practice. Areas of weakness in current in-training evaluation models include the psychometric properties associated with the tools, namely their questionable reliability and validity. Unsystematic observation and documentation of student performance, lack of rater consistency, homogeneity of the population of interest, small sample sizes and factors relating to occasion of testing and timeliness of evaluations all contribute to low reliability of in-training evaluation scores. Also, content specificity, lack of discrimination between items (with the correspondingly high item-total or item-global rating score correlations) and low correlations with other forms of assessment suggest that the validity of interpretations based on in-training evaluation scores is questionable. Given the challenges associated with current in-training evaluation practices, their meaningfulness as summative or formative assessment tools must be reconsidered.

The infrastructure within which the ongoing assessment of the students' clinical competence operates, may also be considered a weakness. Hunt (1992) identified dysfunctional characteristics of prevailing clinical evaluation systems. Among the concerns were faculty with inadequate time for interaction and observation of students; non-standardized forms for collecting evaluation information; evaluation forms lacking in some important content domains; clerkships without clear objectives to indicate core mastery-level material; tardiness of evaluation forms (30% of forms were more than 2 months late); and high turnover for clerkship coordinators and other staff responsible for administering student evaluation methods.

We have chosen to focus on suggested new models of in-training evaluation rather than other objective assessment strategies of clinical competency. An overall system for the assessment of clinical competency will be necessary with the integration of objective and subjective testing methods where appropriate (educationally and psychometrically). We feel, however, that the continuous assessment of practice performance offers opportunity for meaningful improvement. Our current system of in-training evaluation is considered to lack sufficient evidence of reliability and validity to make it defensible under formal challenge. As we look to in-training evaluation to assess the undergraduate student, the resident and the practicing physician, there will be a need to develop effective, evidence-based models.

A NEW PARADIGM FOR IN-TRAINING EVALUATION

Criteria for successful in-training evaluation

Work done by Turnbull et al. (1998), Short (1993) and Hunt (1992) has outlined a framework for improved programs of in-training evaluation. The issues that they identify tend to converge on the following criteria. A successful in-training evaluation program:
1. Includes the systematic observation and documentation of student performance in real clinical settings (i.e., continuous performance assessment);
2. Assesses student performance in a variety of learning domains. This requires that the approach be flexible, so that relevant practice behavior may be evaluated in a variety of circumstances;
3. Is a consistent or reproducible measure of student clinical competence in an applied, patient care setting;

4. Yields an accurate interpretation of a student's current level of competence;
5. Is feasible to implement at the time of student performance, minimizing the need for excessive resources from students, raters or administration;
6. Assesses content areas relevant to developing medical trainees. Measures of performance should come as close as possible to representing what professionals should know and be able to do in the "real world"; and
7. Integrates effectively with other methods for the assessment of clinical competency.

While not essential from an evaluative perspective, effective systems of in-training evaluation must also:

8. Clearly outline expectations and standards (general as well as rotation-specific) for performance at a given level of training and the requirements for promotion; and
9. Be viewed as an important tool (by both students and faculty) for decision-making regarding promotion, identifying learning needs and providing feedback to students.

What would an appropriate model look like?

In an effort to develop a system of ongoing performance assessment, in-training evaluation must be integrated with other appropriate objective measures of clinical ability. Multiple-choice examinations, short-answer questions, the triple-jump, chart-simulated recall and the OSCE may all have their place in measuring the specific objectives reflective of clinical competency in a given situation, depending upon the context and resources available. As stated, however, in-training evaluation has a unique role, as it has the greatest potential to evaluate many of these additional and very important competencies required for future practice. The criteria defined for effective in-training evaluation, however, require that we develop a new paradigm or model.

Drawing upon the industrial model of performance assessment, we propose that the unit of assessment for in-training evaluation be the behavior or constellation of behaviors required for the management of a particular patient. These activities should be objectively documented on an ongoing basis by multiple observers who bring unique perspectives to the measurement of the learner's performance. The objectives of a clinical rotation can be refined into specific agreed-upon behaviors and evaluated in a standardized manner by different observers. In circumstances where this approach was introduced, a sufficient number of objective assessments have yielded reliability estimates of approximately 0.8 (Turnbull et al., 2000). We do not propose devoting further time to the development of items or rating scales.

The content validity of such an approach is determined by the acceptability of the assessment standards. While there are no criterion (predictive) validity studies to support this approach, it must be pointed out that these are often also unavailable for other more costly, structured methods. Feasibility, however, limits this approach. While these behaviors are observed on an ongoing basis, most clinical supervisors do not take the time to document them in an objective fashion. Where this has been introduced successfully, assessment was integrated into the day-to-day clinical practice of trained physicians and allied health professionals.

In one circumstance, a brief rating scale pertaining to five or six domains was introduced into the admitting history and physical form used by clinical clerks on a medical rotation (Turnbull et al., 2000). Patient encounter cards listing a brief series of rating scales documenting patient management strategies were also used. In addition, nurses and patients completed evaluation forms assessing domains of competence relevant to their own perspective. The information based on each patient encounter was gathered on computer scannable forms and was collected by students in a clerkship log. At the completion of a rotation this information was scanned into a final summary profile representing all information, from all sources, collected in an objective fashion. Consequently, it was shown that a minimum of seven or eight pieces of information would provide information comparable in reliability to that of a high-stakes OSCE examination (reliability of 0.7). In addition, this system of in-training evaluation provided opportunities for immediate feedback and highlighted the importance of input from patients and nurses, as well as from faculty.

Similar methods have been incorporated in other domains such as anesthesia report cards pertaining to the management of each case or the addition of a voice prompted resident evaluation system that supplements the surgical dictation by a staff surgeon at the end of the case (Fung Kee Fung, 1997). The priority here is that relevant clinical behaviors be assessed on an ongoing basis. Historically, this information was lost, because it was not gathered *at the time* in an objective fashion, making in-training evaluation more subjective and unreliable. These alternative approaches allow one to capture this information from multiple sources in a feasible and more objective fashion.

When integrated with other objective measures of clinical competency, this approach to in-training evaluation provides the opportunity for a more comprehensive evaluation of the skills believed to be required for the future practice of medicine in a defensible and accountable fashion while maximizing individual feedback in a timely fashion.

A FUTURE AGENDA FOR RESEARCH IN PERFORMANCE ASSESSMENT

Many questions remain for a future research agenda. The answers to these questions will definitively clarify the role of in-training evaluation in the measurement of clinical performance.

Issues of reliability

1. What models will encourage raters to distinguish between rating scale items and between performances? Is lack of discrimination caused by training, teacher-evaluator role or the problem of the evaluation environment-support, time and recognition?
2. How many observers, what type of observers and how many evaluations are necessary to establish a reliable measure of clinical performance?
3. What is the required number of observations necessary to identify generalizable skill sets? How many of these skills are necessary for the future practice of medicine?

While classical psychometric techniques for assessing reliability remain the popular choice, it is important to note that other models, such as generalizability theory, have applications in studies of in-training evaluation. One benefit of generalizability theory is that different sources of measurement error may be investigated in one study. In addition, it allows the researcher to explore various decision options (e.g., varying the number of raters and cases) in relation to the psychometric properties of the tool.

Issues of validity

1. What are the fundamental, behaviorally-based components of clinical competency necessary for the future practice of medicine?
2. Can a similar method to that described for in-training evaluation demonstrate criterion (predictive) validity?
3. What degree of correlation with other assessment strategies commonly used in the assessment of clinical competency is acceptable? How are these other methods best integrated into the overall system of performance assessment?

While the classical conceptions of validity (content-, criterion-, construct-related) continue to be applied in in-training evaluation studies, it is important to note that alternate conceptions of validity (e.g., unified theory of validity, consequential validity) exist and may be explored in the areas of medical education research (e.g., Moss, 1998; Maguire, Hattie, & Haig, 1994).

Issues of feasibility

1. What are the limits to feasibility? What models would enhance the environment for assessment and the quality of information obtained?
2. What is a reasonable standard of accountability, given the limits of feasibility?

CONCLUSION

The difficulties with our existing evaluation methods are not necessarily with how they are structured and implemented but with the use that we, as medical educators, make of the results. In evaluating the overall performance of an individual, multiple methods of assessment must be used in an integrated fashion based upon their relative merits. Existing models of in-training evaluation, unfortunately, do not have the ability to permit meaningful decisions pertaining to the clinical performance of an individual and are not accountable or defensible. A new approach to in-training evaluation is required that takes into consideration the day-to-day evaluation of continued practice performance in a more objective fashion by multiple observers. As we look to in-training evaluation to measure many of the essential qualities necessary for the future practice of medicine, and as we link this to the process of licensure and re-licensure, there will be a need for us to develop methods which are psychometrically rigorous, feasible and accountable. It is anticipated that these methods will also motivate and enhance learning.

REFERENCES

Butterfield, P. S., & Mazzaferri, E. L. (1991). New rating form for use by nurses in assessing residents' humanistic behavior. *Journal of General Internal Medicine, 6,* 155-161.

Crocker, L., & Algina, J. (1986). *Introduction to classical and modern test theory.* Fort Worth: Harcourt Brace Jovanovich College Publishers.

Cronbach, L. J. (1971). Test validation. In R. L. Thorndike (Ed.), *Educational measurement* (2nd ed., pp. 443-507). Washington, D.C.: American Council on Education.

Eldin, M., Magzoub, M. A., Schmidt, H. G., Abdel-Hameed, A. A., Dolmans, D., & Mustafa, S. E. (1998). Student assessment in community settings: a comprehensive approach. *Medical Education, 32,* 50-59.

Fisher Jr., W. P., Vial, R. H., & Sanders, C. V. (1997). Removing rater effects from medical clerkship evaluation. *Academic Medicine, 72*(5), 443-444.

Foldevi, M., & Svendin, C. G. (1996). "Phase Examination" an assessment of consultation skills and integrative knowledge based in general practice. *Medical Education, 30*(5), 326-332.

Fowell, S. L., Southgate, L. J., & Bligh, J. G. (1999) Evaluating assessment: The missing link? *Medical Education, 33*(4), 276-281.

Fung Kee Fung, M. P., Parboosingh, I. J., Temple, L. M., Guy-d'Anjou, C., Haebe, J., & Lussier, R. (1997). Development of a computerized telecommunications system for in-training evaluation of residents in a laparoscopic educational program. *Obstetrics and Gynecology, 90*(1), 148-152.

Gray, J. D. (1996a). Primer on resident evaluation. *Annals of the Royal College of Physicians and Surgeons of Canada, 29*(2), 91-94.

Gray, J. D. (1996b). Global rating scales in residency education. *Academic Medicine, 21*(1 Suppl.), S55-63.

Haber, R. J., & Avins, A. L. (1994). Do ratings on the American Board of Internal Medicine resident evaluation form detect differences in clinical competence? *Journal of General Internal Medicine, 9,* 140-145.

Hastings Center Report (1996). *The goals of medicine: setting new priorities.* Special Supplement. Briarcliff Manor, New York.

Henkin, Y., Friedman, M., Bouskila, D., Kushnir, D., & Glick, S. (1990). The use of patients as student evaluators. *Medical Teacher, 12*(3/4), 279-289.

Holmboe, E. S., & Hawkins, (1998). Methods for evaluating the clinical competence of residents in internal medicine: a review. *Annals of Internal Medicine, 129*(1), 42-48.

Hull, A.L., Hodder, S., Berger, B., Gindberg, D., Lindheim, N., Quan, J., & Kleinhenz, M. E. (1995). Validity of three clinical performance assessments of internal medicine clerks. *Academic Medicine, 70*(6), 517-522.

Hunt, D. D. (1992). Functional and dysfunctional characteristics of the prevailing model of clinical evaluation systems in North American medical schools. *Academic Medicine, 67*(4), 254-259.

Kane, M. T. (1992). The assessment of professional competence. *Evaluation in the Health Professions, 15,* 163-152.

Littlefield, J. H., DaRosa, D. A., Anderson, K. D., Bell, R. M., Nicholas, G. G., & Wolfson, P. J. (1991). Assessing performance in clerkships: accuracy of surgery clerkship performance raters. *Academic Medicine, 66*(9), S16-S18.

Maguire T., Hattie J., & Haig B. (1994). Construct-validity and achievement assessment *Alberta Journal of Educational Research, 40*(2), 109-126.

Maudsley, R. F. (1999). Content in context: medical education and society's needs. *Academic Medicine, 74*(2), 143-145.

McCrae, H. M., Vu, N. V., Graham, B., Word-Sims, M., Colliver, J. A., & Robbs, R. S. (1995). Comparing checklists and databases with physicians ratings as measures of students' history and physical-examination skills. *Academic Medicine, 70*(4), 313-317.

McGuire, C. (1993). Perspectives in assessment. *Academic Medicine, 68*(2), S3-S8.

McManus, I. C., Richards, P., Winder, B. C., & Sproston, K. A. (1998) Clinical experience, performance in final examinations, and learning style in medical students: Prospective study. *British Medical Journal, 316*(7128), 345-350.

Medical School Objectives Writing Group (1999). Learning objectives for medical student education – guidelines for medical schools: report I of the Medical Schools Objectives Project. *Academic Medicine, 74*(1), 13-18.

Messick, S. (1995). Validity of psychological-assessment – validation of inferences from persons' responses and performances as scientific inquiry into score meaning. *American Psychologist, 50*(9), 741-749.

Miller, G. E. (1990). The assessment of clinical skills/competence/performance. *Academic Medicine, 65*(Suppl.), S63-67.

Moss, P. (1995). Themes and variations in validity theory. *Educational Measurement Issues and Practice, 2,* 5-13.

Neufeld, V. R. (1993). Demand-side medical education: educating future physicians for Ontario. *Canadian Medical Association Journal, 148*(9), 1471-1477.

Neufeld, V. R., & Norman G. R. (Eds.). (1985). *Assessing clinical competence.* New York: Springer.

Neufeld, V. R., Maudsley, R. F., Pickering, R. J., Turnbull, J. M., Weston, W. W., & Brown, M. G. (1998). Educating future physicians for Ontario, *Academic Medicine, 73,* 1133-1148.

Norcini, J. J., & Shea, J. (1992). The reproducibility of standards over groups and occasions. *Applied Measurement in Education, 5,* 62-72.

Pangaro, L. (1999). A new vocabulary and other innovations for improving descriptive in-training evaluations. *Academic Medicine, 74*(11), 1203-1207.

Pearson, S., Rolfe, I. E., & Henry, R. (1998). The relationship between assessment measures at Newcastle Medical School (Australia) and performance ratings during internship. *Medical Education, 32,* 40-45.

Ramsey, P. G., Carline, J. D., Blank, L. L., & Wenrich, M. D. (1996). Feasibility of hospital-based use of peer ratings to evaluate the performances of practicing physicians. *Academic Medicine, 71*(4), 364-370.

Ramsey, P. G., Wenrich, M. D., Carline, J. D., Inui, T. S., Larson, E. B., & Logerfo, J. P. (1993). Use of peer ratings to evaluate physician performance. *Journal of the American Medical Association, 269*(13) 1655-1660.

Regher, G. (1996). Issues in cognitive psychology: implications for professional education. *Academic Medicine, 71*(9), 988-1000.

Schmidt, H. G., Norman, G. R., & Boshuizen, H. P. (1990). A cognitive perspective on medical expertise: theory and implication. *Academic Medicine, 65,* 611-621.

Short, J. P. (1993). The importance of strong evaluation standards and procedures in training residents. *Academic Medicine, 68*(7), 522-525.

Smith, R. M. (1993). The triple-jump examination as an assessment tool in the problem-based medical curriculum at the University of Hawaii. *Academic Medicine, 68*(5), 366-372.

Societal Needs Working Group, CanMEDS 2000 Project (1996). Skills for the new millennium. *Annals of the Royal College of Physicians and Surgeons of Canada, 29*(4), 206-216.

Speer, A. J., Solomon, D. J., & Ainsworth, M. A. (1996) An innovative evaluation method in an internal medicine clerkship. *Academic Medicine (Suppl.), 71*(1), S76-S78.

Stillman, P. L. (1991). Positive effects of a clinical performance assessment program. *Academic Medicine,* *66*(8), 481-483.

Tamblyn, R., Benaroya, S., Snell, L., McLeod, P., Schnarch, B., & Abrahamowicz, M. (1994). The feasibility and value of using patient satisfaction ratings to evaluate internal medicine residents. *Journal of General Internal Medicine, 9,* 146-152.

Thomas, C. S., Mellsop, G., Callender, K., Crawshaw, J., Ellis, P. M., Hall, A., Macdonald, J., Silfverskiold, P., & Romansclarkson, S. (1993). The oral examinations – a study of academic and nonacademic factors. *Medical Education, 27*(5), 433-439.

Turnbull, J., Gray, J., & MacFadyen, J. (1998). Improving in-training evaluation programs. *Journal of General Internal Medicine, 13*(5), 317-323.

Turnbull, J., MacFadyen, J., Van Barneveld, C., and Norman, G. (2000). Clinical work sampling: A new approach to the problem of in training evaluation. *Journal of General Internal Medicine, 15,* 556-561.

Van der Vleuten, C. P. M. (2000). There is a paradigm shift in medical education assessment from quantitive to qualitative. Is medical education able and prepared to make such a move? Paper presented at the 9th International Ottawa Conference on Medical Education. Capetown, South Africa.

Van der Vleuten, C. P. M., Norman, G. R., & de Graaff, E. (1991). Pitfalls in the pursuit of objectivity: issues of reliability. *Medical Education, 25,* 110-118.

Weaver, M. J., Ow, C., Walker, D. J., & Degenhardt, E. F. (1993). A questionnaire for patients' evaluations of their physicians' humanistic behaviors. *Journal of General Internal Medicine, 8,* 135-139.

25   Combining Tests and Setting Standards

JOHN NORCINI AND ROBIN GUILLE
American Board of Internal Medicine

SUMMARY

In testing, the area of standards and standard-setting remains relatively unsettled. The chapter begins with definitions of scores and standards, and describes norm-referenced score interpretation, domain-referenced score interpretation, relative standards, and absolute standards. It then reviews the work related to the credibility of standards and outlines some of the more common standard-setting techniques used with MCQ-based tests and clinical examinations. Finally, because it is sometimes useful to combine scores from several related assessments, information is presented on when and how to do so.

THE NATURE OF SCORES AND STANDARDS

Among the areas of work in testing, both in and out of medical education, standards and standard-setting remain relatively unsettled. In part this is due to the arbitrary nature of standards, but it is also a result of confusion over terminology (Norcini, 1992). One writer's absolute standard is another's criterion-referenced scoring and both have been called content-based approaches. In contrast, there is norm-referenced scoring, a term which is frequently used interchangeably with relative standards.

As a consequence of this lack of consensus about terminology and the confusion it causes, it is not possible to describe standards and approaches to standard-setting, without first defining terms. Therefore, using a previously devised framework, this chapter begins with a definition of scores and standards and then describes the types of score interpretation and standards (Norcini, 1992).

International Handbook of Research in Medical Education, 811–834.
G.R. Norman, C.P.M. Van der Vleuten, D.I. Newble (eds.)
© 2002 *Dordrecht: Kluwer Academic Publishers. Printed in Great Britain.*

Definition of scores and standards

Scores

A score is a number or letter that represents how well an examinee performs along the continuum of the construct being assessed. In medicine, it is the degree of medical correctness for a response or group of responses. A score is the numerical answer to the question, "How good is the examinee's performance from the perspective of the patient?"

Scores can often be based on the actual responses of the examinees, and multiple choice questions (MCQs) are a good example of this. Since such items are written to have one clearly correct response, the score on each item is dichotomous (0 or 1), and performance on the entire examination can be captured by simply counting the number right.

In item formats that attempt to reproduce complex clinical situations with high fidelity, scores may involve some form of weighting and they are often based on an interpretation of the responses of the examinees. For example, in an oral examination with live patients, scoring might use weights when there is a desire to capture degrees of correctness. Moreover, this type of examination will likely require interpretation on the part of the examiner because several courses of action could lead to the same patient outcome and the connection between an examinee's behavior and the patient's responses may not always be obvious. This requires the examiner to interpret the examinee's actions in the broad context of the interaction and make judgments about whether they are correct.

Regardless of whether it is weighted or unweighted, based on the actual responses of examinees or an interpretation of those actions, a score reflects the degree of medical correctness from the perspective of the patient.

Standards

A standard is a statement about whether an examination performance is good enough for a particular purpose (e.g., to provide safe and effective care). It is expressed as a special score that serves as the boundary between those who have met the standard and those who have not.

Standards focus on the examinees' performances and judge them against a specific social or educational construct (e.g., the competent practitioner, the student ready for graduation). Therefore, standards are based on judgments about how much the examinee needs to know for a certain purpose, rather than the patient outcomes that form the basis for scoring. For example, the scoring of a standardized patient examination should not change whether it is taken by fourth year medical students or third year residents – the right things to do for the patient are independent of the examinees. However, the standard should differ depending on whether the test is being used to identify students who satisfactorily complete medical school or third year residents who are finishing postgraduate training (i.e., it makes sense to require higher performance from the latter).

Because standards refer to social constructs and are based on educational judgments (rather than being derived from the scientific-medical evidence that forms the underpinnings of scoring), they are arbitrary. There is no such thing as the "true" standard and it is not possible to collect data that support the use of one standard to the exclusion of all others (Glass, 1978; Popham, 1978; Kane, 1994). Thus, for any given test there are a sizable number of acceptable alternatives.

This arbitrariness is both good and bad. On the one hand, it permits considerable latitude in choosing a method and a standard, because it is difficult to mount a significant argument that a specific pass-fail point is incorrect. On the other hand, it is more difficult to build a body of evidence that favors a particular standard over its reasonable alternatives.

Types of scores and standards

Scores

Scores can be interpreted from a norm-referenced or domain-referenced perspective. They are interpreted from a norm-referenced perspective when they provide information on how an examinee performs against others who took the test. For instance, when a rank or percentile is reported, it tells the examinee how he or she did relative to the other examinees. It does not provide information on how much of the content or domain the examinee knows.

In contrast, scores are interpreted from a domain-referenced perspective when they provide data on an examinee's performance relative to the test content. For instance, scores are often reported as the percentage of questions an examinee answered correctly. This provides the examinee information on how much of the material he or she knows. It does not provide information on how the examinee performed relative to the other examinees.

Standards

Standards are relative or absolute. Standards are relative when the decisions are based on a comparison among the performances of examinees. For example, in the past it was routine practice for many licensing and certifying boards in the United States to set the pass-fail point at one standard deviation below the mean score of a reference group. Examinees needed to perform just better than the worst 15% of the reference group.

Standards are absolute when the pass-fail decision is based on how much the examinee knows. For example, to pass a test an absolute standard might require examinees to know 70% of the material or correctly answer 70 of the 100 questions.

CHARACTERISTICS OF A CREDIBLE STANDARD

Since standards are an expression of a social construct, it is not possible to determine whether a particular standard is "correct" or valid in the classic scientific sense (Kane, 1994). Instead, it is important to develop a body of procedural evidence and outcomes data that speak to the issue of credibility. Specifically, standards need to be set by the right number and kind of standard-setters, the method to set them must meet certain criteria, and the outcomes of applying the standard should be reasonable (Norcini & Shea, 1997).

Standard-setters

Standards are always set by people and their work needs to be sensitive to the purpose of the test, the nature of the test material and the quality of the examinees. The best way to ensure these sensitivities is to pick the standard-setters with care.

In a low stakes testing situation, such as an examination at the end of a course, the standard-setter is typically the faculty member who teaches the course. This traditional method of setting standards has some serious drawbacks. The faculty member has a conflict of interest in that he or she is responsible for both the education and the evaluation of the examinees. Moreover, a standard set by a single person is likely to vary in stringency over time and course content. Despite these problems, the faculty member represents all of the important considerations in setting the standard, since he or she knows the purpose of the test, understand the content, and is familiar with the examinees. In addition, this time honored method of standard-setting is efficient and it has credibility with students and the public.

In a high stakes testing situation, setting standards is more complex and it would not be credible to rely on a single faculty member. Using certification as an example, it is essential to include a number of judges in the standard-setting exercise. They will improve the reproducibility of the standards and reduce the effects of differences in stringency over time and test forms. Likewise, it is essential to ensure racial, ethnic, geographical, and gender balance and to avoid the inclusion of any participants who have a conflict of interest or who would detract from the defensibility of the standard.

The exact mix of qualifications in the group of individuals who set standards for a high stakes certifying examination is of considerable importance. Clearly all of those involved in the standard-setting process should be knowledgeable in the content area of the examination and probably certified in it. Academic appointments are valuable because they imply that some of the standard-setters are involved in the educational process, and so are knowledgeable about the competence of the examinees. Engaging practitioners is also of importance since they practice the profession and thus are experts in the content of the test. Finally, some of the participants should be recognized as leaders within the profession, since it will lend credibility and defensibility to the final result.

If the important attributes of the field or profession are represented in the standard setting group, it will likely be large enough to generate reproducible results. From the perspective of reproducibility alone, research reports indicate that as few as eight experts would be sufficient (Brennan & Lockwood, 1980; Norcini, Lipner, Langdon, & Strecker, 1987; Plake, Impara, & Potenza, 1994). Nonetheless, a larger number accrues additional credibility to the final result.

There are a variety of efficient ways of collecting standard-setting judgments that enable the inclusion of larger numbers of experts in the process. When a number of judges are available, they can be broken into several groups, each of which makes judgments about part of the examination (Norcini, Shea, & Ping, 1988). This uses less of each judge's time and minimizes negative group effects (e.g., domination of the process by one or two powerful participants). Likewise, it is possible to have a relatively short meeting of the judges (say 1-2 hours) and ask them to complete the task after the meeting. Research has shown that they set similar standards, while again minimizing negative group effects and making efficient use of the judge's efforts (Norcini, Lipner, Langdon, & Strecker, 1987).

Even if they cannot participate directly in the standard-setting process, it is desirable to incorporate the judgments of as broad a group as possible. One way to accomplish this is to provide the standard-setters data that are based on the judgments of others. It is important to note that the data should be used to inform, not dictate the standard. For example, if standards are being set for an objective structured clinical examination given at the end of medical school, it may be useful to provide the standard-setters aggregated data on the performance of students who received marginal ratings during their clinical rotations. Or, standard-setters for a certifying examination in internal medicine might be given information on the performance of the group of candidates who were rated as barely competent at the end of training by their program directors (Norcini & Shea, 1997). This effectively extends the number of participants in the standard-setting exercise and its reasoned use will significantly enhance the credibility of the results.

Criteria for methods of setting standards

There are many thorough reviews of the advantages and disadvantages of the most popular standard-setting methods (e.g., Berk, 1986; Meskauskas, 1976; Shepard, 1980, & 1984; Livingston & Zieky, 1982) and brief descriptions of several methods follow this section. Although these are very helpful, there is no definitive and substantive way to make a distinction among methods because, in the end, all standards are arbitrary. Therefore, the exact method chosen to set standards is less important than the fact it meets several criteria designed to lend credibility to the final result. Specifically, the method should (1) produce standards consistent with the purpose of the test, (2) rely on informed expert judgment, (3) demonstrate due diligence, (4) be supported by a body of research, and (5) be easy to explain and implement.

Lockwood, 1980; Kane & Wilson, 1984). Although not necessary routinely, some studies have actually compared the estimates of judges over groups and time (Norcini & Shea, 1992). They found that the standards were very similar over different groups (usually varying by only 1-2%) and for the same judges on two occasions, 2 years apart.

Third, it is important that the method for setting standards not foster the influence of unrelated social factors (Fitzpatrick, 1989) or non-substantive differences in the level and type of expert specialization (Busch & Jaeger, 1990; Norcini, Shea, & Kanya, 1988). Studies of Angoff's method reveal that it is robust in this regard. Standards are similar over different groups of judges (Norcini, Lipner, Langdon, & Strecker, 1987; Norcini & Shea, 1992) and work in medicine and teaching indicates that, within broad definitions, level and nature of specialization does not matter (Norcini, Shea, & Kanya, 1988; Busch & Jaeger, 1990). When there are concerns about particular judges, van der Linden (1982) and Kane (1987) have proposed methods that determine inconsistent or biased performance.

Finally, the method should be sensitive to differences in test difficulty and content. Therefore, it is not surprising that, for Angoff's method, there is considerable evidence of a correlation between the judgments of the standard-setters and actual item difficulty. Likewise, Shea, Reshetar, Dawson, and Norcini (1994) found that the standard-setters' judgments varied by the nature of the content as well as by item difficulty.

Methods that are easy to explain and implement

The credibility of a standard is enhanced if the method used to set it is easy to explain and implement. For standard-setters, it decreases the amount of training required and increases the likelihood that they will comply with instructions. For examinees and other users of the test, it enhances credibility by rendering the process understandable and assuring them that everyone is treated the same way.

Some of the recent standard-setting methods have employed sophisticated statistical models to alter the judgments of experts (Jaeger, 1995). Unless there is overwhelming evidence of significant benefit, however, such methods may be counterproductive for three reasons. First, they require the user to argue that the judgments of the experts are so unreliable that they need to be "corrected" in some fashion; this may undermine the argument that the standard-setters are experts. Second, the nature of the correction is unlikely to be accessible to examinees and standard-setters, so they may not understand what has been done and why. Third, these corrections are unlikely to make a substantive difference in a standard that is arbitrary anyway.

Realistic outcomes

If a standard produces outcomes that are not realistic (i.e., broadly consistent with the expectations of the examinees and users), it will not be viewed as credible regardless of the standard-setters and the method they used. Given that there are legitimate alternatives to any standard, building a case for one of them requires evidence that it (1) is viewed as correct by stakeholders, (2) produces pass rates that have reasonable relationships with contemporaneous markers of competence, and (3) is related to later performance.

Gathering the opinions of stakeholders about the "correctness" of a standard forms the most direct test of how realistic it is. Examples of this type of work with physicians and nurses include Norcini, Shea, and Webster (1986), Fabrey and Raymond (1987), and Orr and Nungester (1991). For instance, Norcini et al. (1986) focused on the internal medicine certifying examination and surveyed groups of examinees, practicing physicians, directors of training programs, nurses, and hospital administrators. Their responses reflected an accurate understanding of the pass rates and support for the "correctness" of the standard (78-89% of the respondents thought the standard was "about right").

A comparison of the pass rates of various groups with a set of expectations about performance, what Kane (1994) calls *"validity checks based on external criteria"*, constitutes the second form of evidence for realistic outcomes. A match between performance and expectations will add credibility to the result. Mismatches by themselves will not invalidate a standard, but they raise questions that need to be addressed, and they identify a group likely to mount a challenge to the examination.

For example, if a clinical skills examination is administered at the end of medical school, there are at least two pass rates that would be of interest. First, it is reasonable to expect that the educational process has been effective and only a few students would fail the examination. If the total group pass rate is low, it may reflect a problem with the standard (or the education) and it merits additional attention. Second, it is reasonable to expect that students who have done well in their clerkships should also do well on the examination. Consequently, there should be a very high pass rate among the best students based on clerkship grades and a lower (but still high) pass rate for those students with lower clerkship grades.

Finally, there should be a relationship between a passing or failing performance and later educational and practice outcomes. Although the types of study that would support this notion have enormous intuitive appeal, they are very difficult to do well (Shimberg, 1981; Kane, 1994). There are few well defined educational or practice outcomes and measuring them poses several serious problems.

Nonetheless, an example of this type of evidence can be found in the work of Ramsey, Carline, Inui, Larson, LoGerfo, and Wenrich (1989) who compared certified and non-certified internists on a variety of educational and practice measures. Certified internists had some advantages in preventive services, patient outcomes, and measures of medical knowledge and judgment. Although this study

4. Select a sample of examinees in the region where the cutting score might be.
5. Give the judges the responses of one examinee to the entire test.
6. Ask the judges to decide (by consensus or majority) whether the examinee should pass or fail.
7. If pass, choose another examinee with a lower score; if fail, choose another examinee with a higher score.
8. Repeat steps 5 to 7 until the judges are moving in a small range of scores.
9. Some possible cutting scores (there are many) include the mean of the last 10 passing examinees and the mean of the last 10 failing examinees.

Advantages and disadvantages

These methods have two advantages in common. First, educators are comfortable making the types of judgments required by the methods and they find the process intuitive and convincing. Second, since the judgments are based on the actual test performances of examinees, it informs expert judgment with knowledge of how examinees actually did on the test.

The Contrasting-Groups method has an additional advantage. Because the process yields distributions of passers and failers, it allows the final standard to manipulate the number of false positive and false negative decisions. For example, if the standard is set at the point of least overlap between the distributions it will roughly equalize the false positive-false negative rates. However, if the standard is set at the score that fails all examinees classified as failers by the judges, then it minimizes false positives.

The methods have three disadvantages in common. First, they are time-consuming and it is difficult for the judges to review an examinee's entire test and make an unbiased judgment about the skills of examinees. Second, judgments must be made about a large number of test takers to create reliable passing scores; this is particularly true for the Contrasting-Groups method. Finally, the actual decision about the process for choosing the passing score can be very subjective.

Absolute standards: judgments about individual test items

Methods

In these methods, the standard-setters make judgments about the difficulty and importance of each question on the test. The two most popular of these methods are Angoff's method (1971) and Ebel's method (1979).

Steps in Angoff's method

1. Select the judges.
2. Discuss the purpose of the test, the nature of the examinees, and what constitutes adequate and inadequate skills/knowledge.

3. Define the "borderline" group, a group that has a 50-50 chance of passing.
4. Read the first item.
5. Each judge estimates the proportion of the borderline group that would get it right.
6. The ratings are recorded for all to see, discuss, and change as appropriate.
7. Repeat steps 4 to 6 for each item.
8. Calculate the passing score by averaging the estimates of all judges for each item and summing the items (see Table 1).

Steps in Ebel's method

1. Select the judges.
2. Discuss the purpose of the test, the nature of the examinees, and what constitutes adequate and inadequate skills/knowledge.
3. Define the "borderline" group, a group that has a 50-50 chance of passing.
4. Build a classification table for items based on categories such as item difficulty and importance (see Table 2).
5. Judges read each item and assign it to one of the categories in the classification table.
6. Judges estimate the percentages of items in each category that borderline test takers should answer correctly.
7. Calculate the passing score by averaging the estimates of all judges for each category, multiply it by the number of items, and sum for all of the categories.

Table 1. Calculation of the passing score for Angoff's method

Item	Raters					Average
	1	2	3	4	5	
1	.80	.95	.85	.90	.85	.87
2	.30	.40	.35	.35	.40	.36
3	.50	.60	.55	.60	.60	.57
4	.70	.70	.70	.70	.70	.70
5	.75	.85	.80	.85	.80	.81
6	.40	.85	.80	.75	.80	.72
7	.50	.90	.55	.60	.60	.63
8	.70	.80	.75	.75	.70	.74
9	.45	.55	.50	.45	.45	.48
10	.60	.70	.65	.65	.70	.66

Cutting Score 6.54 (65%)

Advantages and disadvantages

One of the strengths of these methods is that they focus detailed attention on the content of the test questions. They are relatively easy to use and there is a considerable body of published work supporting their application. Moreover, they have been used frequently in high stakes testing situations and they are the most popular of the methods currently available.

The chief disadvantage of these methods is that the concept of a borderline group is foreign to many judges and they often feel they are "pulling numbers out of the air." These methods can also be tedious to apply to very long tests.

Table 2. Calculation of the passing score for Ebel's method

Category	Percent Right	No of Questions	Expected Score
Essential			
Easy	95	3	2.85
Hard	80	2	1.60
Important			
Easy	90	3	2.70
Hard	75	4	3.00
Acceptable			
Easy	80	2	1.60
Hard	50	3	1.50
Questionable			
Easy	70	2	1.40
Hard	35	1	.35
Number of Questions		20	
Cutting Score		15 (75%)	

Compromise methods: judgments about examinees and test content

Methods

As the name implies, these methods are a compromise between relative and absolute standards. Consequently, standard-setters make judgments, both about groups of examinees and the content of the test. The most popular of these methods is Hofstee's method (de Gruijter, 1985).

Steps in Hofstee's method

1. Select the judges.
2. Discuss the purpose of the test, the nature of the examinees, and what constitutes adequate and inadequate skills/knowledge.
3. Review the test in detail.
4. Ask the judges to answer four questions:

   a. What is the minimum acceptable cut score?
   b. What is the maximum acceptable cut score?
   c. What is the minimum acceptable fail rate?
   d. What is the maximum acceptable fail rate?
5. After the test is given, graph the distribution of scores and select the cut score as described by de Gruijter (1985).

Advantages and disadvantages

This method has the advantage of being very easy to implement; standards can generally be set in one hour. In addition, the standard-setters are comfortable with the judgments they are asked to make.

One disadvantage of this method is that the cut score may not be in the area defined by the judges' estimates. When this happens, the standard becomes the maximum or minimum acceptable pass rate. In addition, while it would be acceptable on occasion, this method would not be the first choice in an ongoing high stakes testing situation. Its efficiency may cause some loss of credibility and the procedure is subject to some of the same concerns as the relative standard-setting methods.

METHODS FOR SETTING STANDARDS ON CLINICAL EXAMINATIONS

Some of the methods developed for use with multiple choice questions can be applied, without change, to clinical examinations. In other instances, modification to the methods is required. This section reviews some of the methods applied to clinical examinations.

Relative standards: judgments about groups of test-takers

The methods that produce relative standards and require judgments about groups of test takers, the fixed percentage and reference group methods, can be directly applied following the steps outlined above. They will require no additional effort on the part of the judges.

Absolute standards: judgments about individual test takers

The methods that produce absolute standards and require judgments about individual examinees, the Contrasting-Groups and Up-and-Down methods, can also be directly applied following the steps outlined above. The experts' judgments should be based on the devices used to generate examinees' scores including ratings, checklists, post-encounter paperwork, and the like. Judgments should not be based on videotapes or direct observation, unless they are being used to generate the scores as well. The task of the judges applying these methods is much more complex than with MCQs and it is difficult to do well. They must retain all the information about all the interactions of a single candidate and then repeat this task for many different examinees.

One way to make the task more manageable is to make the judgments on a case by case (or problem by problem) basis and then combine the results over all cases on the test (Clauser & Clyman, 1994). When doing this, it is essential that the judges focus on the standard-setting question (i.e., whether a performance is good enough for a particular purpose, like graduating from medical school) not the scoring question (i.e., whether the examinee's performance is medically correct). The latter judgments should have been incorporated in the scoring algorithms.

Mills, Jaeger, Plake, and Hambleton (1998) have proposed three variations on the Contrasting-Groups method. The Sorting, Analytic Judgment, and Integrated Judgment methods are used to make broad statements about the quality of examinees. They all require judges to sort a sample of examinees' performances into two or more categories. In the example used in the study, students were divided into the categories, "below basic, basic, proficient, and advanced". They then further divided each category into three subcategories, the extremes of which were considered boundaries. These boundary subcategories were then used to derive the score that separates examinees into groups. The three methods differ according to whether the judgments were made about the whole test or portions of it, and exactly when the discussions occurred among the judges.

All of the methods presented to this point assume that the pass-fail decision is based on a compensatory model: examinees can compensate for poor performance on some problems or cases with good performance on others. A class of profile-based standard-setting methods has recently been proposed to handle conjunctive models (e.g., where examinees need to achieve minimal scores on certain critical cases or groups of cases as well as an acceptable score overall). In the Dominant Profile method, Putnam, Pence, and Jaeger (1995) ask judges to work together until they reach consensus about a minimally acceptable profile of scores. In the Judgmental Policy Capture method (Jaeger, 1995), a group of judges individually rate several profiles of performance (e.g., a pattern of scores). Empirical methods, such as multiple regression, hierarchical cluster analysis, or factor analysis, are used to derive a single policy or set of pass-fail rules for the test.

These new variations are still experimental and need to be applied with care. First, some of them require dozens of experts to have days of discussions and/or consider a large number of performance profiles. For most practical applications, it is unrealistic to ask experts to devote several days of their time to a process that will produce a result that is substantially indistinguishable from the result of a briefer, but still rigorous process.

Second, when the methods are applied to a single test, they permit the judges to develop weights for the various exercises, which changes the blueprint of the examination. For example, judges may require a specific performance for a particular patient, assign weights to the ordering of certain tests, devise rules that assign values to linked combinations of therapies, and/or alter the blueprint of the exam to stress certain diseases that they believe are more important. In fact, these decisions should have been made as part of the test construction and scoring processes. This confusion about the scope of the standard-setting process underscores the importance of (1) considering standard-setting implications when making decisions about test content and scoring, (2) ensuring that the standard-setting method selected is congruent with those decisions, and (3) explaining both these points to the experts who actually set the standards.

Table 3: An application of Angoff's method to the history checklist

Checklist Items	Weight Times Angoff Value
Description of pain	3 x .90 = 2.7
Associated symptoms	3 x .80 = 2.4
Previous episodes	3 x .70 = 2.1
Associated with exertion	3 x .90 = 2.7
History of blood pressure	3 x .60 = 1.8
Smoking	3 x .80 = 2.4
Family history of heart disease	3 x .90 = 2.7
Cholesterol	3 x .30 = 0.9
Medications	3 x .40 = 1.2
Provide probable diagnosis	3 x .80 = 2.4
Explain hospital safest	3 x .10 = 0.3
Family history of diabetes	2 x .50 = 1.0
Explain GI/cardiac pain are similar	2 x .50 = 1.0
Diet	1 x .40 = 0.4
Total possible score	38
Passing score	24

A sample history checklist for an SP with unstable angina. Each item on the checklist is given a weight of 1, 2, or 3 for a total of 38 points. To derive the standard, treat the average judgments as though they are an examinee's responses. Multiply the judges' averages by the weights and sum the products. Add the results for all the cases to derive the standard.

Third, some of the methods, especially those that produce relatively complex decision rules, are heavily based on the discussions and interactions that are idiosyncratic to a particular group of experts. Consequently, it is essential to determine if the rules the methods generate are replicated over time and by independent groups, as are the standards resulting from the more straightforward methods now used. Moreover, scores are typically aggregated across problems or cases in a straightforward fashion and then a single standard is applied. Some of the newer methods will result in conjunctive rules that make the pass/fail decision contingent on performance on a single, relatively unreliable exercise or case. Conjunctive rules require that each component is sufficiently reliable for decision-making.

Finally, the use of sophisticated statistical methods to derive standards may adversely affect the credibility of the result. They simultaneously require the user to claim the special expertise of the standard-setters but then change their judgments because they contain errors or do not fit particular mathematical models. Simpler methods enhance the ability to train the content experts to apply the method and make it easier to explain the results to examinees and other users of the results.

Table 4: An application of Ebel's method to the history checklist

Checklist Items	Weight Times Ebel Value
Description of pain	3 x .65 = 1.95
Associated symptoms	3 x .65 = 1.95
Previous episodes	3 x .65 = 1.95
Associated with exertion	3 x .65 = 1.95
History of blood pressure	3 x .65 = 1.95
Smoking	3 x .65 = 1.95
Family history of heart disease	3 x .65 = 1.95
Cholesterol	3 x .65 = 1.95
Medications	3 x .65 = 1.95
Provide probable diagnosis	3 x .65 = 1.95
Explain hospital safest	3 x .65 = 1.95
Family history of diabetes	2 x .55 = 1.10
Explain GI/cardiac pain are similar	2 x .55 = 1.10
Diet	1 x .35 = 0.35
Total possible score	38
Passing score	24

An application of Ebel's method to categories of items within a case. For all checklist items with a particular weight (e.g., all items weighted 3) the judges estimate the proportion of borderline examinees who would respond correctly. For each weight, average their judgments. To derive the standard, multiply the judges' averages by the weights and sum the products. Average the cases to derive the standard.

Absolute standards: judgments about individual items

The methods that produce absolute standards and require judgments about individual questions, Angoff's and Ebel's methods, can also be applied directly to cases or problems treated as items. For example, in Angoff's method the judges would be asked, "what score on this case would you expect the borderline examinee to get?" For Ebel's method, the cases or problems could be categorized in the same fashion as the MCQs and then judges could be asked, "what score on this category of cases would you expect the borderline examinee to get?"

It is also possible to collect judgments, with some modification, for individual items within cases or problems. Tables 3 and 4 illustrate applications of Angoff's and Ebel's method to a portion of a hypothetical standardized patient checklist. Application of Angoff's method in this fashion is very tedious and probably unnecessary. Ebel's method is less tedious, but it requires blanket judgments for sets of items that are not always alike.

Compromise methods: judgments about examinees and test content

The methods that produce compromise standards and require judgments both about groups of examinees and test content, such as Hofstee's method, can be directly applied following the steps outlined above. It does not require more effort to set standards on a clinical examination than an examination consisting of multiple choice questions.

COMBINING TESTS

Sometimes it is useful to combine several, related tests. If they all measure the same thing, treating them collectively will produce a very reliable result. It has the same effect as lengthening the test.

If the tests measure somewhat different concepts, treating them collectively will allow the development of a single score or decision that reflects a more complex construct. Whenever tests that measure different concepts are combined to predict a single criterion, they are called a *battery*. A test battery is preferable to a single test in this case because it can produce more reliable results and it permits the inclusion of different item formats that cannot be administered simultaneously (e.g., standardized patients and multiple choice questions, Anastasi, 1988).

For example, an examination for graduation from medical school might require assessments of clinical skills and medical knowledge. A standardized patient examination would be best to assess history taking and physical exam skills, while a test based on multiple choice questions is best to assess medical knowledge. To accommodate both of these formats in a single examination would be cumbersome, it would create logistic problems, and it would force a reduction in the number of test questions because of examinees' fatigue. Therefore, separate tests combined after administration are preferable.

When tests can be combined

A combined score is most useful when making a pass-fail decision, because its use promotes consistent decision making. This single score is an estimate of the test taker's ability along the construct measured by the battery. In the previous example, the combined score for the battery is the student's estimated achievement at the end of medical school.

Although the combined score should be used in decision making, individual test scores should also be reported to examinees and other stakeholders. It provides a richer profile of the individual, thus allowing an understanding of strengths and weaknesses that can, in turn, lead to continuing improvement of the individual and the educational program.

The rules for combining test scores should be devised and communicated to examinees before the tests are administered. This assures that examinees know how to focus their study efforts and the users of the scores understand their meaning. It also permits the development of predictions of performance on the combined test. For example, the student's grades during clerkship rotations might be predictive of performance on the standardized patient examination. This information, in advance of test administration, could be used by faculty and students to design a remediation process that would improve chances of success.

The length of combined tests

The more items on a test, the more reliable it is. However, there are practical constraints such as the resources to develop test material and examinee fatigue. Moreover, beyond a certain point, gains in reliability are minimal and not worth the effort to acquire them. Therefore, it is not necessarily advantageous to combine a large number of tests that measure the same concept. Combining tests should be considered only when one or more of them is too short to stand reliably on its own.

For a battery that combines measures of different constructs, there is also a practical limit on the number of tests that can reasonably be combined. In fact, combining many more than four tests measuring different concepts becomes unwieldy (Cronbach, 1990). Under such circumstances, it is helpful to identify only the most fundamental concepts and focus on them. For example, it may be better to devise a single test for knowledge of internal medicine rather than separate tests for cardiology, gastroenterology, endocrinology, and the like.

Rules for combining tests

There are two models for combining scores from different tests: compensatory and non-compensatory. In a compensatory model, test takers are allowed to make up for poor performance on one test in the battery with good performance on others. The most straightforward way to combine test scores in a compensatory fashion is to simply sum them. However, many users multiply each test score by a constant number or *weight* before summing them, which is an attempt to increase the relative importance of some of the tests in the combined score.

There are a variety of methods for generating weights. The most common is to ask experts in the field to use their judgment in selecting the weights. A second method is to develop the weights by selecting a criterion and applying a statistical technique such as multiple regression. Either method is acceptable, although the estimation of weights by experts is probably more credible. In neither instance, however, will the weights make a substantial difference in the scores of examinees. There is considerable work indicating that, as long as the signs of the weights (positive or negative) are correct, their magnitude makes little difference in the validity of the combined score (Dawes & Corrigan, 1974; Wainer, 1976).

In a non-compensatory model, test takers are required to perform to a standard on one or more of the tests in the battery. So, for example, the clinical skills and medical knowledge tests each have their own standard and, to graduate, a student must pass both tests. Therefore, good performance on the clinical skills test cannot make up for poor performance on the medical knowledge test, and vice versa.

There are any number of ways to combine tests in a non-compensatory fashion. For example, it is possible to set standards or score the battery based on a pattern of results. To pass, students may need to obtain very high grades on the history component of the standardized patient examination, less well on the physical exam component, but very well on the medical knowledge test.

Here are three different examples of passing rules:
1. "Pass" if the student scores greater than 80 on the clinical skills exam and greater than 70 in medical knowledge, otherwise "Fail".
2. "Pass" if candidate scores greater than 150 on both tests added together, otherwise "Fail".
3. "Pass" if candidate's total score is greater than 230, where the total score is equal to 2 times the clinical skills score plus the medical knowledge score, otherwise "Fail".

Example 1 is a non-compensatory model: the hurdle for clinical skills is 80 and the hurdle for medical knowledge is 70. This is also known as the method of multiple cutoff scores. Example 2 is a compensatory model where the candidate can make up for poor performance on the medical knowledge test with good performance on the clinical skills examination. Example 3 is also a compensatory model but here the clinical skills exam has twice the weight of the medical knowledge examination.

Simply doubling the weight is unlikely to have the desired effect and it would be more useful to actually double the length of the standardized patient examination.

Clearly, a mixed compensatory and non-compensatory model can also be developed. For example, a non-compensatory model may be used as a first stage and a compensatory model is used as a second stage. Multiple cutoffs are first applied to produce a field of candidates eligible for stage two scoring. In stage two, a weighted score could be developed and one of the standard-setting methods described above could be applied.

RECOMMENDATIONS FOR FUTURE RESEARCH

- Study methods for setting standards on clinical examinations.
- Study means for making the standard-setting process more efficient.
- Study the effects of group interactions on standards.
- Study the effects of expertise and content on standards.
- Study the effects of mixed compensatory and non-compensatory models.

IMPLEMENTATION GUIDELINES FOR SETTING STANDARDS: STEPS IN THE PROCESS

1. Decide on the type of standard: relative or absolute.
2. Decide on the method for setting standards.
   a. It should produce standards that are consistent with the purpose of the test.
   b. It should produce standards that are based on informed judgment.
   c. It should require due diligence.
   d. It should be supported by a body of research.
   e. It should be easy to explain and implement.
3. Select the judges.
   a. Select an appropriate number (at least 6-8 for high stakes testing).
   b. Select the characteristics the group should possess.
   c. Develop an efficient design for the exercise.
4. Hold the standard-setting meeting.
   a. Make sure all judges attend throughout.
   b. Explain the procedure and educate the judges about the consequences of their decisions.
   c. Discuss the purpose of the test, the nature of the examinees, and what constitutes adequate and inadequate skills/knowledge.
   d. Review the test in detail.
   e. Practice with a few items, cases, or examinees.
   f. Give feedback at several intervals.
5. Calculate the standard.
   a. Decide how to handle outliers, missing data, etc.

b. Ensure that the standard is reproducible.

c. Have a compromise standard available if possible.

6. After the test:

a. Check the results with stakeholders.

b. Check to see if the pass rates have reasonable relationships with other markers of competence.

c. Check to determine if the results related to future performance.

REFERENCES

Anastasi, A. (1988). *Psychological testing* (6th ed.). New York: Macmillan.

Angoff, W. H. (1971). Scales, norms, and equivalent scores. In R. L. Thorndike (Ed.), *Educational Measurement*. Washington, DC: American Council on Education.

Berk, R. A. (1986). A consumer's guide to setting performance standards on criterion-referenced tests. *Review of Educational Research, 56*, 137-172.

Brennan, R. L., & Lockwood, R. E. (1980). A comparison of the Nedelsky and Angoff cutting score procedures using generalizability theory. *Applied Psychological Measurement, 4*, 219-240.

Busch, J. C., & Jaeger, R. M. (1990). Influence of type of judge, normative information, and discussion on standards recommended for the National Teachers examinations. *Journal of Educational Measurement, 27*, 145-163.

Clauser, B. E., & Clyman, S. G. (1994). A contrasting-groups approach to standard setting for performance assessments on clinical skills. *Academic Medicine, 69*, S42-S44.

Cronbach, L. J. (1990). *Essentials of psychological testing* (5th ed.). New York: Harper Collins.

Cross, L. H., Impara, J. C., Frary, R. B., & Jaeger, R. M. (1984). A comparison of three methods for setting standards on the National Teachers Examination. *Journal of Educational Measurement, 21*, 113-129.

Cusimano, M. D. (1996). Standard setting in medical education. *Journal of Educational Measurement, 21*, 113-129.

Dawes, R. M., & Corrigan, R. (1974). Linear models in decision making. *Psychological Bulletin, 81*, 95-106.

De Gruijter, D. N. M. (1985). Compromise models for establishing examination standards. *Journal of Educational Measurement, 22*, 263-269.

Ebel, R. L. (1979). *Essentials of educational measurement*. Englewood Cliffs, NJ: Prentice-Hall.

Fabrey, L., & Raymond, M. (1987). Congruence of standard-setting methods for a nursing certification examination. Paper presented at the annual meeting of the National Council on Measurement in Education, Washington, DC.

Fitzpatrick, A. R. (1989). Social influences in standard setting. *Review of Educational Research, 59*, 222-235.

Glass, G. V. (1978). Standards and criteria. *Journal of Educational Measurement, 15*, 237-261.

Jaeger, R. M. (1989). Certification of student competence. In R. L. Linn (Ed.), *Educational Measurement* (pp. 485-514). New York: American Council on Education and Macmillan.

Jaeger, R. M. (1995). Setting performance standards through two-stage judgmental policy capturing. *Applied Measurement in Education, 8*, 15-40.

Kane, M. (1987). On the use of IRT models with judgmental standard-setting procedures. *Journal of Educational Measurement, 24*, 333-345.

Kane, M. (1994). Validating the performance standards associated with passing scores. *Review of Educational Research, 64*, 425-461.

Kane, M., & Wilson, J. (1984). Errors of measurement and standard setting in mastery testing. *Applied Psychological Measurement, 8*, 107-115.

Livingston, S. A., & Zeiky, M. J. (1982). Passing scores: A manual for setting standards of performance on educational and occupational tests. Educational Testing Service. Princeton, NJ.

Meskauskas, J. A. (1976). Evaluation models for criterion-referenced testing: Views regarding mastery and standard-setting. *Review of Educational Research, 45*, 133-158.

Mills, C. N., Jaeger, R. M., Plake, B. S., & Hambleton, R. K. (1998). An investigation of several new methods for establishing standards on complex performance assessments. Paper presented at the annual meeting of the American Educational Research Association, San Diego, CA.

Norcini, J. J. (1992). Approaches to standard-setting for performance-based examinations. In R. M. Harden, I. R. Hart, & M. A. Mulholland (Eds.), *Approaches to the assessment of clinical competence Part 1* (pp. 32-37). Dundee, Scotland: Centre for Medical Education.

Norcini, J. J. (1999). Standards and reliability: When rules of thumb don't apply. *Academic Medicine, 74,* 1088-1090.

Norcini, J. J., & Shea, J. A. (1992). The reproducibility of standards over groups and occasions. *Applied Measurement in Education, 5,* 63-72.

Norcini, J. J., & Shea, J. A. (1997). The credibility and comparability of standards. *Applied Measurement in Education, 10,* 39-59.

Norcini, J. J., Lipner, R. S., Langdon, L. O., & Strecker, C. A. (1987). A comparison of three variations on a standard-setting method. *Journal of Educational Measurement, 24,* 56-64.

Norcini, J. J., Maihoff, N. A., Day, S. C., & Benson, Jr., J. A. (1989). Trends in medical knowledge as assessed by the certifying examination in internal medicine. *Journal of the American Medical Association, 262,* 2402-2404.

Norcini, J. J., Shea, J. A., & Kanya, D. T. (1988). The effect of various factors on standard-setting. *Journal of Educational Measurement, 25,* 57-65.

Norcini, J. J., Shea, J. A., & Ping, J. C. (1988). A note on application of multiple matrix sampling to standard-setting. *Journal of Educational Measurement, 25,* 159-164.

Norcini, J. J., Shea, J. A., & Webster, G. D. (1986). Perceptions of the certification standards of the American Board of Internal Medicine. *Journal of General Internal Medicine, 1,* 166-169.

Orr, N. A., & Nungester, R.L. (1991). Assessment of constituency opinion about NBME examination standards. *Academic Medicine, 66,* 465-470.

Petersen, N. S., Kolen, M. J., & Hoover, H. D. (1989). Scaling norming and equating. In R. L. Linn (Ed.), *Education measurement* (pp. 221-262). New York: American Council on Education and Macmillan.

Plake, B. S, Impara, J. C., & Potenza, M. T. (1994). Content specificity of expert judgments in a standard-setting study. *Journal of Educational Measurement, 31,* 339-347.

Popham, W. J. (1978). As always provocative. *Journal of Educational Measurement, 15,* 297-300.

Putnam, S. E., Pence, P., & Jaeger, R. M. (1995). A multi-stage dominant profile method for setting standards on complex performance assessments. *Applied Measurement in Education, 8,* 57-84.

Ramsey, P. G., Carline, J. D., Inui, T. S., Larson, E. B., LoGerfo, J. P., & Wenrich, M. D. (1989). Predictive validity of certification by the American Board of Internal Medicine. *Annals of Internal Medicine, 110,* 719-726.

Shea, J. A., Reshetar, R. A., Dawson, B. D., & Norcini, J. J. (1994). Sensitivity of the modified Angoff standard-setting method to variations in item content. *Teaching and Learning in Medicine, 6,* 288-292.

Shepard, L. A. (1980). Standard setting issues and methods. *Applied Psychological Measurement, 4,* 447-467.

Shepard, L. A. (1984). Setting performance standards. In R. A. Berk (Ed.), *A guide to criterion-referenced test construction* (pp. 169-198). Baltimore: Johns Hopkins Press.

Shimberg, B. (1981). Testing for licensure and certification. *American Psychologist, 36,* 1138-1146.

Smith, R. L., & Smith, J. K. (1988). Differential use of item information by judges using Angoff and Nedelsky procedures. *Journal of Educational Measurement, 25,* 259-274.

Van der Linden, W. J. (1982). A latent trait method for determining intrajudge inconsistency in the Angoff and Nedelsky procedures. *Journal of Educational Measurement, 19,* 295-308.

Wang, M. W., & Stanley, J. C. (1970). Differential weighting: A review of methods and empirical studies. *Review of Educational Research, 4,* 663-705.

Wainer, H. (1976). Estimating coefficients in liner models: It don't make no nevermind. *Psychological Bulletin, 83*(2), 213-217.

26 Licensure and Certification

W. DALE DAUPHINEE
Medical Council of Canada

SUMMARY

This chapter addresses the issues of licensure and assessment from two perspectives. The concepts and processes of licensure are traced from their beginnings to the present time. The other perspective deals with the approach to assessment for licensure and certification.

The first portion of the chapter begins with a historical survey of the origins, including debates and socio-political changes from which current notions of licensure and certification emerged. This background identifies the reasons why society and the courts have directed that the processes be conducted as they are today. Principles and policies do not occur in a social vacuum. Hence the key principles and societal values, as well as their social conduct, are identified, thereby demonstrating the iterative development of licensure and certification over time.

The second portion of the chapter reviews key concepts and notions that underlie the assessment processes used in licensure and certification. They too are iterative in their development. Attention has been focused on key articles and writings that delineate that which is acceptable by current standards.

Each one of those methods thereby informs the reader about the critical concepts, principles and possible shortcomings of current assessment methods, hopefully directing users to the most suitable approaches to the evaluation of physicians for licensure and certification.

INTRODUCTION

"License n. official permission to own/to do something/carry on a trade."
(Concise Oxford Dictionary)

"Certificate n. a formal document attesting to a fact/fulfillment of requirements."
(Concise Oxford Dictionary)

International Handbook of Research in Medical Education, 835–882.
G.R. Norman, C.P.M. Van der Vleuten, D.I. Newble (eds.)
© 2002 *Dordrecht: Kluwer Academic Publishers. Printed in Great Britain.*

The words license and certificate are frequently used in daily conversation. We speak of "a license to operate an automobile", or, "a physician's certificate excusing one from school". But in the field of health professional education and training, these two commonly used words have taken on very specific and different meanings. When health professionals speak of license, they refer to the outcome of the process of licensure and when they speak of certificate, they refer to the outcome in a certification process. Both processes represent forms of assessment and credentialing, designed to identify each individual's competence in a particular area of practice, and are usually based on predetermined criteria. Nielsen differentiates the two processes by denoting licensure as being mandatory and certification as being voluntary (Nielsen et al., 1990). Mueller has used two very simple headings to convey the basic notions of medical licensure and certification (Mueller, 1985). Licensure and license: the privilege to practice medicine; certification: the mark of special competence.

In the western world, particularly in North America, the two words refer to two distinctly different processes. In the fields of medicine and nursing, for example, licensure refers to the basic qualification process that must be successfully completed before entering the practice of that profession. It is mandatory. Mueller notes that

"... licensure is the process by which society, acting through a government agency or an agency authorised by government, grants permission to an individual to engage in a given occupation or use a particular title." *(Mueller, 1985, p. 311)*

In contrast, certification refers to another level of qualification, typically in a specialty or even sub-specialty of medicine or nursing, but it may or may not be required as a prerequisite for licensure. In this instance, Mueller quotes from a National Board of Medical Examiners' glossary that defines certification as

"... the process by which a governmental agency or an association grants recognition to an individual who has met certain predetermined qualifications specified by that agency or association." *(Mueller, 1985, p. 318)*

In this chapter, these words will refer to the basic qualification required to practice a health profession (licensure) and the attestation of specialized competence in a particular area or subset of clinical practice in one of the health professions (certification). It must also be recognized that, in some jurisdictions, the process of "registration" is synonymous with licensure. Examples are the United Kingdom and Australia.

An appreciation of the history of licensure and certification is necessary in order to understand their evolution as professional and legal tenets and to correctly apply them to current measurement and legal processes. As will be seen, licensure, in particular, is anchored in concepts of regulation dating back to ancient times. The current notions of certification and licensure grew out of years of practical politics that led to the underlying but not explicitly defined social contract that health professionals have with society. Of the two, certification is a more recent concept, having grown out of increasing self-awareness of the profession as the hospital developed in the late 1800s and provided a new focus to health care in America (Stevens, 1971).

DEVELOPMENT OF THE CONCEPTS

History of licensure

To pursue the origins and evolution of the notion of licensure, one must begin in ancient times and travel through the centuries to the Middle Ages when, according to Sigerist, medical licensure became common in Europe (Sigerist, 1935). Thus, the trail of developments starts in the time of Hammurabi, through antiquity to the first medical legislation in the West by King Roger of Sicily in the thirteenth century and onward through influence of the Church, the Medieval Guilds and the early universities.

Many begin the story of licensure with Hammurabi. It is clearly documented that Hammurabi's Code listed fees for successful therapies but also punishments for treatment failures. However, we know very little about either the extent or manner in which the laws were enforced. Clearly, they were not developed or imposed from within the profession. The ancient Greek practitioners were faced with a different approach. Burns has argued that the Hippocratic Treatise *Law* was

> "a principal mode of social evaluation, its absence would have meant that there was no generally accepted standard of professional reputation in the Greek city-states." *(Burns, 1977, p. 1)*

In fact, Burns notes that there were no state penalties for unethical practitioners, whom he viewed as *"those who were ignorant"*. There was only the penalty of dishonor. This notion introduces the idea of the ethic of competence, which other authors have proposed as possibly the main contribution of Hippocratic oath, and by implication, the immorality of ignorance.

But the "anatomy" of the ancient licensure laws and requirements does not provide the underlying ideas and concepts, such as competence, that are so pivotal to the notion of licensure today. To develop the significance of the concept of competence, one needs to examine more closely the early Greek times and acquire another view of the significance of Hippocrates. The notion of the inappropriateness of ignorance in the practitioner has been proposed as a fundamental contribution of the Hippocratic period of medicine. Jonsen has suggested that the Hippocratic maxim *"be of benefit and do no harm"* implied the imperative of competence (Jonsen, 1990). Jonsen believes this to be the major contribution of the Hippocratic period and its oath.

By medieval times, when medicine was adopted as a university subject and as a guild activity in the Middle Ages, competence became an explicit virtue.

Competence at that time implied the mastery of knowledge of theories and practitioner observations that were "enshrined" in the writings of the classic medical authors. This was the context of the Greek millennium (500 BC to AD 500) and was to be carried for the next thirteen hundred years when medicine retreated to the monasteries and when monks and other clergy, while still referring to the Greek sources, wrote in Latin. Thus, Latin was the language of medicine until the sixteenth century.

The next stop on the trail of the concept of licensure takes one to medieval medicine which can be divided into two periods: the so-called dark ages, or the period of monastic medicine, and the second half or scholastic period. The significance of the monastic period is that it was the last refuge of learning when the knowledge of medicine became the realm of the priests. The distinction between their religious and medical roles was clear: medicine was only accessory to their sacred mission (Ackerknecht, 1982). A good example of this relationship is Hildegard of Bingen, a twelfth-century abbess, whose music is currently experiencing a revival on Compact Disc amongst early music lovers. She emphasized that it was important to strengthen the body to withstand attacks by the devil! (Ackerknecht, 1982). Following the Council of Clermont in 1130, the practice of medicine by monks was forbidden, as it was seen to be in conflict with the monks' primary role and medicine fell to the secular clergy. The significance of this change was that medicine was to be taught in schools and the newly emerging universities in the cities of the later Middle Ages, hence the name – the scholastic period. It also marked the influence of Arab authors on medicine and, with it, came the medical lore of Greek Medicine. Thus it is not surprising that Salerno near Arab Sicily became the first outstanding medical medieval university in Europe, followed by others like Montpelier, which was close to Spain (Ackerknecht, 1982).

The universities provided the scholastic standards that had not hitherto existed and which would dominate Europe for the foreseeable future. The idea of setting standards was thus linked to centers of learning and universities, but not in the formats of learning and discovery as we know it today (Ackerknecht, 1982). The study of medicine remained centered in the library and not the laboratory.

The legal regulation of the profession appears again in the Middle Ages when the title of "doctor" first appears. King Roger II of Sicily introduced the first instance of legislation dealing with the practice of medicine in 1140, and it included the need for examinations. King Frederick II expanded the scope of that legislation in 1224. It has been suggested that medical standards in the form of a licensure decree from Frederick II came only after a medical curriculum was defined and established at Salerno (Hartung, 1934). But most Western political authorities did not have licensure policies, which can be considered surprising as other laws did emerge at that time (Burns, 1977). An explanation is that there were no structures or organizations to monitor or develop the criteria for standards or, for that matter, even to interpret them in their application.

This latter point requires emphasis, as one takes a journey through the history of regulation. To be effective, any regulatory body or political authority must develop linkages between its infrastructures that establish criteria or standards; that in turn monitor the processes; and then administer them. Otherwise, any law or regulation is inoperable and therefore socially meaningless. As will be discussed later, the interplay of the authority given via the state and the profession's obligations to regulate itself or be regulated is critical. One without the other is insufficient.

Although rare, by the late 1280s, similar laws did exist in other areas of Italy and in certain German speaking states. Later, French kings began to issue decrees that supported regulatory efforts of the medical faculties such as at Paris, while Montpelier had licensure carried out as a joint responsibility of the church officials and the faculty itself (Burns, 1977).

Often, the licensure of physicians and surgeons differed. For example, surgeons were often members of guilds and were considered craftsmen. In part this may have been due to the fact that the church did not approve of monks and clerics being involved with the shedding of blood, for the reasons noted previously following the ruling of 1130. Thus the surgeons were neither university graduates nor ecclesiastics. Physicians were treated differently as early as the thirteenth century when their licensure often evolved from faculties in the universities. A good example was Salerno, the first faculty to license physicians (Derbyshire, 1979). At that time, surgeons were trained via a system of apprenticeship and had to pass examinations before joining a surgical guild. If there were too few for a surgical guild, they might join other guilds like the blacksmiths because they made their own instruments!

Thus one has seen the evolution to the guilds: from professional education and licensure being monitored via the church and later the universities to the origin of licensure in the late Middle Ages.

The first provision for licensure in England occurred in 1511, beginning with examinations administered by the local Diocesan bishop and then, in 1518, to one of self-regulation by the Royal College of Physicians, after which Parliament confirmed its charter in 1522. Licenses also existed for midwives. The principle was simple, to quote Burns: *"Any person had the right to practice medicine and a person had the right to seek medical attention from another person"* (Burns, 1977, p. 10).

And the principle of individual liberty remained paramount in England well into the nineteenth century. In 1858, the Medical Act required that a person proclaiming to be a physician had to demonstrate evidence of appropriate qualifications from educational institutions in order to have one's name entered in the national registry as a qualified physician. Thereby, patients and society could differentiate who was qualified and who was not.

This was a significant development. It pointed out that while an act gives authority to the professions to self-regulate, it clearly requires a reciprocal demonstration or submission of evidence to justify designating an individual as a qualified physician. Clearly, a bargain is implied and under the purview of parliament or another legislative body, the act or regulation also serves to ensure that the public's interest in the bargain is maintained by the profession.

In North America, professional accreditation began with the Medical Practice Act in Virginia in 1639 and was followed in 1649 by an attempt to regulate "Chirurgeons, Midwives and Physitians" by law in Massachusetts (Shyryock, 1967). The first medical licensing legislation, in what was to become Canada, was enacted by the Intendant Ingot in Quebec in 1750 (Kerr, 1979). The North American scene was different in its orientation than in England. The states brought forward more restrictive forms of laws to deal with medical licensure. In 1772, New Jersey and later in 1808, the Territory of Louisiana passed laws that restricted the practice of medicine to those physicians who were examined by the local medical society in the case of New Jersey, and by a medical committee in New Orleans (Burns, 1997). Again, whether or not these laws were effective is not clear.

The partnerships that were emerging between states and the profession in the United States of America grew until the time of President Jackson. At that time, objections to regulation in American society increased, in rhetoric, as McGuire has pointed out, remarkably similar to that heard recently: restraint of trade; protecting the economic interests of special groups or private associations; inhibiting the introduction and application of unorthodox ideas or treatments (McGuire, 1997). And so the trend continued until the mid-eighteenth century when licensure was non-existent in the United States of America. The consequences were significant: medical degree "factories", fraudulent therapy claims, and purchasable degrees, to mention but a few examples. As will be described later, the founding of the American Medical Association (AMA) in 1847 became the turning point. One of its principal objectives was to push for structures and mechanisms that could establish and apply badly needed standards in medical practice and education. However, another critical event was a Supreme Court decision in 1889. In Dent versus West Virginia, the Court upheld the state's requirements for training and credentialing for medical licensure. Thus ended an era wherein any person could claim the constitutional right to practice a profession, regardless of qualification or preparation. In America, the tide had turned!

The other jurisdictions that greatly influenced western medicine were the German states and Austria. Sigerist summarized the approach to licensure in Prussia and Austria (Sigerist, 1935). Until 1725, a Masters degree from a medical faculty was sufficient to practice in Prussia. Starting in 1725, an individual with a Masters degree had to take a course in anatomy and pass a "casus medico-practico" with the state board of health. Thus it was that the right of licensure passed from the university to the state. In reality, all physicians were examined twice: for their medical degree and then by the state for a license. After unification, a state license gave the privilege of licensure in other states in Germany. However, it was also decided that the most qualified, namely the university professors, should constitute the state board of examiners which in effect avoided the previous two examination formats. Thus after seven hundred years, there was a return to the format of Frederick II. In Austria, in 1749, the right to examine for licensure was taken from the universities and was given to the state director of studies, even though the examinations were still given by university faculty.

The intent of this section has been to establish certain principles that lie behind modern licensure of physicians and provide a model for other professions. The ethic of competence begins early in the time of Hippocrates. Later, a clearly implied tension between the two notions of self-interest and moral obligations of monastic influences characterized an evolving professional creed in the Middle Ages. The evolution of three elements has been traced: the fundamental notion of competence; the tension of self-interest and altruism; and their linkage with the application of laws by the state to regulate the profession or ensure protection of the public by national registration mechanisms. The role of universities in the survival of medical knowledge, such as it was, has been identified, as has been their role in setting standards in Middle Ages. And finally the role of the guilds was outlined. All of these influences come to bear on the contemporary notion of licensure in many parts of the world: particularly in North America, Australasia and much of Europe.

Finally, the interplay of forces that have led to self-regulation has been identified. It requires more than altruism, professional creeds and the ethic of competence. It requires a bargain with society, variously defined by law or regulation on behalf of society, to accomplish the terms. As will be noted in the next section, there are many variations and many social and cultural influences that will define those bargains in each jurisdiction.

Influences on professional regulation

Having described the historical elements of medical licensure as a form of professional regulation that is shared by many professions, it is important to appreciate the current notions of this regulation from three perspectives: as legal processes; as sociological phenomena; and as a professional obligation. As has been cited, the beginnings of self-regulation began in England with the Royal College of Physicians in the sixteenth century. However, other models exist besides the self-regulatory model. One could outline the possible models of regulation as: self-regulation; state regulation; and economic models. As has been developed earlier in this review, regulation of the profession is complex in its history and in the interplay of the various socio-economic influences. Perhaps one should not imply that there are distinct models, as much as there are variations amongst which many influences are variously dominant within any national or local framework. And in reality, these relationships are continuing to evolve today. A wonderful example of the interplay of these influences is offered in Klein's discussion of the recent evolution of the profession and the state in the National Health Service in the UK, subtitled "the politics of the double bed" (Klein, 1990).

One of the most widely applied approaches to medical licensure is self-regulation. It is being challenged in many jurisdictions, not because of the concept, but rather because of loss of trust in its current effectiveness or the issue of increasing costs (Stacey, 1997; Cruess & Cruess, 1997). The concept of medical self-regulation has been reviewed by Stacey (Stacey, 1997). She notes that most professions are not self-regulated and in fact almost no examples exist that are "pure" self-regulatory. The formal characteristics of a self-regulated profession are beyond the scope of this overview but have been well reviewed again by Stacey (1997) and by Cruess and Cruess (1997). But the main point to be emphasized is that wherever the concept of self-regulation is put forward, the notion of what MacDonald has called the "regulative bargain" must be explicitly understood and honored (MacDonald, 1995). The privilege of self-regulation is granted in return for the promise of a physician's special obligation towards the client, to be trustworthy and, for the common good of society, to be honest and upright citizens. Ethicists would emphasize the notions of doing good (beneficence) and causing no harm (maleficence) as part of the special obligations (Cruess & Cruess, 1997). In return, the profession is "granted" certain privileges: a near monopoly in the market place, autonomy in practice, and the facility to regulate their conditions of work and practice (Stacey, 1997). Stacey goes on to note that, as part of the bargain for these special privileges, professionals must promise to be competent and trustworthy, such that all who seek their advice and counsel, can do so with confidence (Stacey, 1997). Thus, the promise commits all who enter the profession to be well prepared and competently trained. This is the "regulative bargain" for the privilege of self-regulation.

Other models include greater involvement of either the state or of economic influences. But even within the self-regulatory model, both of these factors have impacts. The relatively recent book edited by Hafferty and McKinley examines these aspects (Hafferty & McKinley, 1993). Their book offers several case examples, by country, to illustrate these relationships. In particular, Chapter 2 on Medical Profession and the State, by Frenk and Ruran-Arenas, is an excellent politico-sociological analysis of these changing relationships as the world moves towards a more global economic system, and as the state becomes increasingly involved in regulation, financing and delivery of care (Frenk & Ruran-Arenas, 1993). They define a framework based on the political and economic dimensions versus the type of relationship between the professional (internal) factors and external factors, like relationship with the state or market forces. Thus, the state has a strong political influence in Scandinavian countries but is challenged with a strong and powerful professional association; whereas in France and most other western European countries, the state political power is weaker and the role of professional associations is powerful, but in these times of change, the latter may be susceptible to weakening. The economic influences in the United States of America under managed care are another example of a changing picture of professional regulation. While the traditional models of regulation: self-regulation and state regulation (and combinations thereof), may be seen as in evolution, there is new emphasis on economic considerations with state, and maybe even state-professional collusion.

Thus, while one may think of pure models of regulation like self-regulation and a state-directed approach, as seen in the Soviet bloc in the previous century, the influences emerging from changing economic and political structures, as well as fiscal policies, are making for more complex inter-relationships. The impact of the European Community is a perfect example. The reality is that no model is pure. There are only gradations of influences and power in the regulatory mechanisms of most western nations. In the United States of America, which appears to be "pure" self-regulatory, the influence of the state in issues is clear. For example, the direct financing of aspects of medical education and medical research and, indirectly, education via teaching hospitals, has had a major impact on the profession in terms of numbers and types of physicians and, therefore, the profession's ultimate influence.

To return to Stacey's viewpoint, there is good evidence that "*the kind of state and its surrounding culture influenced the way professions arose and the amount of self-regulation achieved*" (Stacey, 1997, p. 21). For example, attitudes towards commerce matter, as we see in the United States of America around the patenting of genes by physician scientists. A key notion has been raised by Stacey that "Strong state control does not necessarily mean lack of self-regulatory power." The nature of the state can influence or "modify" the self-regulatory process by the ways in which it is promoted or curtailed. Thus, she notes that being too near to the state can be as deleterious as being too near commerce, and both can lead to "malfunction" of the self-regulatory processes. These are complex inter-relationships and each context must be viewed separately. As a wise person said about medical schools, if you have seen one medical school, you have seen one medical school. The proof is in the specifics, the checks and balances, not in the generalizations from applications of models elsewhere.

Possible confounders in the self-regulation process

While many authors would extol the virtues of self-regulation and the advantages of its natural tensions of self-interest and altruism, there is need to consider the down sides: possible misuses and the powerful responsibilities that are inherent in a self-regulating profession. They are potential confounders in the licensure process too, if it is abused for other interests. Two possible and oft cited co-founders reflect the possible intrusion of excess self-interest in licensure and regulation: entry control and boundary drawing. As one considers licensure and certification process in a self-regulatory environment, it is crucial to appreciate potential misuses of the process.

Again Stacey has offered a concise and clear view of these issues (Stacey, 1997). Her outline of possible arguments against professional self-regulation focuses on *entry control* and *boundary drawing* as misdirected examples of self-regulation. The best example of entry control is the exclusion of women from entry into medicine for years in countries like the United Kingdom, United States of America and Canada. While the rationale was supposedly scientific (on the basis of female physiology), it was not defensible. The issue of boundary drawing is interesting as it is often more subtle. It has been argued that professional privilege has been used to place other health professions in a subordinate relationship with medicine: nursing being an example. It is postulated that the same relationship developed with other emerging health professions over the years. Midwives would be an example. But, even within the profession, the issues of territoriality in special competencies can result in defining boundaries that were not the intent of the regulatory bargain. Some examples of these latter problems will be noted in the discussion of the evolution of certification.

In some cases it can be pointed out that there can be collusion with other agencies, including payers and the state to serve another master's interests. These are interests that must be recognized as not part of the "bargain". In fact, some argue that by delegating the power over the process of regulation to professional associations or structures, is a potential source/opportunity for collusion. The voluntary turning over of the responsibility to associations, like Boards or Councils, has been described as having the fox guard the hen house! A particular proponent of that view is Morrison (Morrison, 1992). His arguments about collusion are worthy of noting. In particular, the questioning of the benefits to society in terms of the public's perception of the quality of medical service is a significant challenge to the medical profession and, for that matter, any regulated profession.

Origins of specialty certification

The notion of the certification of medical specialists, as it has been defined for this review, is clearly tied to the development of specialty training and practice in the United States of America. Specialty certifying boards "*... are distinctly American, forged by a distinctly American history*" (Stevens, 1999, p. 9).

After the Civil War a profound change came over American medicine. The War had slowed any national approach to problems like medical associations, as one might obviously expect. There was nothing that was the equivalent of the Royal Colleges in Britain. Yet, there were pressures for national academies (Stevens, 1971). Even after the founding of the American Medical Association (AMA), the notion of establishing a national academy of medicine or a similar structure was considered but did not happen. At the same time, independent of the tensions in the country, an important sociological phenomenon appeared during the last half of the nineteenth century in the United States of America. Stevens has referred to it as the "growth of self-awareness": a desire for "*comparative distinction among his peers*" (Stevens, 1971, p. 34). There also emerged a push for more scientific medicine and standardization, the culmination of which is best represented by the Flexner Report on Medical Schools in 1910 (Flexner, 1910). But the standardization was also symbolic of an AMA desire for egalitarianism: a trend to see a common standard for entry into practice and, once that was attained, all physicians were to be seen as equal. But there were British influences. There, although a common standard was being established, once institutional appointments were sought, additional qualifications mattered. Those who finished the core medical program then chose to be a surgeon or a physician, in order to be different from the general practitioner. As Stevens has put it, though there was a common pathway through a national registry, there was not standardization.

However, the lack of Royal Colleges, or their equivalent, in the United States of America, meant that American medicine was less hospital-based and surgeons and physicians did not automatically belong to different groups. Thus the stimulus for and response to specialism was to be different in the United States of America. The influence of Americans traveling to Germany and Vienna for extra training was to have an impact. Issues first arose around the advertising of specialist's skills in the 1850-1860s. Yet there was a gap developing between the potential of medical science and the knowledge typically applied in the field. A new technical medical elite was emerging and debates continued around whether a specialist was one who, by self-imposition, restricted practice to a narrow area or not. Specialist associations began to appear in the late 1880s, starting with the American Ophthalmological Society in 1864. In the 1870s, larger hospitals began to recognize specialist interests in the outpatient departments, beyond the previously existing inpatient units, such as maternity or children's wards. Doctors were often designated as a surgeon or physician. The great American specialty clinics began to emerge: Mayo, Ochsner, etc. The emergence of the battle over the status of these specialty clinics came much later in America because hospitals were slower to develop than in Europe. The establishment of outpatient clinics in Britain resulted in a feud between specialists and generalists that was eventually resolved when the notion of a referral system between specialists and general physicians became formalized between 1880 and 1914 (Stevens, 1986).

As events moved to the early twentieth century, many of the reforms that the AMA had sought to achieve were accomplished. Standardization was then evident. The licensing authorities had formed a national organization. The Flexnor Report had been published in 1910. The National Board of Medical Examiners (NBME) had been formed in 1915. These changes leading to standardization were accomplished mainly by the use of strict state controls (Stevens, 1971). By World War I, licensure was state based and the AMA was pursuing an egalitarian approach (Stevens, 1986). Unlike the United Kingdom, where specialism was manifest through the Royal Colleges, an extension of the old guilds, analogous structures did not formally exist in the United States of America. They would take a few decades to evolve.

But another era was about to begin with the appearance of new organizations that would lead directly to the birth of Specialty Boards in the United States of America.

The influences in the United States of America would differ from the United Kingdom. Surgeons were already developing a high profile in the United States of America, unlike the United Kingdom where physicians were held in higher regard than surgeons. American physician groups followed another route to "elevate their status": the model of the German clinics that emphasized careful investigation, logic, and exact methods. William Osler symbolized the physicians' challenge to the impressive practicality of surgery at that time, by emphasizing facts (pathology) and skills (diagnostic acumen) (Stevens, 1986).

The greater status of the surgeon compared to the physician in the United States of America was typified by the founding of the American College of Surgery in 1913: the first national elite in the United States of America that was comparable to the Royal Colleges in Britain. Its membership was focused on the medical schools and their distinguished faculty, again as had happened in Germany. They did not focus on the politics of regulation initially (Holden, 1979). The first elite group of physicians had organized themselves as the Association of American Physicians in 1885. They focused on the promotion of learning and improvement of medicine through scientific research, but they were not politically active. However, in his presidential address in 1885, Osler did call for the recognition of internal medicine as a specialty. Even with the emergence of the American College of Physicians in 1915, the formal recognition of Internal Medicine as a specialty was to wait until 1936 with the founding of the American Board of Internal Medicine (Stevens, 1986).

In the meantime, the major impetus for specialty certification in the United States of America really arose out of the need to define and to regulate the practice of surgery (Holden, 1979; Stevens, 1986). Without the events in Britain that regulated surgery by the recognition of the specialty via the Royal College and hospital appointments, this fell to the American College of Surgeons and was echoed by the appearance of the American Board of Ophthalmology in 1917 (Stevens, 1986).

Another impetus arose out of the AMA Council on Medical Education in 1920. It formed 15 specialty subcommittees from specialty societies and university groups to set criteria for the quality of undergraduate and postgraduate medical education (Stevens, 1986). Many of these committees would in time serve as the nidus for their particular specialty boards.

Other specialty boards were to follow in the 1930s (Stevens, 1971; Holden, 1979). Stevens notes that the boards served two broad goals:
1. To establish standards of quality in fields that were targets for general practitioners.
2. To establish monopolies on emerging specialists' techniques.
Overall, the intent was to establish certification requirements that would in turn raise their member's prestige above that of the generalists and assure them of opportunities and significant roles in the medical schools.

The subsequent evolution of the Specialty Boards in the United States, including the overall role of the American Board of Medical Specialties, has been well described by both Stevens (1971) and Holden (1979).

Developments of specialty certification in other countries followed similar lines. In Canada, one Royal College was founded in 1929 with two sections, surgery and medicine, but within those structures, it now certifies specialists in over 51 fields. In Australasia, there are some 16 separate Colleges that certify in the various specialties.

In Germany, which we have noted had a great influence on the development of institution-based specialty practice and training in America, certification is accomplished via Facharzt Prüfung and additive certificates. This system of "certification" is university-based and is skill- and procedure-oriented.

Current approaches and trends in regulation

Building on the previous discussion of regulation, it is worthwhile to examine some current trends in regulation. The reader is referred to Klein (1993) for an overview. The case studies in the same book by Hafferty and McKinlay (1993) are drawn to the attention of the reader as well. While primarily a sociological view of the profession of medicine that reassesses its recent dominance, the case studies provide a good background for emerging issues related to the profession's current interactions with the state and society in many sectors of the world.

Klein's analysis is sociological, but with a political perspective. He focuses on the relationship between the state (government) and the profession: identifying the resources which each commands/influences and the institutional structures/framework in which the group/organization functions. Using the distinction between diffuse and concentrated influences and interests, he notes four basic models.

1. The American model demonstrates a concentrated profession and a diffuse state influence. The inability to mobilize forces politically to deal with any opposition (e.g. insurance industry or certain sectors of the profession) to national health plans is an example.
2. Britain could be characterized as concentrated state and concentrated profession influences. In this instance one sees mutual accommodation as an operating mode, for example, over health policies.
3. France has a diffuse profession pitted against a concentrated state influence. Often government gets its way, but interestingly, the public's philosophy about health matters prevails and guides the final policy decisions.
4. The fourth model is a diffuse state and a diffuse profession. That results, as Klein notes, in uncoordinated policy making.

There are variations on these models and other influences worth noting. For example, which stakeholders does government see as "at the table"? In many countries like France, the United Kingdom, Germany and Canada, the medical

individual has attained basic qualifications before entering the practice of medicine. Perhaps the best discussion of the intent of the license is covered in the first of Sir Donald Irvine's articles on "the performance of doctors" (Irvine, 1997). He defines three characteristics of a medical professional: expertise, ethics and service. Currently, there is great interest not only in the entry-level qualifications of physicians, but in a more careful assessment of the on-going performance of doctors (Irvine, 1997; Dauphinee, 1995). In fact, Irvine calls for a new agreement between the profession and society with respect to the changing times and the demand and need for greater accountability. This will be discussed in more detail shortly.

However, this brief account of the changing demands on the profession serves to focus on the types of licensure and on the approach to assessment used in two contexts: initial and on-going assessment.

Licensure is given to those who meet the qualification requirements. These requirements may vary from circumstance to circumstance, and from one jurisdiction to another. However, certain generalizations can be made to provide guidelines to the reader. License usually refers to an entry-level license to practice medicine without restrictions in regard to location or type of practice. Additional requirements may exist in certain jurisdictions with regard to more specialized types of practice, but in most jurisdictions the issuance of a license is typically based on the initial processes that assess candidates' abilities for unrestricted general medical practice.

Furthermore, in many jurisdictions, pre-licensure registration with local licensing authorities may be needed, depending on the geographic circumstances and the temporal position of the individual in the educational process. Thus, students in medical school or individuals in a postgraduate training program may need to have an "educational" license or be on an "educational" or "provisional" register with the local licensing authority to be "eligible" for patient contact. Similarly, "restricted" licenses or "limited registration" mechanisms often exist for those physicians who may in some way not meet all requirements for the usual license or unrestricted license. In those circumstances, not surprisingly, these individuals are referred to as holding a permit, registration, or license that is "restricted" or "limited". The restrictions imposed on such individuals are typically with respect to location of practice or scope of practice. Thus, an individual may be fully qualified as a specialist in another part of the world but comes to another jurisdiction to work in a narrowly focused area. That practitioner's practice could be "restricted" to a specific field and in a specific location until such time as he or she takes the steps necessary to meet the requirements for the unrestricted license. Typically, many variations exist with respect to the types of restricted license, depending on the need and purpose. For example, visiting clinical professors, who are fully qualified in their country, could be registered on a temporary register while teaching at a medical school in another country.

The length of licensure is typically for life, barring problems with expertise (competence), fitness to practice, or other misconduct findings. Sanctions from disciplinary actions by the licensing process and decisions by the courts or other judicial bodies may also influence licensure process in most jurisdictions, particularly if it involves criminal acts. In such cases a hearing must be conducted by the licensing authorities, as the actions of another body do not automatically dictate the licensure processes. However, licensure for life has changed in many jurisdictions and now on-going requirements have been added that must be met regularly. The detailed consideration of these "maintenance" requirements is beyond the scope of this review, but the approach to the on-going assessment of practicing physicians will be covered shortly.

The assessment of any physician for licensure entails two distinct processes. The first is the credentialing process that in turn involves two steps: verification of all documents as authentic and valid; and the assessment by credentialing agents that the documentation and training meets the criteria of the licensing bodies to which the physician is applying. The second process involves the formal assessment of the individual's attributes such as skills, attitudes and knowledge. The credentialing process, including certain verification steps and an assessment of all previously held credentials, will not be covered in this chapter. One aspect of the process that is topical is the role of possible reciprocity and/or mutual recognition by one jurisdiction of another jurisdiction's process as equivalent to theirs. While it is beyond the primary purpose of this chapter, suffice to say that reciprocity and mutual recognition can be fraught with legal challenges if the criteria for such arrangements can be deemed as discriminatory against the individual or if they are not applied equitably to all graduates of all jurisdictions. The administrators of licensing processes are advised to be aware of local and national jurisprudence in this regard when considering such regulations or agreements. There are standards and legal principles that should guide such processes. When in doubt, one should seek appropriate legal counsel.

Finally, other considerations may impact significantly on the approach to both credentialing and assessment for licensure. A set of principles that are widely applied across the western world are the notions of "fairness" and "equitable process". In the eyes of the courts and human rights tribunals, the application of these principles can focus on any of three areas: access to the assessment process; conduct of the assessment process; and the opportunity to appeal the conduct of the process. In each instance, the test before the courts or tribunals will focus on whether or not the processes were equitable and fair. Another recent issue has appeared. The definition of what constitutes exclusive or uniquely medical "acts" varies from jurisdiction to another. In this way, laws and legislative requirements may influence the nature of entitlements under the local legislation that defines the licensing authority's mechanisms to license physicians.

Principles and approaches to assessment for licensure

Most of the approaches to assessment for licensure can be divided into one of three formats:
1. Relying on a medical school based assessment for licensure with regular accreditation of the medical schools;
2. Relying on medical school based assessment for licensure without accreditation of schools;
3. Relying on a combination of accreditation of medical schools with exit examinations of all medical graduates that are set by an external agency.
Frequently, the assessment of candidates who have graduated outside the local jurisdiction, such as from another country, must be integrated into the system. In most cases, those candidates are accepted based on the confirmation of their diplomas and other training requirements whereafter they enter the "normal" assessment pathway like all other "internal" graduates. In other instances, the internationally trained medical graduate undergoes both an independent written assessment process of medical knowledge and a period of retraining or integration that typically involves an assessment of skills and overall clinical performance. There are other variations in approaches that may be hybrid in nature but, for the purposes of this discussion, the focus will be on the assessment procedures used in these three primary approaches.

Before discussing the methods used in assessment for licensure, a further word about the assessment of internationally trained graduates is necessary. By "international medical graduate", one refers to those individuals who have received their medical education and maybe postgraduate medical training outside the licensing country. This designation is typically independent of citizenship. Thus a citizen of country A may be trained and educated in country B, but when returning to country A, that graduate will be considered an international graduate.

In North America the approach to international graduates is similar. Although both Canada and the United States of America are federations, and the granting of licenses is a state or provincial matter, a national assessment process exists that is usually recognized by all jurisdictions. If an individual is a medical graduate of a Liaison Committee on Medical Education (LCME) accredited medical school in either country, that individual can enter a standard process in either country. In Canada, for example, those graduating from a non-LCME school must take a medical knowledge screening examination first (Medical Council of Canada, 1999). That step was used in the United States of America previously, but has been superseded by the integrated United States Medical Licensing Examination process in 1992, and internationally educated physicians can enter the assessment process even while still in medical school overseas if they may be thinking of coming to the United States of America for postgraduate training (Educational Commission for Foreign Medical Graduates, 1999).

In the Australasian context, the overall approach is similar in New Zealand and Australia, although the specifics differ. In each instance, local graduates of nationally accredited medical schools are not required to take any external examinations prior to licensure but all internationally trained physicians must undergo an assessment process of both knowledge and clinical skills, as well as certain other training requirements, before licensure is offered (http.//www.amc.org.au/ assess.asp).

In the United Kingdom the situation is similar in principle to the Australian system. However, the process does involve different steps: recognition of the degree and training by the General Medical Council, then the successful completion of postgraduate training requirements and then successful passing of certain examinations. Currently, the clinical assessment of their process is being revised (http://www.pgmd.man.ac.uk/overseas/registration_with_the_general_me.htm).

The impact of the European Community (EC) is worth noting as it may encourage precursor models that could lead to mutual recognition methods on an international scale. This is particularly topical in an era of economic globalization wherein pressure for globalization of licensure standards may increase. To date the consequence of the EC has been to open doors to more physician movement across national borders but often additional criteria exist for licensure. Karle and Nystrup (1995) have noted that a report proposing a common European general examination for licensure was presented to the Advisory Committee on Medical Training of the European Union in 1992, but no action has been taken to date. Readers are referred to their web site (http://e.lio.se./UEMS/publicat.html).

Whatever the approach used to assess international medical graduates, certain broad principles appear to have been established in many jurisdictions that one is advised to apply when undertaking the assessment of such individuals. In some instances, principles of law are involved and others involve standards for testing that are widely accepted by the measurement bodies. They can be summarized as a series of questions that any assessment agency must ask itself.

1. Is the process being applied fairly and equitably to all candidates?
2. Are the same standards applied to all candidates with respect to the determination of content, the assessment methods and the methods used in setting the passing mark?
3. Does equity of access exist for all candidates at each level of the assessment process?
4. Does the process discriminate against any group other than for reasons of ability?

The answers to these questions should be: "Yes" for items 1-3; and "No" for item 4.

Methods of assessment in current use

Other chapters have covered the specific details of the various methods of assessment. The purpose of this section is to present the methods in the context of licensure to explain why they must address different needs and to note the recent evolution of the development of assessment for licensure. Thus, commonly used methods will be identified and their purpose and advantages/disadvantages will be noted only in the licensure context.

The goal of assessing clinical competence implies certain notions and principles that should be explicitly clear to those involved in the creation and administration of tests, before undertaking either the development of an examination or reassessment of an existing examination system. This is particularly key in a high stakes situation like licensure.

Recent developments in the assessment of professional competence in general, without regard for the particular needs for licensure, have been reviewed by Van der Vleuten (Van der Vleuten, 1996). He begins by addressing the traditional notion of competence and how it was approached in the immediate post-World War II era beginning in the 1950s. An implicit assumption was made that competence was an "aggregate" of latent traits or attributes, from which emerged an approach to assessing competence wherein each trait was typically measured by one or more distinct methods. But this was not to be the answer as neither a consensus on the traits nor the best methods could be established. Part of the new understanding of the difficulty of the approach came from studies of those same methods. Van der Vleuten reviews several methods: multiple-choice questions (MCQs), written simulations, learning process measures and live simulations from the perspectives of reliability and validity of the methods as well as educational consequences (Van der Vleuten, 1996). However, before commenting on his analysis of these issues, it would be worthwhile to look at a framework for assessing the methods and procedures used to measuring competence for licensure. For that, one can turn to the views of Kane.

Kane has put forward a framework for thinking about the strengths and weaknesses of methods used to assess professional competence (Kane, 1992). His concluding comments are key: *"The choice of method for evaluating professional competence involves a series of trade-offs. As we move from performance testing to simulations to objective tests, our observations become more standardized but less realistic"* (p. 180).

In drawing conclusions about candidates' competence based on test results, he suggests that at least three inferences need to be made for the interpretation of each assessment procedure: evaluation, generalization and extrapolation. The first inference is the evaluation of the performance: is it good, bad or borderline. The second inference is the generalization of the observed to other situations: can observation of two cases of fracture in the lower limb be used to generalize to all fractures? The third inference is extrapolation from the testing circumstance to the actual world. For any testing method, ideally all three criteria should be strong. So for the ultimate validity of a procedure and its defensibility, Kane calls for the greatest attention to be paid to each method's weakest links in the chain of inferences. For example, in performance testing, evaluation and generalization are weakest. For objective testing, extrapolation is weakest. For simulations, any link can be weak, depending on the situation. Thus, the weaknesses determine the plausibility of the "chain of inferences" made from each application of a method. As he points out, it is hard to win if only one method is used.

Overall, the methods in use in the last decade have emphasized the assessment of medical knowledge, including basic science knowledge; the assessment of clinical decision-making; the assessment of clinical skills; and the assessment of clinical performance. The formats have included: the use of written tests for the assessment of knowledge and clinical decision-making; the use of oral examinations and objective structured clinical examinations (OSCEs) for the assessment of clinical skills and decision-making; and the use of ratings for in-training assessment.

Figure 1 summarizes the development and state of these methods currently, using Van der Vleuten's classification system.

Van der Vleuten's analysis follows the classification used by him in an earlier publication (Van der Vleuten & Newble, 1994). After reviewing each area, he identifies the reliability and validity issues that should guide the test developer and outlines a different view of the underlying concepts that should direct test development today. He goes on to offer suggestions, based on consistent findings arising from work published in the field. The key concepts in the literature that should apply to all high stakes assessment processes are summarized as follows.

Reliability issues

"The variability of performance of candidates across tasks, originally found in problem-solving research appeared to be one of the most consistent findings in the measurement of clinical competence" (Van der Vleuten, 1996, p. 48). Van der Vleuten notes that this conclusion does not appear to apply to fundamental communication skills. In all other situations that view is operative: oral examinations, chart audits, MCQs, patient management problems (PMPs), practice performance – even in other disciplines such as law or mathematics. Thus certain examinations with a small number of items or cases produce an unstable or unreliable score. Certain less efficient methods, like Objective Structured Clinical Examinations, often require hours of testing, depending on the context or purpose. Sources of variability, other than the candidates' ability, can challenge the reliability of the measure and must be anticipated. That includes some that may be dealt with by other measures. For example, the problem of rater variability can be dealt with in part by some standardization and structure. But even that cannot be assured if it is not monitored or searched for by measurement techniques, as we will note shortly.

One approach is to use large numbers of items or cases with a good test design. The principle is to design the test to deal with areas of variability – such as an adequate sample of the situations or items to minimize the effect (Swanson, 1987; Van der Vleuten, 1996). Thus in a clinical test, one may employ strategies whereby situations are sampled widely to deal with the content specificity issue which is inherent in the candidate and using one examiner, rather than two or more per station or case. The reason is that the variability in the candidate's ability between cases is greater than the variability between examiners, if structures and guidelines are in place to guide the assessor/observer. In cases without standardization, and using global methods, such as clinical ratings in clinical rotations, the methods can be "hopelessly" unstable. This has been reviewed by Gray (Gray, 1998).

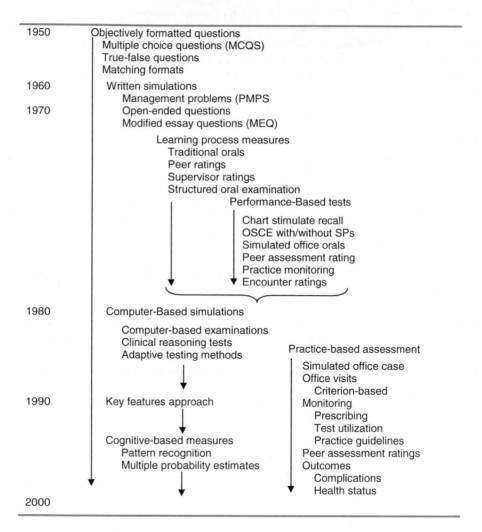

Figure 1. Historical representation of the application of assessment methods for licensure (adapted from Van der Vleuten and Newble, 1994)

Validity issues

A key consideration is the validity of the process. Validity refers to the notion that an examination process should do what it is intended to do. In particular readers are reminded of the importance of three specific validity issues that are often neglected in planning a defensible assessment process for licensure or any other high stakes process. The traditional unitarian view that validity applies mainly to the interpretation of test scores has been challenged by LaDuca (LaDuca, 1994). His view is that, in assessment for professional licensure, additional issues arise. He raises three modifications to traditional test strategies in order to establish a valid process. They are: a theory of professions must be incorporated into the development process; the importance of test design must be enhanced in the licensure context; and the concept of construct validity must be expanded to include the special features of the content that are inherent in the professional licensure testing. His concerns can be addressed at certain key points in the process in the following ways.

1. Does the assessment process follow content in keeping with a practice model for that profession or discipline? This is a step that is often addressed inadequately, or is completely neglected in many circumstances.

2. Is the need for standards for development of test scores and standard-setting (determining the passing score) handled separately? Norcini has addressed this issue (Norcini, 1994). McGuire has referred to this as psychometric due process (McGuire, 1997).

3. Is the interpretation of test scores validated sufficiently that it can support the interpretation of the test scores? This issue has been covered thoroughly in the context of licensure examinations by Kane (1994).

When deciding if a test measures what it is supposed to measure, one needs criteria and standards. Van der Vleuten decries the lack of good research in the field. However, he feels some developments are worth noting.

- The trait approach, as noted, has not been supported by empirical research.
- The use of correlation studies between certification examinations and performance in the real world of practice has found relationships, but without differential method interactions.
- It is difficult to make causal inferences from correlation data. A high correlation between two methods does not mean that the same construct is being measured. In fact, what one is measuring depends more on the task presented in the test item or instrument than on the characteristics of the specific assessment method. This is illustrated by the example of MCQs. MCQs do not measure knowledge because one must pick one of five possible responses. MCQs measure knowledge because the problem posed stimulates the candidate's recall and use of organized factual knowledge. The MCQ can also measure problem solving if the item involves a case that requires a management decision. The candidate then must focus on the solution (diagnosis) and the needed action steps such as

management. Thus, what is asked during the use of any method is more important than the method used (Van der Vleuten, 1996).

- The trivialization of complex clinical issues because it is easier to use rigid checklists in the name of objectivity may sacrifice the validity of the test for no gain. We will return to this point shortly in a test development context.

Feasibility

The issue of feasibility has been well covered by Neufeld several years ago (Neufeld, 1985). The important considerations include the following. Is the cost of the method reasonable? Are the logistical and scheduling steps manageable and reasonable? Is the maintenance of the test material simple and reasonable in cost and human resources? Frequently, small bodies find such costs prohibitive. New technology may be too costly even for larger bodies. Where such problems arise, working with others in consortia may be a solution. This issue must be considered very early. Often the use of expert opinion or the use of piloting will assist inexperienced groups before the damage is done.

Educational consequences

This is critical as licensure and certifying assessments can drive the educational process in the wrong direction. Again Neufeld (1985) emphasizes the importance of considering appropriateness of the setting and of the method proposed, and being aware of the strengths and weaknesses of each. In the end, it is key to recall that there are invariably side-effects and it is important that they be minimized. Often the literature is helpful, as are experts in assessment, in anticipating these problems.

More modern view of competence

Van der Vleuten has pointed out some developments that support a current model of competence (Van der Vleuten, 1996). Expertise is strongly linked to knowledge. But how the knowledge is accumulated and retrieved is important and these processes differ greatly between novice and experts (i.e. fully trained physicians, not experts in the academic sense or subspecialty sense). Furthermore, as physicians become more experienced and specialized, the expertise may be highly individualized.

This framework explains many previously surprising results: there are no underlying constructs but rather expertise is developed by states or steps that are restricted to specific areas of meaningful experiences and knowledge. This notion is critical to how we assess competence. For a careful analysis of the issues raised in studies comparing testing formats, the reader is referred to Norman et al. (1996).

The overall assessment of competence is complex and not a matter of selecting from a set of testing options. It requires building an assessment program from the ground up, as will be outlined now.

Guidelines on how to design and build an assessment process

The use of currently accepted methods without regard for the overall plan or goals of the assessment process is not defensible in court or in most appeals processes in many licensure bodies (McGuire, 1994). To avoid such risks, there are some basic principles and guidelines that must be followed before deciding on which methods are best suited. For a comprehensive overview, readers are referred to the paper on the guidelines for developing procedures for assessing clinical competence by Newble et al. (1994). Assuming that the basic purpose/goal of the assessment has been established, such as that which is required for licensure, Newble and colleagues have outlined four topics that must be addressed for effective, efficient and defensible procedures for assessing basic clinical competence. They can be summarized as follows.

1. Define what is to be tested in three steps
   a. Identify the clinical problems that the candidate should be able to handle to some defined level of resolution;
   b. For each problem define the clinical tasks in which the candidate is expected to be competent;
   c. Prepare a blueprint to guide the selection of problems to be included in the assessment procedure.
2. Select the test methods and format, utilizing the following three steps:
   a. Test methods should strive for a representation of reality (fidelity) that is appropriate to the clinical tasks being posed;
   b. The clinical tasks being posed should determine the method by which it is to be tested;
   c. There must be recognition of the practical constraints in selecting the optimal examination methods.
3. Address issues of test administration and scoring in six steps:
   a. Decide the level of efficiency needed in the particular testing environment. For example, to shorten testing time, one can use the multiple hurdles approach, as is often done by certifying boards, or use adaptive testing or sequential testing methods;
   b. Decide how the candidate's performance on the test is to be recorded or captured. For example, there are technical issues and cost issues when you must decide whether or not to use checklists and raters on an OSCE;
   c. Determine a method to assign scores to the cases and/or elements within the cases (meaning an item or set of items or a station) or problems;
   d. Take appropriate steps to ensure that the examination provides an unbiased measure of the candidate's performance;
   e. Evaluate the need for equating scores across different examinations. The key notion is to ensure that the scores on any two examinations using the same blueprint are interchangeable;
   f. Review the procedure to ensure that trivialization of the real tasks or challenge has not occurred;

4. Address the setting of standards of performance in two steps. Standard setting means the process of determining the score needed to pass the test or examination:

a. Determine the type of standard desired and then the appropriate standard setting method;

b. Develop procedures for effectively communicating the results of the test.

These topics and the sub-steps constitute a "checklist" of issues that any high stakes examination process must address to be defensible. They are applicable in all circumstances but merely addressing them without meeting certain validity standards is not sufficient. A set of publications by Norcini (1994), Kane (1994) and LaDuca (1994) are recommended to readers as the bases for dealing with the basic validity issues in the licensure context.

In summary, the fact remains that there is no examination for all seasons. Anybody faced with a high stakes situation in a professional context must first address the issues noted by Newble et al. (1994) by designing the set of instruments using the appropriate methods. That includes addressing the following points: content design; scoring; monitoring the quality of the items or cases; setting the passing score; deciding on the methods to report the results; and offering possible appeal mechanisms. The article by Newble et al. is intended to look at the challenge of designing an assessment process, rather than an assessment of the individual methods. The latter are covered in other chapters.

Possible methods

As noted, recent methods and developments in licensure assessment are summarized in Figure 1. It highlights the trend to more objective testing since the 1960s. Then one saw the development of simulations in the 1960s and 1970s that have now moved on from written to computer-based systems. The focus on ratings of learning processes emerged in the 1970s. Many of the developments that took place at that time in the United States of America, have been nicely described by McGuire (McGuire, 1995). This was followed by the appearance of the performance-based testing methods in the late 1970s and 1980s, perhaps best characterized by the OSCE with or without standardized patients. More recently, the focus has moved to assessment methods in practice and the possible monitoring or even reassessment of practitioners for the maintenance of licensure. Those methods include direct monitoring of prescribing; office visits utilizing criteria; peer and patient ratings of practice performance; and the emergence of outcomes of care. Most of these individual methods are covered in other chapters in this book.

All of the cited methods have strengths and weaknesses. However, a few general principles are critical to direct the test developer away from rocky shoals. They are: the need for test equating; the verification of objectivity; and the notion that reliability and validity are properties of particular interpretations of candidates' performances on a specific examination, not inherent properties of the format. Another critical issue is the setting of standards where there is often confusion between setting a passing score (the correct meaning) and a general notion of maintaining standards of practice.

The need for test equating has been alluded to previously. Equating refers to the need to establish for any test, given repeated use of the same blueprint, but with different versions of items or cases, that any two versions of the test are equivalent. And they may be, but it should be documented, not assumed on circumstantial evidence such as a stable passing rate from administration to administration. This is especially true in high-stakes, career determining assessments as in licensure or certification. There are ways to ensure equivalency. One is test equating using item response theory, but this approach requires large candidate populations to adequately calibrate the items (Lord, 1982). This is not always possible in jurisdictions where examinations are given to dozens of candidates instead of hundreds of candidates. Another method is to repeat items and determine if the test results are comparable, but this has limitations and should only be used as an alternative approach (Kolen & Brennan, 1995).

A word about objectivity is needed. As Norman et al. (1991) have pointed out, there can be a certain amount of self-deception when planning tests, that can only be addressed by proper analysis. One of those is the notion of objectivity. In particular, the authors remind test developers not to confuse the pursuit of objectivity (that is the empirical demonstration that a measurement is free of subjective influences) through studies of reliability, with the actual steps of objectification (such as the use of behavioral checklists that appear to be objective) that one may need to create when developing an examination. They review evidence that shows so-called more objective-appearing methods are not necessarily more reliable than the so-called subjective methods. The key notion is that in any assessment method, despite any intuitive comfort that one may have in one's desire for objectification, a method should only be labeled as objective based on their demonstrated superiority to other existing methods and their appropriateness to the specific situation being assessed. This is particularly a challenge during performance based methods of assessment such as Objective Structured Clinical Examinations. The use of global rating scales on Objective Structured Clinical Examinations appears to be subjective and the use of checklist appears to be more objective. Yet examples exist in the literature wherein the opposite is true (Regehr et al., 1998; Cunnington et al., 1996). The proof is in the study of each instance, not in the generalization from other applications of the method!

Regarding the myth of the reliability and validity of a specific technique, Christine McGuire has said it best (McGuire, 1995):

".... reports of the so-called reliability and validity of a technique are at best indefensible over generalisations, and, more often than not pure nonsense. Reliability and validity are properties of a particular interpretation of performance on a specific examination; they are not attributes of a generalised technique or a test format." *(p. 739)*

She goes on to note that the only characteristics that can reasonably be assessed to a format are its inherent limitations, as well as its potential when properly developed and used (McGuire, 1995).

Issue of standards

There is no notion about which there is more confusion among non-psychometric professionals than standards. The confusion often revolves around two issues: the use of the word "standard" in different contexts; and the lack of clarity about the steps involved in establishing the "score" as opposed to the "pass-fail point". On the latter point, Christine McGuire has described the state of the art for licensure and certifying processes as follows.

> "We have, fortunately, lost much of our blind faith in the sacred numbers we once used to determine the passing score (e.g., 70%) and/or the failure rate (e.g., 10%) on our examinations – but we still need to learn how to set performance requirements consistent with the actual demands of health care delivery in the real world." *(McGuire, 1995, p. 739)*

Recently, Norcini has addressed the issue of standards as it specifically relates to licensure and certifying examinations (Norcini, 1994). He starts by defining the words that are frequently heard and often misused, and proceeds by differentiating between standards and scores. Often the word "standards" is used to refer to what a practitioner needs to know, but at other times, how much the practitioner needs to know. Norcini suggests that the first meaning – what the practitioner needs to know – can be used to refer to scores which differentiates it from how much the practitioner must know, which relates to the standards.

   The appropriate approach to a given situation in practice is often referred to as the "standard of practice". But in testing, the standard of practice becomes important when the process has to make decisions about the degree of appropriateness or correctness of the responses during the scoring process. Thus, scoring requires the identification of what is good or what is not and weighting each action, aggregating the weights and, in the end, the candidate's performance is expressed as a score. Thus the *"content decisions about correctness of responses, their values or weights, and how the weights are aggregated will be referred to here as scoring"* (Norcini, 1994, p. 162). He goes on to point out that one source of confusion between scores and standards is the incorrect notion that, whenever judgment is required, one is speaking of standards. This notion comes from the MCQ where the simple best answer format suggests that scoring is just a matter of counting the correct answers! In most other situations, testing is a lot more complicated, so in those instances, experts are asked to make judgments about correctness of the response.

   In contrast, standard refers to how much a practitioner needs to do to care appropriately for a situation and the patient's needs. Thus, standard deals with "how much care is enough" (Norcini, 1994). This focus on how much is enough is a key issue in licensure and certification processes because to quote Norcini again, *"it defines the boundary of the profession"* (pp. 162-163). He suggests that standards in this instance differ from scores in two ways. Standards are based on educational and social judgments, rather than content judgments needed to define scores. Thus, the correctness of the response is independent of who takes the test. The standards might differ as to how many correct responses are needed to pass between two groups of candidates: one junior to the other. The second difference relates to the fact that standards are arbitrary. Norcini quotes Sheppard who noted that there is no such thing as a "true" standard (Norcini, 1994). Why? The answer is that proficiency in a group of professionals is distributed continuously and, therefore, no single point delineates who is competent and who is not. Hence, more than one standard to pass an examination process could be defined depending on the circumstance (level of training) but in either case, a rational argument would be needed to defend the standard.

Having tried to clarify the concepts and nature of scores and standard setting, the next issue is the methods. Typically, one speaks of relative and absolute methods. These issues are well covered in the chapter on standard setting in this book. In particular, an excellent discussion of current standards and the related issues is available in Cusimano's review in *Academic Medicine* that is specifically aimed at the clinical examination setting (Cusimano, 1996). For a more detailed review on setting standards specifically on credentialing examinations in the health field, the reader is referred to Meskaukas (1986) and to Bowmer et al. (1994).

Other issues

The issue of "representativeness" of the tasks to the actual practice content and environment has been addressed in earlier comments referring to the work of LaDuca and need not be repeated, except to remind readers of its great importance in high stakes examinations.

It is critically important to note that there are measurement standards that have been developed by the American Psychological Association which reflect the state of the measurement "art". They should be standard guidelines for any high stakes type examinations like those used in licensure or certification and are almost certain to be applied in any legal challenge. We will comment further on that issue in a later section.

New developments and implications

New developments are occurring daily in the field. For an introductory overview, readers are referred to McGuire (1995) for her comments on the evolution of these measurement tools. Dauphinee and Norcini have provided an overview of the current directions of developments in the field of assessment (Dauphinee & Norcini, 1999). Within that same issue of *Advances in Health Sciences Education*, there are excellent perspectives on the field as it applies to five critical areas of development:

1. Use of outcomes (Tamblyn, 1999);
2. Use of peer assessment ratings (PARS) of performance (Ramsey & Wenrich, 1999);
3. Application of computer-adaptive testing methods (Zara, 1999);
4. Application of intelligent authoring systems (Sumner et al., 1999); and
5. An analysis of the measurement issues around the use of Objective Structured Clinical Examinations in high stakes situations (Swanson et al., 1999).

For the purpose of this review, we will focus on four areas of development:

- Performance-based assessment
- Adaptive methods
- Use of multi-media
- Practice-based assessment.

Performance-based assessment

The use of performance-based assessment methods has characterized many of the developments in the late 1980s and 1990s. Its origins are probably quite simple – a push for authenticity. Although there is no set definition of performance-based testing, Swanson and colleagues have noted that a *"common theme is an emphasis on testing complex, higher order knowledge and skills in the real world context in which they are actually used"* (Swanson et al., 1995, p. 5). Typical examples are noted in Figure 1. This article reviews four so-called performance-based assessment methods used in assessing health professionals. Again, the reader is referred to other chapters dealing with the specific methods, but a brief review of Swanson and colleagues' analysis serves this chapter's purpose: to define issues crossing the whole field of assessing for licensure and certification. They identify eight lessons.

Lesson 1: The fact that candidates are tested in realistic performance situations does not make the test design or sampling simple or straightforward. Sampling must consider issues of context (situation/task) and construct (knowledge/skill) – as well as complex interactions between these elements. Even if tasks are identified, it may not be sufficient as not all tasks are performed in the same way in all contexts.

Lesson 2: No matter how realistic a performance-based assessment is, it is still a simulation, and examinees do not behave in the same manner as in the real world and in practice.

Lesson 3: High fidelity performance-based assessment methods often yield "rich" and interesting data on the candidates; scoring those data can be problematic. Two examples illustrate: use in oral examinations and in patient management problems.

Lesson 4: Regardless of the method, performance in one context (typically a patient case) does not predict performance in another context. In-depth assessment in a few cases results in scores that are not sufficiently reproducible for use in high-stakes tests as in licensure.

Lesson 5: Correlation studies of the relationship between performance-based test scores and other testing methods aimed at other performance skills have produced variable results that are difficult to interpret. Validation should focus on threats to the validity, not their relationship to other assessments.

Lesson 6: Performance-based methods are complex and very complicated to administer, such that multiple forms and administrations may be needed in licensure and certification settings. This poses a challenge for security and test equating because the number of items available for comparison may be relatively small.

Lesson 7: Since all high stakes tests like licensure examinations, may influence teaching and education programs, developers must monitor for unintended consequences and effects.

Lesson 8: Neither traditional methods nor performance-based tests are a panacea. Select methods based on skills to be assessed and use a blend of methods.

The principal type of simulation used in Objective Structured Clinical Examinations has been standardized patients. The issues of standardized patients and Objective Structured Clinical Examinations are well covered in chapter 21. However, the assumption that simulations are limited to the use of standardized patients is not realistic. With the coming of new technologies, and the development of multi-media and virtual environments, one can foresee the day when many other methods could be introduced into the OSCE format. In particular, the assessment of surgical and technical skills, or the assessment of gynecological and urological examinations, would be of particular interest. These developments raise two questions: are the maneuvers and required performances sufficiently described that programmers or producers can produce these products (Hoffman & Vu, 1997). A second issue is the question of how much fidelity is needed to measure effects needed in the licensure and certification context. Elaborate and highly scripted simulations are expensive and time consuming. They perhaps are of value in teaching and formative assessments contexts. But for licensure and certification, the question must always be asked: is the expense and testing time required for detailed multi-media simulations needed for high-stakes assessment necessary. A recent review by Reznick illustrates what can be done with low-tech solutions in the assessment of surgical skills (Reznick, 1998).

Adaptive testing

Adaptive testing methods are those in which the test material is altered based on the performance or content orientation of the candidate. Currently, such methods are used to decrease testing time by adapting MCQ items to the candidate's performance on the previous item or series of items. To understand the conditions for using adaptive methods and the need to calibrate items, the reader is referred to the 1993 paper by Hambleton and Jones that compares classical test theory with item response theory in their application to test development, including adaptive format. Adaptive methods are used in many settings now, although they are only just beginning to appear in high-stakes medical assessments. For example, the nurses have used adaptive methods in their MCQ licensure examinations in the United States of America for some time now (Zara, 1999). The Medical Council of Canada has field-tested a computer-based adaptive MCQ type examination for two years and it is due to be introduced on its Qualifying Examination, Part I in late 2000. Adaptive approaches have also been proposed for other formats such as the OSCE. Such experiences are few and those that have existed have proven administratively difficult (Dauphinee et al., 1998). In the case of the MCQ, the approach is greatly facilitated by their administration by computer, as all items must be calibrated using item response theory approaches before they can be used. The computer enhances the administration by being used for the analysis and by being programmed to choose the right item based on its characteristics and the candidate's characteristics.

Multi-media

We have already raised the fidelity issue surrounding the use of multi-media based high tech methods on licensure and certification examinations. This is not to argue against them but merely to point out that feasibility in terms of the costs of development and testing time are important considerations for any licensure or certifying organization thinking about venturing into this arena.

Practice-based assessment

The whole issue of practice-based assessment has pushed its way into the foreground of the measurement agenda for two reasons. The recent events around the competency of certain pediatric cardiac surgeons in the United Kingdom and the changes in the regulations in many licensure communities have moved the licensing bodies to administer assessments of the practicing doctor. The second new influence is the decision of the American Board of Medical Specialties to equate certification with the need to maintain lifelong competency (Nahrwald, 1999). Whatever the reasons, the issue of monitoring and assessing the performance of practicing physicians is a here and now challenge for many bodies. Suffice to say that certain assessment approaches are increasingly being used in this challenge. They include:

- Peer assessment ratings: peers are asked to assess the performance of a local colleague on a number of parameters. The work at the American Board of Internal Medicine is noteworthy as is the work on behalf of the Alberta College of Physicians and Surgeons in Canada (Ramsey & Wenrich, 1999; Fidler et al., 1999; Hall et al., 1999).
- The monitoring of physicians in practice is new, especially by licensure bodies, but such developments are now appearing. Typical approaches include monitoring prescribing practices; utilization reviews; patient assessment ratings; peer assessment ratings; and practice profiles (Dauphinee & Norcini, 1999).
- Office visits, with the inspection of charts by peers using pre-set criteria on a random basis, is used in certain licensure jurisdictions (McAuley et al., 1990).

- Case-based assessments are now being used in assessing physicians who are reported or are identified in other monitoring or screening procedures (Southgate & Dauphinee, 1997).
- The use of outcomes has emerged in the United States of America in several forms such as doctors' report cards. Their use has not been primarily associated with licensure or certification procedures.
- A promising development is the use of adaptive methods applied to questionnaires assessing functional status of patients. This method would allow patients' functional and quality of life measures to be standardized and adaptable such that all patients could complete an on-line assessment at the end of each office visit, thereby giving an ongoing measure of a therapeutic program's success. Whether such measures would be part of the maintenance of competence assessment or in-training assessment of potential certificants is too early to say. But it is a method worth watching (Dauphinee & Norcini, 1999).

The issue of re-examination versus maintenance of competency strategies has come to the forefront in the United States of America. There are currently 18 out of 24 Boards in the American Board of Medical Specialties that require re-certification in the form of written assessment of knowledge. Some are open book examinations and generally the passing rate is high (over 95%). It is said that the scope is too narrow and the notion of competency should involve a wider definition. This implies a multidimensional approach. The new position paper of the American Board of Medical Specialties defines the notion of competency and six general components to that definition (Nahrwald, 1999). The implication is that there will be indicators of these components that must be addressed in the future re-assessment of certificants, in addition to the test of knowledge. It is likely that an educational component will be identified such that continuing medical educational criteria will need to be met to maintain one's specialist status. That approach is now being introduced in Canada by the certifying Colleges and has been used by one certifying College in New Zealand and Australia (Newble et al., 1999). The notion of offering feedback from such monitoring and in practice assessments is viewed by many as an excellent way in which to direct learning and to enhance the physician's performance.

TYPES AND APPROACHES TO ASSESSMENT FOR CERTIFICATION

Overview

The purpose of certification, as we have defined it for this chapter, is for "an agency or association to grant recognition to an individual who has met certain qualifications specified by that agency or association". These forms of recognition most often deal with qualifications that are post-licensure.

The significance of certification must be acknowledged as it has many consequences to the holder. The holder is now "certified" as having achieved a certain standard of additional competence that is important in terms of professional status and in terms of assuring the public. The status of certificant or Fellow, for example, has major economic consequences too. A physician's appointment on staff at a hospital or at other institutions may be conditional on being certified as a specialist. It can be recalled in an earlier section, the status of Fellow offered major entitlement in the early days of the Colleges in England. That is true to a greater degree in the United States of America now than in the immediate past. Until recently, being Board eligible (meaning a physician has been in an approved program and has met all requirements, but has not taken the final certification examinations), was usually sufficient to receive appointments as a specialist and to be compensated as a specialist. Currently, Board eligible may not be sufficient to receive institutional appointments in the newly competitive environment of managed care. As a result, the American Board of Internal Medicine has noted that the proportion of Internists without the certificates, but being Board eligible, has been falling for several years.

As implied there are economic consequences for individuals wanting to be reimbursed as a specialist. The status of being Certified or a Fellow or whichever other designation one may receive is significant in another sense. As some jurisdictions move to require physicians to remain in good standing, either by examination, by educational credits or to document one's competencies in several broad categories, the maintenance of one's certification status becomes critically important. In turn, this change in the definition of re-certification places a major responsibility on certifying bodies to ensure that their processes for maintenance of certification are educationally and psychometrically sound. Not to do so will invite legal challenges as the stakes become higher. These obligations mean that many of the issues raised earlier regarding the validity and reliability of the assessment processes at entry to practice will apply to assessment at all subsequent stages of a physician's career.

Approaches to assessment for certification

There are three general types of approaches to assessment for this process, even though, in some jurisdictions, the process may not be referred to as certification. But in principle, since these exceptions do observe the process and intent of certification as we have defined it, they will be considered as certification processes for the purpose of this discussion. They are the North American approach such as used in Canada and the United States of America; the British approach such as used in the United Kingdom and Australasia; and the European approach such as used in countries such as Germany and the Netherlands.

The North American approach

This approach to assessment for certification involves three distinct assessment processes: accreditation of the training program and its processes; the assessment of in-training performance; and a summative assessment. The process of accreditation of training programs is carried out by bodies independent of the training program and against pre-set criteria. In the United States of America, that is done by the Accreditation Council on Graduate Medical Education as well as by the individual Certifying Boards. Programs in the United States of America need not be under university sponsorship and control. They can be hospital-based. In Canada, the accreditation process for specialty training programs is carried out by one body, the Royal College of Physicians and Surgeons of Canada, but all programs are required to be under university control and therefore the university has responsibility for its quality and its compliance with the pre-set criteria for accreditation. The second component is the assessment of the in-training performance of the individual candidate. Typically, that is done by ratings by supervisors or senior peers and is reported in a final assessment form either each year or at the end of the program. Other requirements may also be defined such as observation of specified skills by supervisors. Often a mid-point assessment of knowledge is required. In the end, depending on the specialty and jurisdiction, a summative assessment is carried out and may involve several steps. They include: summative assessment of in-training reports; written assessment either terminally or at some other time during the training period; and an exit assessment that may involve written examinations, Objective Structured Clinical Examinations, oral examinations, or various combinations thereof. The recent piece by Cassie et al. (1998) deals with these steps and requirements.

The "British" approach

This approach is administered through the Royal Colleges, of which there may be several (16) as in Australasia, or relatively few. Often more than one specialty, as thought of in the American context, may be linked under one College. In this approach, the steps of program accreditation are less formalized, as candidates may often move around within teaching institutions, and the pre-set requirements for areas to be covered are less specific. After a minimal number of years or time in specified rotations are fulfilled, the candidate may sit the final assessment. The final assessment typically involves written assessments and a clinical assessment, such as a clinical oral or set of orals in various topics. At the end of the process, one is entitled to be called a Member or Fellow of the particular Royal College.

The "European" approach

This approach is less rigid and typically involves a pivotal role for an approved trainer or department head. Once in a program, the trainee has to meet specified consultative and skills experiences which must be approved by the trainer or department head. After the in-training requirements are met, the candidate then can enter the final assessment process which may involve written materials and clinical assessments. Again the clinical assessment often comes in the form of clinical oral examinations. In some instances, the final clinical assessment is based on the trainer's attestation of competency.

The processes obviously differ and each has strengths and weaknesses. One can only ever assess any particular application of a measurement process, as we have pointed out before in the previous section. However, a few points of caution can be raised about some of the methods used in many of these approaches. They include the following. The use of oral examinations is fraught with problems of reliability, if not structured and monitored carefully. The use of in-training reports taken weeks after the specific encounters can be very unreliable. The use of skills or cases approved and assessed by only one individual can lead to bias, or even discrimination.

In summary, the mechanisms by which one can obtain specialty certification vary from one jurisdiction to another, as they do in the licensure processes. While we have outlined some of the general approaches, explicit note should be made of the various mechanisms used:

- By regulated and/or monitored assessment in accredited training programs followed by or in combination with examinations;
- By years of training in specified programs plus examinations;
- By challenge examinations with or without successful completion of acceptable training programs;
- By designation via accredited programs that can award certificates of special competence (often used in sub-disciplines or in technical areas of a specialty);
- By election, based on distinguished performance in the field concerned.

Typically most processes involve two elements: clinical experience with some form of assessment plus an exit process, that often involves examinations or other forms of assessment.

None of these approaches is necessarily better than another, as the validity of the processes always depends on the specific application. Generally speaking, the more that pre-set criteria are established and applied by trained assessors, either in the accreditation or the examination process, the more likely one is to create a valid assessment program that is fairly applied and defensible. Similarly, the fact remains that no one method is able to stand alone, as has been alluded to in the writings of Van der Vleuten (1996). Therefore, combinations of valid and reliable methods will yield the most defensible approaches, bearing in mind that each approach itself must be monitored and assessed to show that it does what it is supposed to in a fair, valid and reliable manner.

Methods of assessment currently in use

Many of the methods used in licensure are also used in certification processes. The general concerns regarding the issues of validity, reliability and the need for an assessment plan as outlined still apply to the certification processes.

In the case of certification, certain processes may receive more emphasis than in licensure, due to the specificity, higher skill levels and longer training periods in many more varied situations. Thus, while the methods listed in Figure 1 are valid methods to be used in certification, additional demands are made of these methods in postgraduate specialized clinical training. To illustrate, the Boards and Colleges often require their external evaluation methods to be added to those of the internal systems that may exist at the training site. Furthermore, the standards for successful completion may be different or additive to those developed and used locally. Internal program requirements in turn may utilize methods that are not required by the certifying body as part of the internal in-training assessment. Typical examples may be tests of knowledge assessment or local assessments of clinical or procedural skills. Case records may be required for internal purposes, but not for external requirements.

Frequently used assessment methods used in specialty training include:
- Global rating scales of clinical performance over specified training periods;
- Oral examinations;
- Written assessments including essay, short-answer and MCQ questions;
- Objective Structured Clinical Examinations, with or without standardized patients, even using technical props as proxies for surgical skills;
- Computerized assessment using MCQs or visual materials, with or without multi-media;
- Combinations of several of the above.

Whatever the method used, there are a number of issues that require special attention in the certification context. These are above and beyond the classic properties of any assessment method: reliability, validity and feasibility, which we have addressed. The additional problems are:
- The concept inherent in any assessment process is to recall that there are three distinct foci to any assessment process: structures to ensure quality; processes to promote quality and outcome variables to measure the product's ultimate effectiveness (Donabedian, 1967). One of the last or least accessible elements is measuring outcomes, although some pioneering work in Canada by Tamblyn et al. (1996) is trying to address the issue.
- The quality of training, including the need to accredit programs, is a long established procedure. Thus one of the first approaches is to assess the structures by which programs are run and administered. This is a critical step in postgraduate education.
- Process steps focus in the quality of the educational program and the mechanisms to ensure standards of training are actually observed. The same

would apply to the quality of the examinations. To that end, there are criteria and standards about assessment tools developed by the American Psychological Association and other bodies which serve to establish acceptable processes for high stakes processes like licensure and certification examinations. We will return to these issues of standards in the next section.

- Another area of process in need of attention is human rights. Human rights challenges are increasingly frequent around the issues of fairness and access, particularly in North America for individuals with disabilities. Again, this is beyond the scope of this chapter, but it is advisable to be aware of the jurisprudence in this field.
- Finally, the issue of outside training and the problem of equivalencies of training in jurisdictions where different standards may exist, often is a major challenge to Boards and certifying agencies. In the absence of international standards, the issue can only be resolved on a case by case basis, if at all. Again, the resolution usually rests with the assessment of process, rather than a magic bullet like a challenge examination, as was often done in the past.

The actual approach to designing the content for certifying examinations as part of an assessment program has been well described by Dauphinee et al. (1994). They outline three basic steps in the process of determining content: define the problems to be handled by the candidate at what level of resolution for the level of training, define the tasks for each problem and again the level of resolution expected, and develop a test blueprint. These steps are not unique to certification but are often neglected, especially by smaller certifying organizations. Yet they are the essence of demonstrating that the test is "practice related", a useful criterion for all examination bodies to bear in mind as a bottom line, in case of challenge or appeal.

STANDARDS FOR TESTING

It has been pointed out that, when one speaks of testing for licensure or certification, one is not attempting to indicate a construct as one does in aptitude or intelligence testing (Jaeger, 1991). Jaeger goes on to point out that licensure or certification assessments are really applications of testing. For example, the applications are part of the screening process prior to issuing a license.

As such, there are different psychometric investigations needed to "scrutinize" tests used in both licensure and certification. Among the most important considerations are: test validation; a determination of measurement reliability; and the development of standards of acceptable practice or performance.

As a guide to these challenges, standards have been developed by the American Psychological Association, in association with the American Educational Research Association and the National Council on Measurement in Education. The previous edition, called the *Standards for educational and psychological testing,* was published in 1985. As we go to press, the latest version has just been released for publication (APA, 1999). Thus, one cannot understate the importance of these standards. They set out the level of the bar for test developers and there are specific sections that are either particularly important for licensure and certification testing, or that specifically address licensure and certification. These standards are critical for the test developer or administrator, as they set the gold standard by which any agency should expect to be judged in a legal challenge to its testing procedures.

The 1985 version has two chapters that are especially relevant to the validity of licensure and certification examinations. They deal with "Validity" and with "Professional and Occupational Licensure and Certification". As Jaeger again suggests, these sections "contain standards that apply inclusively or specifically to such tests". For example, in the first chapter on Validity, there are some 25 standards of which two are critical to licensure and certification testing. Thus, to claim validity on content-related evidence, there are requirements about this to be carried out and justified in relationship to how the test is to be used. Or if panels of judges are to be used to justify content validity, there are standards related to the judges' qualifications.

Similarly, in the chapter on Professional and Occupational Licensure and Certification, again five standards are offered and, equally importantly, explanations accompany the standards in order to assist the reader.

The purpose of this brief commentary is not to review the guidelines. It is to emphasize that such standards exist and are being revised as we write. They are not road-blocks. They are road maps that users can use to stay clear of trouble and to ensure that the user can offer fair, valid and reliable tests in the certification and licensure processes.

CURRENT AND FUTURE CHALLENGES

What are the current and future challenges that confront licensure and certification bodies with respect to their assessment and evaluation procedures and methods? At the micro level, many are technical and inherent in the specific designs and applications in which they are used. Those challenges and issues have been raised in the earlier sections and in the chapters of this volume dealing with the specific methods and applications.

On the other hand, at the macro and policy levels there are challenges facing the licensure and certification communities. These issues can be grouped around seven headings.

- The variability in the quality of the application and the measurement instrumentation.
- The impact of technology and telemedicine.
- The challenge of outcomes-based assessment.
- The impact of new socio-economic drivers.
- The challenge of mutual recognition.
- The redefinition of the exclusivity of certain traditionally medical acts.
- The alternatives to licensure.

In each of these instances, the licensure and certification communities must regard these challenges as opportunities. The pressures for change, and in particular the impact of technologies, dictate that agencies assess and define their values and their missions such that there is a context for the development of policies and implementation steps to anticipate the new order.

Variability of quality

There are no internationally defined standards for the quality of instrumentation and application of measurement procedures used for licensure or certification. Yet, such standards do exist through associations like the American Psychological Association or the American Educational Research Association, as was pointed out in the previous section. Why is this issue important? It is not a case of imposing one jurisdiction's "procedures" on another. It is a case of needing to observe similar standards for assessment as we enter the area of globalization and increase mobility of health professionals. Currently, one of the major impediments is variable quality in training standards, particularly for specialty certification, and in the quality of assessment procedures used at all levels of professional assessment. All agencies should monitor and judge the quality of their procedures, using recognized standards.

Impact of technology and telemedicine

The new electronic technologies are having a major impact on licensure and certification from two perspectives. The first is from a practice or training perspective. The use of telemedicine and related technologies has a critical impact on the application of licensure and certification in regions remote from the point of origin. Is the specialist certified according to the standards of jurisdiction wherein the patient resides? How does the agency protect the patient's interests and how does the patient address any harm originating from outside the area via telemedicine? There are other issues: informed consent, security of information and privacy issues, and invasive procedures executed over distances, to mention a few. To work to maximal benefit and maintain accountability, certain performance standards are needed. The opportunities have been reviewed by Eliasson (1998) in his article appropriately entitled *"Performance Improvement in Telemedicine"* . He outlines an approach to the performance improvement and standards challenges, based on their experience with telemedicine in the United States of America military through the Walter Reed Medical Centre.

The application of new technologies in actual assessment and evaluation procedures is moving quickly. Current applications in adaptive testing and the use of multimedia have been mentioned earlier. Regarding the development and application of the new electronic technologies in assessment, the biggest challenge is the cost. Most certifying bodies are relatively small and therefore the costs are enormous proportionally (Dauphinee, 1998b). In addition, as we look forward to the use of virtual environments, the principal limitation is the lack of definition of essential elements and steps needed to begin to develop a virtual environment or reality. Hoffman and Vu (1998) have outlined those challenges. Even if agencies and interested parties do meet such challenges and develop the definition of essential elements needed to advance these technologies, so they can be made and the products turn out to be affordable, two other things must happen. There is need for underwriters of the initial developmental costs and much more collaboration and networking amongst agencies with an interest in these new methods will be essential.

Challenge of outcomes-based assessment

The move to outcomes-based assessment is moving forward at two levels. The first is the need to consider the predictability of many of our current methods regarding practice patterns. Tamblyn has been a leader in that challenge and her early results suggest that may be possible (Tamblyn, 1994, 1999). This approach may have its greatest impact in the area of monitoring and enhancing physicians' practice patterns and habits. Recent experiences in Canada illustrate the key elements of this approach: linking the monitoring of practice patterns and assessments to feedback to the physician and then academic prescribing or enhancement (Dauphinee, 1999).

The second level is the monitoring of patient outcomes by newly developing technologies that utilize modern psychometric methods such as item-response theory in the same manner as in adaptive MCQ testing. The work of Bjorner and Ware illustrates this opportunity (Bjorner & Ware, 1997). The day is nearing when adaptive on-line instruments utilizing calibrated items can be administered after each patient's visit, thereby offering the means to assess practice outcomes, including during training, based on measure of functional status and quality of life. These measurements may turn out to be much more sensitive to the impact of health care than traditional measures like death rates and complications (Dauphinee & Norcini, 1999).

The impact of new socio-economic drivers

There are several emerging socio-economic factors that are delineating new challenges for licensure and certification systems. The most obvious two have been the impact of managed care in the United States of America and the European Community in Europe. Each offers a different dilemma. In Europe, the need for "community" wide standards for assessment around licensure and certification is clear, if the market forces are to mean anything. In contrast, in the United States of America, the impact of managed care has been to promote existing certification standards, as has been noted earlier. In either event, the lessons are that the economic shifts and globalization of workforces mean that some old barriers are now being challenged and found wanting. In other areas, good assessment systems are being used to establish standards. This leads to a related challenge: mutual recognition of qualifications.

Mutual recognition

The classic mutual recognition problem is how to establish the basis for equivalency of qualification across both national and international borders? The traditional approach earlier in this century was to accomplish this by agreements or understandings of "reciprocity". This was common amongst many British Commonwealth countries. However, human rights challenges in several jurisdictions have defeated such "old boys'" agreements. The situation is that the older methods of reciprocity are no longer acceptable, but alternative approaches have been slow to evolve until very recently. A series of international conferences have occurred and are continuing in an attempt to begin to establish two things: international postgraduate training databases with mutually acceptable standards for collecting the data; and analogous training standards and criteria for licensure between partnered countries. If successful, these initiatives may offer the means by which licensure and certifying agencies can apply standards using the similar terminology and criteria.

Redefinition of medical acts

The down-delegation of traditional medical acts has been observed over several decades; for example, the use of nurse practitioners in the United States of America. While this approach has been introduced widely throughout the world, a new view of licensure has been seen recently. The old view states that the profession of medicine has a social contract with society that implies exclusivity of certain acts and self-regulation, but in return, certain of society's conditions must be met by the profession. The new view is that many so-called medical acts need not be so and that they could be the purview of other professionals if appropriately trained. The economic and technical imperatives would be removed from several acts, thereby allowing open competition to meet certain of society's "health needs". In some jurisdictions, this view is ingrained in legislation. One example is in the Canadian province of Ontario where the Health Professions Act has "de-listed" certain medical acts. It has opened the way to other providers such as nurse practitioners (College of Physicians and Surgeons of Ontario, 1996).

Alternatives to licensure/certification

Finally, certain authors have openly challenged the notion of licensure and certification. The purpose is not to argue their respective views, but to point out that there are "other" views. One of the most interesting was put forward by Stewart in New Zealand (Stewart, 1998). He argued for: the abolition of licensure and certification; opening of the posts and roles to other providers (issue of contestability); requiring all information about providers to be made public; absence of any requirements of providers except for the need to provide information and compliance with public policies and interests; and that all providers were responsible for all consequences for failure to meet standards of care. This is an interesting idea but who would establish and administer these standards? One could call this "the open market–public beware model".

Another perspective is the appearance of competing criteria that could be surrogates for current certification processes. The recent initiative of the American Medical Association with its American Medical Accreditation Program has been seen by some as a surrogate to the current Specialty Boards (Kassirer, 1997).

In Europe, Karle and Nystrup have argued for a comprehensive evaluation system instead of the Board examinations, as seen in the United States of America (Karle & Nystrup, 1995). Their points are well taken but suggest that the United States of America Board system is based on examinations only, which is not valid. The American system has other components such as in-training reports, requirements for in-training assessment besides ratings of individual's rotations, program accreditation standards, as we have pointed out earlier.

In terms of the traditional view of certification, of even more interest is the move of the American Board of Medical Specialties to redefine their roles as promoting competence in the form of six broad competencies, outlined in a position paper entitled "Concept of the Maintenance of Certification" (American Board of Medical Specialties, 1999). While approved at their Board meeting in mid-1999, if the 24 Boards implement this policy change, they would require evidence of maintaining all general competencies at acceptable standards for a certificant to continue to be designated as "certified". Other developments in Canada and in Australasia are emphasizing educational components in their maintenance of certification programs. Thus, while not proposing an alternative, these developments indicate that the traditional view of certification as "for life" is changing. Clearly, the process of accountability will continue to extend into the practice years and not stop at the initial hurtles of licensure and certification, as has been the case for many decades in North America and in Australasia. No doubt this will be only the beginning.

CONCLUDING COMMENTS

This review has been deliberately written from two separate perspectives. One deals with processes and concepts of licensure and certification. The other focuses on the approach to assessment and provides guidance on the nature of those processes used in licensure and certification today.

The first portion has been written with a strong historical perspective. To understand the origins and underlying debates and socio-political changes leading to modern licensure and certification, is to be better prepared if one is involved in either process. With this background comes the tacit knowledge about why society and the courts have influenced and directed that the processes be conducted the way they are today. Principles and policies do not occur in a social vacuum. Thus, the content of the early portion of the chapter has attempted to identify the context of key principles and social values that have directed the changes in the conduct and approach to licensure and certifying processes in an iterative manner for many decades. That suggests that the processes and concepts are not and should not be static. But as we seek better ways and more valid principles, it is still incumbent on each participant to be conscious of how matters came to be as they are today.

In the second portion of the review, the emphasis has been on key concepts and notions that should underlie the assessment processes involved in licensure and certification. They too have an iterative history. There is no attempt to be prescriptive or to discuss specific methods or procedures. The focus has been on a small number of articles and other publications which the authors believe delineate what is acceptable by contemporary standards and to provide the reader with insights as to what is acceptable, desirable and preferable. In many instances we still fall short. To quote Christine McGuire one final time:

> "Most of our official agencies are slowly developing an ever more rational and defensible overall system for setting standards for licensure and certification – but not only do we need to be increasingly rigorous in documenting and applying that system, we need also desperately to explore ways of extending it to resolve the many issues surrounding re-certification of continuing competence." *(McGuire, 1995, p. 740)*

But McGuire is not the first to challenge the licensure and certification communities. Another person considered the issues in a speech to his colleagues many years before. A concluding comment summarizes the challenge facing licensure bodies and all Boards and Colleges dealing with professional standards.

> "The control of the licensing power is the most important function of the medical boards. Acting on behalf of the State, it is their duty to see that all candidates for license are properly qualified. They stand as guardians of the public and the profession, and here their responsibilities are indeed great." *(Osler, 1885, pp. 83-84)*

This quotation is from Sir William Osler's presidential address to the 18th Annual Meeting of the Canadian Medical Association in 1885, entitled: *"On the Growth of a Profession"*. It can be argued that it is equally relevant today.

REFERENCES

Ackerknecht, E. H. (1982). *A short history of medicine* (Chapter 8; pp. 79-80). Baltimore: Johns Hopkins University Press.

American Board of Medical Specialties Record (1999). *Task force moves ahead.* Volume VIII, No. 4, Fall 1999. Evanston, IL: American Board of Medical Specialties.

American Educational Research Association, American Psychological Association, and National Council on Measurement in Education (1999). *Standards for educational and psychological testing.* Washington, DC: APA.

Bjorner, J. B., & Ware, J. E. (1997). Using modern psychometric methods to measure health outcomes. *Medical Outcomes Trust Monitor, 3*(2), 12-16.

Bowmer, I., Davis, W., Des Marchais, J., Gabb, R., Norcini, J. J., & Whelan, G. (1999). Standard setting in certification tests. In D. Newble, B. Jolly, & R. Wakeford (Eds.), *The certification and recertification of doctors: issues in the assessment of clinical competence.* Cambridge: Cambridge University Press.

Burns, C. R. (1977). Introduction. In C. R. Burns (Ed.), *Legacies in law and medicine* (pp. 1-5). New York: Science History Publications.

Cassie, J. M., Armbbruster, J. S., Bowmer, M. I., & Leach, D. C. (1999). Accreditation of post-graduate medical education in the United States and Canada: a comparison of two systems. *Medical Education, 33,* 493-498.

Coburn, D. (1993). Professional powers in decline: medicine in a changing Canada. In F. W. Hafferty & J. B. McKinlay (Eds.), *The changing medical profession. An international perspective* (pp. 92-102). New York and Oxford: Oxford University Press.

College of Physicians & Surgeons of Ontario (1995). *Controlled acts model: a guide for physicians and policy makers.* Toronto: College of Physicians and Surgeons of Ontario.

Cruess, R. C., & Cruess, S. R. (1997) Teaching medicine as a profession in the service of healing. *Academic Medicine, 72,* 941-951.

Cunnington, J. P. W., Neville, A. J., & Norman, G. R. (1996). The risks of thoroughness: reliability and validity of global rating scores. *Advances in Health Professions Education, 1,* 227-233.

Cusimano, M. D. (1996). Standard setting in medical education. *Academic Medicine, 71*(supplement), S112-120.

Dauphinee, W. D. (1995). Assessing clinical performance. Where do we stand and what might we expect? *Journal of the American Medical Association, 274,* 741-743.

Dauphinee, W. D. (1998). Emerging technologies in evaluation: assessing their role in the evaluation of residents. In E. L. Mancall & P. G. Bashook (Eds.), *Evaluating residents for board certification* (pp. 79-96). Evanston, IL: American Board Medical Specialties.

Dauphinee, W. D. (1999). Revalidation of doctors in Canada. *British Medical Journal, 319,* 1188-1190.

Dauphinee, W. D., & Norcini, J. J. (1999). Introduction: assessing health care professionals in the new millennium. *Advances in Health Sciences Education, 4,* 3-7.

Dauphinee, W. D., Fabb, W., Jolly, B., Langsley, D., Wealthall, S., & Procopis, P. (1994). Determining the content of certifying examinations. In D. Newble, B. Jolly, & R. Wakeford (Eds.), *The certification and recertification of doctors: issues in the assessment of clinical competence* (pp. 92-104). Cambridge: Cambridge University Press.

Dauphinee, W. D., Blackmore, D. E., Smee, S. M., Rothman, A., Des Marchais, J., & Reznick, R. K. (1998). Adaptive testing. Report on the results and myths arising from the use of a sequenced OSCE for national licensure. Presented at the Ottawa Conference on Medical Education. Philadelphia, PA.

Derbyshire, R. C. (1969). *Medical licensure and discipline in the United States.* Baltimore: Johns Hopkins University Press.

Donabedian, A. (1967). Evaluating the quality of medical care. In D. Mainland (Ed.), *Health services research* (pp. 166-201). New York: Milbank Memorial Fund.

Educational Commission for Foreign Medical Graduates. (1999). Information Booklet. Philadelphia, PA: (1999). Educational Commission for Foreign Medical Graduates.

Elaisson, A. H. (1998). Performance improvement in telemedicine: the essential elements. *Military Medicine, 163,* 530-535.

Fidler, H., Lockyer, J. M., Toews, J., & Violato, C. (1999). Changing physicians' practices: the effect of individual feedback. *Academic Medicine, 74,* 702-714.

Flexner, A. (1910). *Medical education in the United States and Canada.* Bulletin #4. New York: Carnegie Foundation for the Advancement for Teaching.

Frenk, J., & Ruran-Arenas, L. (1993). Medical profession and the state. In F. W. Hafferty & J. B. McKinlay (Eds.), *The changing medical profession. An international perspective.* New York and Oxford: Oxford University Press.

Gray, J. D. (1996). Global rating scales in residency education. *Academic Medicine, 71*(supplement January), S55-S63.

Hafferty, F. W., & McKinlay, J. B. (Eds.) (1993). *The changing medical profession. An international perspective.* Oxford: Oxford University Press.

Hall, W., Violato Lewkonia, R., Locklear, J., Fidler, H., Toews, J., Jennett, P., Donoff, M., & Moores, D. (1999). Assessment of physician performance in Alberta: the physician achievement review. *Canadian Medical Association Journal, 161,* 52-57.

Hambleton, R. K., & Jones, R. W. (1993). Comparison of classic test theory and item response theory and their application to test development. *Educational Researcher, 22,* 38-47.

Hartung, E. F. (1934). Medical regulations of Frederick the second of Hohetaufen. *Medical Life, 41,* 587-601.

Hoffman, H., & Vu, D. (1997). Virtual reality. Teaching tool of the twenty-first century? *Academic Medicine, 72,* 1076-1081.

Holden, W. D. (1979). The American specialty boards. In T. Samph & B. Templeton (Eds.), *Evaluation in medical education. Past, present, future* (pp. 165-200). Cambridge, MA: Ballinger.

Hubbard, J. P. (1971). *Measuring medical education. The tests and test procedures of the National Board of Medical Examiners* (1st ed.). Philadelphia: Lea & Fibiger.

Hubbard, J. P. (1978). *Measuring medical education. The tests and the experience of the National Board of Medical Examiners* (2nd ed.). Philadelphia: Lea & Febiger.

Irvine, D. (1997). The performance of doctors. I: professionalism and self-regulation in a changing world. *British Medical Journal, 314,* 1540-1542.

Jaeger, R. M. (1994). The psychometric demands of testing for licensure and certification. In D. Laveault, B. D. Zumbo, M. E. Gessaroli, & M. W. Boss (Eds.), *Modern theories of measurement: problems and issues* (pp. 305-335). University of Ottawa: Faculty of Education.

Jonsen, A. R. (1990). *The new medicine and the old ethics.* Cambridge, MA: Harvard University Press.

Kane, M. T. (1992). The assessment of professional competence. *Evaluation & the Health Professions, 15,* 163-182.

Kane, M. T. (1994). Validating interpretative arguments for licensure and certification examinations. *Evaluation & the Health Professions, 17,* 133-159.

Karle, H., & Nystrup, J. (1995). Comprehensive evaluation of specialty training: an alternative to board examinations in Europe. *Medical Education, 29,* 308-316.

Kassirer, J. (1997). The surrogates for board certification. What should the standard be? *New England Journal of Medicine, 337,* 43-44.

Kerr, R. B. (1997). *History of the Medical Council of Canada.* Victoria, Canada: Morris Printing Company.

Klein, R. (1990). The state and the profession: the politics of the double bed. *Canadian Medical Journal, 301,* 701-702.

Klein, R. (1993). National variations on international trends. In F. W. Hafferty & J. B. McKinlay (Eds.), *The changing medical profession. An international perspective* (pp. 202-209). New York and Oxford: Oxford University Press.

Kolen, M. J., & Brennan, R. L. (1995). Introduction and concepts. In M. J. Kolen, & R. C. Brennan (Eds.), *Test equating: methods and practices* (pp. 1-26). New York: Springer.

LaDuca, A. (1994). Validation of professional licensure examinations. Professions theory, test design, and construct validity. *Evaluation & the Health Professions, 17,* 178-197.

Lord, F. M. (1982). Item response theory and equating – a technical summary. In P. W. Holland & D. B. Rubin (Eds.), *Test equating* (pp. 141-148). New York: Academic Press.

MacDonald, K. M. (1997). *The sociology of the professions.* London: Sage Publications.

McAuley, R. G., Paul, W. M., Morrison, G. H., Beckett, R. F., & Goldsmith, C. H. (1990). Five-year results of the peer review assessment program of the College of Physicians and Surgeons of Ontario. *Canadian Medical Association Journal, 143,* 1193-1199.

McGuire, C. H. (1993). Standards in the certification of physicians. In E. L. Mancall, P. G. Bashook, & J. L. Dockery (Eds.), *Establishing standards for board certification* (pp. 3-12). Evanston, IL: American Board of Medical Specialties.

McGuire, C. H. (1995). Reflections of a maverick measurement maven. *Journal of the American Medical Association, 274,* 735-740.

McGuire, C. H. (1997). Physician assessment: a rite of passage or a right to practice. *The Long Term View, 3,* 13-21.

Medical Council of Canada (1999). *Evaluating examination information booklet.* Ottawa: Medical Council of Canada.

Meskaukas, J. A. (1986). Setting standards for credentialing examinations: an update. *Evaluation & the Health Professions, 9,* 187-203.

Morrison, R. D., & Carter, E. A. (1992). Licensure, certification, and registration. In M. D. Alkin (Ed.), *Encyclopedia of educational research* (6th ed., pp. 747-751,). New York: Macmillan.

Mueller, C. B. (1985). Implications for licensure and certification. In V. R. Neufeld & G. R. Norman (Eds.), *Assessing clinical competence* (pp. 311-339). New York: Springer.

Nahrwald, D. R. (1999). ABMS Competencies for maintenance of certification. Presentation at the Annual Meeting of the Royal College of Physicians and Surgeons of Canada, Montreal.

Neufeld, V. R. (1985). An introduction to measurement properties. In V. R. Neufeld & G. R. Norman (Eds.), *Assessing clinical competence* (pp. 39-50). New York: Springer.

Newble, D., & Wakeford, R. (1994). Primary certification in the UK and Australasia. In D. Newble, B. Jolly, & R. Wakeford (Eds.), *The certification and recertification of doctors: issues in the assessment of clinical competence* (pp. 13-18). Cambridge: Cambridge University Press.

Newble, D., Dawson, B., Dauphinee, W. D., Page, G., Macdonald, M., Swanson, D., Mulholland. H., & Van der Vleuten (1994). Guidelines for assessing clinical competence. *Teaching and Learning in Medicine, 6,* 213-220.

Newble, D., Paget, N., & McLaren, B. (1999). Revalidation in Australia and New Zealand: approach of Royal Australasian College of Physicians. *British Medical Journal, 319,* 1185-1188.

Nielsen, B. B., Scofield, R. S., Mueller, S., Tranin, A. S., Moore, P., & Murphy, C. M. (1996). Certification of oncology nurses: a history. *Oncology Nurses Forum, 23,* 701-708.

Norcini, J. J. (1994). Research on standards for professional licensure and certification examinations. *Evaluation & the Health Professions, 17,* 160-177.

Norman, G. R., Van der Vleuten, C. P. M., & De Graaff, E. (1991). Pitfalls in the pursuit of objectivity: issues of validity, efficiency and acceptability. *Medical Education, 25,* 19-126.

Norman, G. R., Swanson, D. B., & Case, S. M. (1996). Conceptual and methodological issues comparing assessment methods. *Teaching and Learning in Medicine, 8,* 208-216.

Osler, W. (1886). On the growth of a profession. *Canadian Medical & Surgical Journal, 14,* 1239-1255.

Ramsey, P. G., & Wenrich, M. D. (1999). Use of professional associate ratings to assess the performance of practising physicians: past, present, future. *Advances in Health Sciences Education, 4,* 27-38.

Regehr, G., MacRae, H. M., Reznick, R. K., & Szalay, D. (1998). Comparing the psychometric properties of checklists and global rating scales for assessing performance in an OSCE format examination. *Academic Medicine, 73,* 993-997.

Reznick, R. K. (1998). A good pair of hands versus a reliable and valid measure of technical skill. In E. L. Mancall & P. G. Bashook (Eds.), *Evaluating residents for board certification* (pp. 73-78). Evanston, IL: American Board of Medical Specialties.

Shyryock, R. H. (1967). *Medical licensing in America: 1650-1965.* Baltimore, MD: Johns Hopkins Press.

Sigerist, H. (1935). The history of medical licensure. *Journal of the American Medical Association, 104,* 1057.

Southgate, L., & Dauphinee, W. D. (1998). Maintaining standards in British and Canadian medicine: the developing role of the regulatory body. *British Medical Journal, 316,* 697-700.

Stacey, M. (1997). The case for and against medical self-regulation. *Federation Bulletin, 84,* 17-25.

Stevens, R. (1971). *American medicine and the public interest.* New Haven and London: Yale University.

Stevens, R. (1986). Issues for American internal medicine through the last century. *Annals of Internal Medicine, 105,* 592-602.

Stevens, R. A. (1999). How are certiciation and professional competence linked? *Professional competence and board certification conference material.* Evanston, IL: American Board of Medical Specialties.

Stewart, R. D. H. (1998). Licensing medical practitioners: is there an alternative? *New Zealand Medical Journal, 111,* 235-236.

Sumner, W., Hagen, M. D., & Rovinelli, R. (1999). Item generating methodology of an empiric simulation project. *Advances in Health Sciences Education, 4,* 49-66.

Swanson, D. B. (1987). A measurement framework for performance-based tests. In I. Hart & R. Harden (Eds.), *Further developments in assessing clinical competence* (pp. 13-45). Montreal: Can-Heal Publications.

Swanson, D. B., Norman, G. R., & Linn, R. L. (1995). Performance-based assessment: lessons from the health professions. *Educational Researcher, 24,* 5-22.

Swanson, D. B., Clauser, B. E., & Case, S. M. (1999). Clinical skills assessment with standardised patients in high stakes tests: a framework for thinking about score precision, equating, and security. *Advances in Health Sciences Education, 4,* 67-106.

Tamblyn, R. (1994). Is the public being protected? Prevention of suboptimal medical practice through training programs and credentialling examinations. *Evaluation & The Health Professions, 17,* 198-221.

Tamblyn, R. (1999). Outcomes in medical education: what is the standard and outcome of care delivered by our graduates. *Advances in Health Sciences Education, 4,* 9-25.

Tamblyn, R., Abrahamowicz, M., Brailovsky, C., Grand'Maison, P., Lescop, J., Norcini, J., Girard, N., & Haggerty, J. (1996). Association between licensing examination scores and resource use and quality of care in primary care practice. *Journal of the American Medical Association, 280,* 989-996.

Van der Vleuten, C. P. M. (1996). The assessment of professional competence: developments, research and practical implications. *Advances in Health Sciences Education, 1,* 41-67.

Van der Vleuten, C. P. M., & Newble, D. (1994). Methods of assessment in certification. In D. Newble, B. Jolly, & R. Wakeford (Eds.), *The certification and recertification of doctors: issues in the assessment of clinical competence* (pp. 105-125). Cambridge: Cambridge University Press.

Willis, E. (1993). Medical profession in Australia. In F. W. Hafferty & J. B. McKinlay (Eds.), *The changing medical profession. An international perspective* (pp. 104-114). New York and Oxford: Oxford University Press.

Zara, A. R. (1999). Using computer-adaptive testing to evaluate nurse competence for licensure: some history and forward look. *Advances in Health Sciences Education, 4,* 39-48.

27 Relicensure, Recertification and Practice-Based Assessment

JOHN CUNNINGTON
McMaster University

LESLEY SOUTHGATE
Royal Free and University College Medical School, University College

SUMMARY

Over the past 25 years the maintenance of competence of physicians in practice has emerged as a central issue in health care. On the basis of public concern there have been increasing calls for the recertification or the relicensure of physicians. Such revalidation of physician abilities must be based (like the original validation) upon evidence that physicians have indeed maintained their competence. Measuring the outcomes of maintenance of competence activity, however, is fraught with scientific, administrative and political difficulties.

One approach to recertification stems from the belief that continuing medical education (CME) is a marker for those who keep up to date. Such an approach has the advantage of being readily acceptable to the profession, as it is perceived to be non-threatening. There is, however, little evidence in the literature to show, (1) that physicians learn from continuing medical education, (2) that they apply the lessons learned in their practices, (3) that improvements can be measured in terms of improved patient care, or (4) that even if these things could be shown they would translate into an appropriate curriculum to ensure ongoing maintenance of competence. In fact there is little or no evidence to suggest that the surrogate outcome of continuing medical education hours translates into maintenance of competence.

Other approaches include revalidation based upon examination and assessment of practice. Recertification examinations have the advantage over continuing medical education of looking at the breadth of practice expectations, and they can define a minimum standard to which all physicians can be held accountable. Studies of certification examinations have shown that test scores correlate well with clinical competency even out to ten years. This makes it likely that recertification examinations will prove to be similarly effective. An ambitious program of

International Handbook of Research in Medical Education, 883–912.
G.R. Norman, C.P.M. Van der Vleuten, D.I. Newble (eds.)
© *2002 Dordrecht: Kluwer Academic Publishers. Printed in Great Britain.*

recertification by examination is being undertaken by the American Board of Medical Specialties and its member organizations.

An alternative approach is assessment of continued maintenance of competence (MOC) by the assessment of what physicians in practice really do or by the outcomes of their patient care. Practice audit by peers is a powerful tool to gather data to ensure maintenance of standards. Supported with tests of competence (such as seeing standardized patients) the evidence of competence, or lack of it, can be strong enough on the one hand to justify restriction of license and on the other to justify public confidence in the revalidation process. The General Medical Council in the United Kingdom and the Royal Australasian College of Physicians, and the programs of the College of Physicians and Surgeons of Ontario, have introduced practice assessment by peers, colleagues and patients.

INTRODUCTION

For much of this century one measure of a modern, civilized society is that its citizens have the right to health care. A corollary to that entitlement is that the practitioners who provide that health care are competent. Since the nineteenth century most developed countries have had mechanisms to ensure that newly qualified physicians have achieved a standard of competence acceptable to the profession and the community. Generally speaking, this translates into two activities: one is the attesting by examination of the satisfactory achievement by the candidate of the standards of the universities, professional organizations and national examination bodies. The second is the use of that information by the licensing authorities to confer a license to practice medicine in a political and geographic area.

For 100 years this process has provided the public with confidence about new health care providers but over the past two decades concerns have been raised about the abilities of physicians in practice. As society has become increasingly aware of the possibility of decline in physician performance, as a consequence of physical or mental illness, cognitive decline, drug and alcohol dependence, laziness, greed or other human frailty through a 30 to 40 year practice lifetime, so concern has increased about assuring that practitioners continue to meet the standard of providing quality care. This chapter is about the challenge that the profession, the educators, the public and the national licensing and certifying bodies are engaged in to ensure that public confidence is well founded.

As a consequence of training and qualifying examinations, it can generally be accepted that those embarking upon practice have achieved a level of performance that we call competence. By contrast, for those in practice the central question is whether they have continued to maintain that competence. Fundamental to the issue of *maintenance of competence* (MOC) is the protection of the public through defining standards of care and ensuring that these standards are met. An additional element is the provision of guidance to the profession regarding the standards and of the requirement and means for those standards to be maintained.

Several issues devolve from the concern of maintenance of competence. One is the definition of competence. While there may be a general sense that we recognize competence when we see it, it is difficult to provide *evidence of maintenance of competence* without measuring competence, and competence is difficult to measure without a clear vision of its nature. To some extent the definition will vary with the purposes of the group doing the defining. However a practical *definition of competence* should incorporate the idea that the physician has the knowledge and skills expected of a professional in a field of medicine and that the physician applies the knowledge and skills in a consistent, responsible and professional manner.

The difficulties of definition multiply as competence to begin independent practice becomes performance in actual practice. Competence is not only maintained, but transformed by clinical experience and the development of expertise (Charlin, Tardif, & Boshuizen, 2000). This transformation presents challenges and opportunities for collecting evidence about the standard of clinical practice that are not applicable to initial licensure.

If society requires maintenance of competence the scientific questions are: What knowledge, skills and behaviors do we measure? And, how do we measure them? There is also the administrative issue of how we attest to their accomplishment. The result is multiple possible combinations of what to measure and how to measure it. In addition, the system of measurement with its problems, and the administrative system testifying to the accomplishment of the objectives, must be considered.

The central scientific question is the *measurement of maintenance of competence*. The options include:

1. The measurement of the *inputs* (the effort) contributing to maintenance of competence, which translates into the measurement of continuing medical education study time and/or content, either voluntary or mandatory, and/or by self-report or by a professional organization.
2. Assessing the *outputs* (the results) of the maintenance of competence activities, which translates into assessing either:
   a. What has been learned, or
   b. What effect the learning has had, either
      i. In changing practice patterns, or
      ii. In changing patient outcomes.

RECERTIFICATION AND RELICENSURE

Before exploring the scientific issues, it is useful to clarify the meaning of the terms recertification and relicensure. Traditionally both licensure (usually undertaken by government sponsored or controlled licensing bodies) and certification (usually undertaken by professional organizations responsible for assessing the quality and adequacy of training, with or without final qualifying examinations) have been valid for life. The awarding of the certificate testified to the accomplishment of the predefined goals and standards. This is analogous to the awarding of a university degree; once you have it, you have it for life. Increasingly, however, both types of organizations have been moving towards time-limited certificates with renewal contingent upon successful completion of some form of mandatory maintenance of competence activity. In the United States, for example, the vast majority of medical specialty boards now require their diplomats to recertify (Norcini & Lipner, 1999). While the American Board of Medical Specialties requires recertification it does not allow its member organizations to rescind initial certificates through the recertification process unless time-limited certificates were issued in the first place (Simon & DeRosa, 1999). In Australia, only the Royal Australian College of Obstetricians and Gynaecologists has a time-limited Fellowship, although other Colleges award certificates of participation in maintenance of standards programs (Newble & Paget, 1999).

In the United Kingdom it will be mandatory from 2002 for all doctors to submit evidence of fitness to practice (maintenance of competence) to the General Medical Council or face referral to the procedures that investigate poor performance. If incompetence is confirmed and remediation is unsuccessful, the outcome will be removal from the register and an inability to work as a doctor. The program is called revalidation: the word has been chosen to emphasize the validity and currency of the doctor's license to practice. But the effect is that all United Kingdom physicians, in every discipline and at every stage of their career, will be subject to periodic relicensure, in addition to any recertification requirements in their own discipline (Southgate & Pringle, 1999).

This fundamental change is taking place at different times, in different ways, and in different jurisdictions, setting the stage for the new concepts of recertification and relicensure.

Recertification is the usual result of the measurement of maintenance of competence activities. It means that the certifying body has designed a mechanism which, when completed by the practitioner, results in affirmation by the certifying body that the physician has satisfactorily demonstrated continued maintenance of competence. In practice the certifying organization will require the physician to meet one of the following goals:

1. The completion of a predefined quantity of continuing medical education (often continuing medical education activities pre-approved by the organization);
2. The passing of a recertifying examination; or
3. A satisfactory outcome to the assessment of the physician's practice (practice-based assessment).

Relicensure is not fundamentally an assessment or measurement procedure, but rather an administrative decision, which confirms that a physician has completed the maintenance of competence activities required by a professional certifying body. Relicensure tends to have a political dimension and results not only from the measurement of the maintenance of competence activity, but also from the interaction of that measurement with other factors.

Generally these issues are determined by local geographic and political considerations. Since they are fundamentally outside the scientific and research agenda they will not be specifically addressed in this chapter except as they directly pertain to the central considerations. A number of external influences on the decision to implement relicensure are:

- the weight of public opinion in favor;
- professional opinion;
- the fears of physicians about the implications of the process leading to resistance to change;
- political necessity and the positioning of governments and their oppositions;
- measurement and administrative options available;
- the number of physicians to be assessed;
- costs and who pays them.

Relicensure versus critical incident review and screening

It is worth pointing out that time-limited certificates for relicensure are not the only possible response to the problem of maintaining standards of care. Instead of relicensure, most licensing organizations deal with the problem in two ways. The first is by adjudicating complaints. This is clearly seen by the public as addressing their concerns, and the result is that a small number of practitioners are identified as having failed to maintain the standard of care, usually in an isolated case. Typically these physicians would either lose their medical license or have it suspended, and/or they would be compelled to upgrade their knowledge and skills upon threat of delicensure.

The other approach is based upon the principle of random screening for a disease we might call dyscompetence (incompetence being too strongly charged a word to be useful). In this model all license holders are made aware that they equally likely to be chosen for review (in practice it is more efficient to target high risk groups, such as older physicians in solo practice) and some form of review, often a practice-based assessment, is used to identify those whose practice is sub-standard. Examples of such programs include the peer assessment program of the College of Physicians and Surgeons of Ontario (McAuley, Paul, Morrison, Beckett, & Goldsmith, 1990). In this program physician assessors are sent into the office of randomly selected physicians. The review consists of an assessment by predetermined criteria of 20-25 randomly selected charts of patients seen in the previous week, followed by a physician interview. While 82% of physicians were found to have neither deficient records nor an unsatisfactory level of care, 15% of the family physicians and 2% of the specialists were found to have serious deficiencies in one or both areas.

Proponents of such programs argue that these kinds of activities raise the standard of care by putting the profession on notice of the requirement to maintain standards, as well as serving a case-finding function for incompetence. Opponents counter that it is just a way of finding the "bad apples", which demeans the profession as a whole. Irrespective of either argument the reality is that random screening is constrained by its resources; only a limited number can be assessed (in Ontario 350 out of 25,000 physicians in the province are assessed annually) and consequently many can escape the screening process and possible detection. In the United Kingdom there is no plan to sample the register; revalidation will apply to everyone. The dangers of demoralizing the competent majority by an emphasis on minimum standards are recognized and present a major challenge for the General Medical Council as it designs the components of the program. Either way, relicensure and recertification are applied equally to everyone. As a result, it is not only more effective at maintaining the standards and protecting the public, but in fact, it is fairer.

The political dimension

Before considering the scientific issues it is appropriate to reflect briefly upon the political issues that drive, determine and constrain the process and the outcomes of maintenance of competence activities. The first is perhaps the question of who is in charge. While it may seem intuitively obvious that some overseeing organization is in charge, this does not reflect the historical background. Until very recently the responsibility for keeping up to date with changes in medical knowledge has rested with the physicians themselves. It was simply expected that keeping up was part of the job and that practitioners would do what was necessary to fulfill their obligations. The assumption of this responsibility by professional organizations has created changes that, while serving the public interest, have created resistance in the profession due to the perceived threat to physician independence and to the loss of individual control. Some measure of the professional resistance to this approach may be inferred from the fact that it was in 1968 that the American Board of Internal Medicine reached the decision to limit the duration of its certificates, but the American College of Physicians refused to endorse it (Benson, 1991). In 1973 the American Board of Medical Specialties adopted in principle, and urged its member boards to implement, voluntary periodic recertification and the establishment of a deadline for recertification. The policy, however, was not adopted until 1978, and it was not until 1993 that all boards were required to establish a plan for recertifying diplomats (Simon & DeRosa, 1999). By now it is clear that individuals are no longer in sole charge of their maintenance of competence activities. Instead, standards are set by the professional organizations.

The question of which professional organization is in charge is a political one. The answer is dependent on the division of responsibilities in differing geographical areas. In some countries this reflects a power struggle between organizations and has led to problems of defining who is responsible for what. However, these issues have been adequately settled in most jurisdictions. In general, the licensing bodies, by virtue of statute, view themselves as being charged with the responsibility of setting and maintaining standards. Depending on their resources and interests, they may be willing to allow the certifying bodies to assume the work and then use the results of that determination to make their own decisions. Complicating problems can arise when organizations such as health maintenance organizations or government agencies impose a third tier of requirement for continuing medical education activity.

Compounding these issues is the question of cost and who pays for maintenance of competence activities. When the task is earning continuing medical education hours the benefits accrue to the physician and it is appropriate for the costs to be borne by the practitioner. But when the issue is one of the development, pre-testing, taking and marking of an examination, the membership of a professional organization can balk, feeling that the requirement is imposed from "outside" and that they are not the direct beneficiaries of the activity. The problem is somewhat relieved if there is the sense that all are contributing equally to maintaining an expensive infrastructure but it is compounded when the maintenance of competence activity is a practice audit. In Ontario, while anyone may be audited, the reality is that most will not get audited in 20 years. The costs of these assessments, which equal approximately $1000 per audit, are borne by the licensing authority, which in the end is spending the monies gathered from physicians in licensing fees. If an individual does poorly in the practice audit, he or she can be referred for individualized testing, which costs in the range of $4000 and is borne solely by the practitioner.

In the United Kingdom the costs of assessing poorly performing doctors are borne by the General Medical Council which is funded by the profession (General Medical Council, 1999). However the United Kingdom Government is also imposing standards for all physicians working in the National Health Service and will bear part of the cost. But this has led to fears that the professionally led regulation of the profession is threatened by state control (Secretary of State for Health, 1999).

All of these issues – power, control, loss of autonomy, fear, and expense – contribute to the resistance to maintenance of competence activities exhibited by the profession. No organization can afford to deal with these concerns by brushing them under the carpet. Managing physicians' concerns is a part of the successful introduction of any maintenance of competence program. Centrally important to physician acceptance of such programs is the active involvement of perceived physician leaders, especially those in the professional organizations, the medical associations and the universities. The involvement of patient groups, community health councils and consumers in the debates with physicians is also an important piece of the jigsaw. Public participation in the detail of physician assessment has been a feature of the General Medical Council work in the United Kingdom and paradoxically has been one of the principal mechanisms for increasing physician confidence in the changes. The wide dissemination of the clear message that such activities are designed to protect the health of the public and that they are the responsibility of a public spirited, self-regulating profession can go a long way in providing the public and professional support required to marginalize individual dissent or disagreement.

MEASUREMENT OF MAINTENANCE OF COMPETENCE

The fundamental measurement options are either the *input* to maintenance of competence, which translates into the measurement of continuing medical education effort, or the *output* of maintenance of competence activities, which means assessing what has been learned, or what effect the learning has had on practice patterns, or patient outcomes.

Recertification by counting CME hours

Time and again, we are told that medical knowledge is rapidly changing and that if we do not keep up we will fall inexorably behind. Therefore it appears to be intuitively obvious that attending a refresher course or update on a topic relevant to one's medical practice is going to keep one up-to-date. In consequence of this obvious "face validity", the measurement of the input to maintenance of competence activity by the counting of continuing medical education hours has become ubiquitous and, in many jurisdictions, mandatory. The other great attraction to this approach is the ease of measurement, which typically is done as hours of continuing medical education attended. With hours of time spent accepted as the standard unit of continuing medical education activity, it is an easy matter for a professional organization to establish criteria for the number of hours required to qualify for recertification. Administrative structures vary. Some organizations use an honor system in which physicians' attendance at continuing medical education events is accepted without question. Others require a record of attendance at continuing medical education events to be kept, allowing for the possibility of audit either at random, or for situations in which concerns have been raised. Examples of such programs include that of the Royal Australasian College of Physicians recertifying program, which is based upon the completion of 500 hours of study time (maximum of 450 hours of continuing medical education) in 5 years (Newble & Paget, 1996).

There are several disadvantages of this approach to maintenance of competence. The one that many of the professional organizations have chosen to address is the question of whether the continuing medical education activity was of sufficient quality to be worth counting. To deal with this organizations requiring such activities have tended to require certain preconditions to be met if credit is to be granted for the activity. Typically these include: that the event has an organizing committee which includes members of the target group; that it undertakes to determine the educational needs of its proposed audience; and that there is assessment of the quality of the presentations and feedback to the presenters. Because of the variability in the types of continuing medical education, both in terms of content and format of presentations, some organizations have also attempted to assign different weights to different activities; for example, the College of Family Practitioners of Canada distinguishes between types of activities, e.g. self study modules (Mainpro-M1 credits) versus self directed reading (Mainpro-M2 credits). By controlling the number and type of credits required for recertification the certifying bodies hope to positively influence the quality of the educational offerings and the individual physician's learning.

In addition to ease of measurement, the other advantage of the "hours of continuing medical education" approach to maintenance of competence is that the profession does not perceive it as threatening. The ground rules are laid out in advance and only those who have not got the common sense to sidestep the net are likely to be caught in its web. The professional organizations, of course, will suggest that continuing medical education is not about identifying incompetence but about raising the educational standard of the whole profession through lifelong continuing education. The trouble with that argument, however, is that what is being measured is a surrogate outcome for learning. There is actually no certainty that anyone is learning anything.

For example, one study that measured physician performance with a test which included standardized patient assessment showed a negative correlation of self-reported continuing medical education hours with competence ($r = 0.30$); the implication being the more the continuing medical education, the lower the competence (Caulford et al., 1994). Of course it could be said that this just underscores the unreliability of self-reporting. However, even if professional organizations are responsible for accrediting the continuing medical education activity and counting the hours "earned", there is little evidence that this translates into lessons learned or practice modified. In fact, much of the evidence suggests the opposite, at least for formal didactic, lecture type continuing medical education, which represents the majority of the educational activities offered by providers or engaged in by physicians.

In 1995 Davis et al. published the results of a systematic review of the effect of continuing medical education strategies (Davis, Thomson, Oxman, & Haynes, 1995). They found that relatively short (1 day or less) formal continuing medical education events such as conferences generally effected no change in physician performance or health care (six interventions demonstrated negative or inconclusive effects).

A second review by Davis et al. (1999) looked specifically at whether conferences, workshops, rounds, and other traditional continuing medical education activities change physician behavior or health care outcomes (Davis et al., 1999).

They conducted a literature search for all randomized controlled trials of educational interventions in which objective determination of performance in the workplace or health care outcomes was obtained. They divided the interventions into didactic (predominantly lectures or presentations with minimal audience interaction), interactive (which used techniques to enhance physician interaction, such as role play, discussion groups, hands-on training, and problem or case solving), or mixed didactic and interactive sessions (the use of both), and they considered the effect to be positive if one or more primary outcome measure related to physician performance or patient health care demonstrated a statistically significant change. Of the four didactic continuing medical education interventions they were able to find in the literature, none was shown to alter physician performance. They concluded that didactic continuing medical education interventions were ineffective in changing physician performance.

This is a profound message, which the medical community has generally ignored. Based upon slowly accumulating evidence, it has been widely suspected that large group didactic continuing medical education teaching sessions are ineffective at creating change. But the providers of continuing medical education have failed to change their product. Perhaps it's not surprising that pharmaceutical companies continue to sponsor lectures announcing the launching of new products, but it should be surprising that the scientific and education based university continuing medical education providers continue to pour resources into expensive and sometimes massive didactic teaching sessions without any evidence for their effectiveness. Part of the explanation probably lies in the fact that this is a multimillion-dollar industry in which any organization that can bring in the registrants can reap the profits. Another factor is that this is the product most familiar and least threatening to physicians. It does not challenge them to take a stand or commit themselves. It is not surprising that they subscribe; it's human nature to be more interested in one's own comfort than in being challenged to learn new ideas or implement new practice patterns. Unfortunately, doing what one prefers may not be educationally valuable. Indeed, one randomized controlled trial of a continuing medical education intervention showed that when the topics were of relatively great interest to the physicians, the study group showed no more improvement than the control group, but when the topics were not preferred the documented quality of care provided by the study physicians rose and significantly differed from that provided by the control physicians (Sibley et al., 1982).

To attempt to deal constructively with this dilemma some organizations have required not just the measurement of the time spent in the activity, but also some assessment by the physician of the lesson learned from the activity, usually in the form of an educational diary or dossier. Examples of such programs include the Royal College of Physicians of Canada's maintenance of competenceOMP program that asks physicians to document not only what they have learned but also how it has affected their practice. Notwithstanding the attractiveness of this approach, there is no evidence to support its effectiveness.

The rush to embrace mandatory continuing medical education by the counting of hours has not been limited to physicians but has been embraced by other health specialties such as physiotherapy, occupational therapy and nursing. In 1996 it was reported that 18 U.S. states required continuing education as a condition for relicensure of registered nurses (Hewlett & Eichelberger, 1996). However, a review by these authors, done as part of a task force carried out by the Mississippi Nurses Association, failed to demonstrate that mandatory continuing education actually translates into changes in practice or health outcomes. They concluded with the seemingly obvious, but widely ignored, recommendation that no state should consider mandating continuing education for relicensure in an effort to improve quality of care provided by registered nurses unless the relationship of continuing education to practice is clearly established.

In spite of the disappointing evidence of effectiveness of traditional continuing medical education, there is some evidence to suggest that well designed, interactive continuing medical education can have an effect on practice patterns and patient outcomes. Models of this type of activity include problem based, small group learning activities, such as described by Premi and colleagues (Premi et al., 1994).

In the study reported above by Davis only six interactive and seven mixed didactic and interactive interventions met the selection criteria. Of the six interactive sessions all measured the impact on physician performance and four of the six demonstrated a significant impact; of the seven mixed didactic and interactive sessions five were positive on measures of physician performance and two of the three that measured impact on health care outcomes demonstrated positive changes.

A comprehensive review of the literature for the United Kingdom Chief Medical Officer (Grant & Stanton, 1999) reached similar conclusions. The United Kingdom government funds continuing medical education for general practitioners and the subsequent report (www.doh.gov.uk/cmo/cmodev.htm) will influence the introduction of planned, accredited professional development for British GPs directed at their needs rather than wants, and delivered using methods likely to be more effective than passing time listening to lectures. All general practitioners will be required to have a formally documented personal learning plan as part of the NHS system of clinical governance now being put into place.

If certifying bodies demanded more interactive continuing medical education and rigorously scrutinized the quality of the educational offerings presented for accreditation they might overcome the reluctance of continuing medical education providers to create the kind of interactive interventions that have been shown to make a difference. However, even if they did, it is not certain that they would be successful in enticing physicians to attend.

But even if it is possible to show that continuing medical education, when optimally designed and carried out, can effect a change in physician behavior and practice outcomes, this does not necessarily mean that the physicians involved are keeping up to the standard of the profession in their field. It might just mean that the physician has learned and applied one important, but isolated, item of practice. In fact, there is simply no evidence to support the contention that physicians, when choosing their continuing medical education activities, can or do design for themselves a curriculum that would keep them up to date in their field. It remains an article of faith that they would do so if given the right opportunities. One prominent educator has written:

> ... it is difficult for me to conceive of a domain of learning where self-direction is less appropriate than in medicine. All professions are defined as such because they possess common and specialized funds of knowledge. To assume that mastery of this knowledge can be left to chance or whim (or what amounts to nearly the same thing – individual self-direction) strikes at the core of professionalism ... the notion that students should be able to formulate their own learning objectives based upon their own interests flies in the face of a lot of knowledge about human foibles and the nature of professions. *(Norman, 1999, p. 888)*

Until there is evidence that self-directed continuing medical education by counting hours is as effective as approaches designed to assess abilities across the breadth of a professional field, such as recertification examinations or practice-based peer review, it will be impossible to justify selling continuing medical education to the public or the profession as an adequate solution to the problem of maintenance of competence. Indeed, as the public becomes more demanding in requiring the profession to give evidence of maintenance of competence in its practitioners, it is likely to become more aware of the weakness inherent in measuring educational inputs by counting hours. The profession courts the charge of having created a system of smoke and mirrors which gives the appearance of protecting the public interest but, in fact, does little more than protect its own members. To obviate such a charge, professional organizations have increasingly taken up the challenge of looking beyond the measurement of continuing medical education inputs. The result is they have been obliged to come face to face with the thorny issue of addressing the outcomes of maintenance of competence activities, the choices being between recertifying examinations and the assessment of physicians' performance in their own practices.

Recertification by examination

Recertification by examination has the advantage that it need not take into account how much effort has, or has not, been put into maintenance of competence activities by either the physician or the continuing medical education provider. The product of that effort and the effort that is put into daily practice is addressed. The goal is to create a convenient, standardized and fair assessment of physician ability that any competent physician will pass without difficulty, and which will reliably distinguish between competence and incompetence. Typically such examinations are organized by professional organizations. The exams may be directed at one or several of the classic educational domains of: knowledge (usually assessed by multiple choice questions); skills, things physicians do, rather than things they know (for example, taking a history or performing a physical examination on a standardized patient often in the form of an objective structured clinical examination); and attitudes (through something that can be directly observed as professional behavior).

All such examinations involve test blueprinting, which means defining the breadth of the domain to be assessed, question construction and testing, standard setting (i.e. defining pass/fail scores) marking and, for a professional organization (as opposed to a licensing body), helping those who fail to improve so that in the end they can meet the standard (Newble, 1994).

Standards for the examination

A central conceptual question that must be addressed by any organization facing the responsibilities of certification or licensure is whether certification and recertification are the same thing or whether there is a difference between them. At the beginning of independent practice there is only competence to certify, whereas later, knowledge and skills are embedded in a context which includes the physician's professional behavior. Should there be one standard for both certification and recertification and, if so, should there be only one test for them both?

A first answer to this question must start from the position that standards are standards and that a professional group must subscribe to a basic minimum standard that all practitioners must meet. Standards at this level are not negotiable. In the United Kingdom, for example, the standard for the general register is known as Fitness to Practise and the common ground for the entire profession is set out in the General Medical Council guidance *Good medical practice* (General Medical Council, 1999). But it is understood that the standards will be expressed differently in the unique clinical practices of beginning and established physicians; they will however be equivalent and capable of assessment.

But the question of whether the same test should be used to measure both certification and recertification is a different one. Test methods can only be selected when the purpose and content of an assessment are defined. The *purpose* of certification is to assure the community that a physician entering practice has met or demonstrated the minimum basic requirements in knowledge, skills, behaviors and judgment, which we can call competence. The *content* of certification is determined by the common and important problems that the physician must be capable of resolving from the first day. When faced with providing certification or licensure to applicants that they have not themselves trained, organizations may use reports generated at the training institution, but typically, in North America (and in many other countries in the case of international medical graduates), they rely upon their own examination, which serves to provide an external guarantee of the candidate's competence.

Fundamentally, such a test can consist of nothing more than a series of multiple samples or biopsies from the field of interest. Certainly, the test design must be broad enough to adequately survey the requisite knowledge, skills and behaviors, and it is the task of the test designers to decide how many test questions are required for the certifying organization to be confident in certifying competence. As only so much information can be gathered in a unit of time, such tests typically require several days of test time, usually composed of at least one or two written papers, and increasingly, some form of performance-based assessment, such as actual or simulated patient encounters. While all possible clinical problems cannot be tested, the sampling will be broad enough for the certifying organization to have a high degree of confidence that all important domains and basic standards have been met.

Recertification has a different purpose and content; the assessment of the actual practice of the doctor within the discipline to which he or she is certified. Recertification starts from a position of confidence that the candidate has already met the high and rigorous standards of the certifying body. The question is not whether this candidate is competent to enter practice, but rather has the candidate kept his previously demonstrated skills up to a sufficient level so that the certifying body can justifiably assure public confidence. For this, the level of evidence need not be as extensive. It should not be necessary to sample so broadly. Fewer questions or test scenarios should be sufficient to distinguish those who have kept up from those who have fallen unacceptably behind. And while some of the support for this point of view can be justified on conceptual grounds alone, some of it is based on psychometric factors.

Simply put, it is the job of any test to discriminate between the performances of those taking it. In a certifying examination there are usually a large number of relatively similar candidates, who by virtue of recent and similar training are reasonably comparable in their knowledge, skills and behaviors. Reliable discrimination between them requires relatively large number of test items. By contrast, recertification typically involves looking at the skills of those who have been in practice for 10, 20 or even 30 years. The passage of time, plus differences in local facilities and practice patterns, results in a highly diverse group. The result is that a test with fewer questions will be sufficient to discriminate between performance in this more heterogeneous group.

Any assessment of competence can be regarded as a diagnostic test to detect a relatively rare disease called "incompetence". As with any test, there are true negatives (competent physicians called competent), true positives (incompetent physicians called incompetent), false negatives (incompetent physicians called competent) and false positives (competent physicians called incompetent).

We can conceptualize two distributions of test scores, one corresponding to truly incompetent physicians, and a second, higher distribution, corresponding to truly competent physicians. Now, for every test, a cut score must be established below which individuals will be declared incompetent and above which they will be declared competent. Depending on the location of the cut score, there will be a greater or lesser risk of false positive and false negative results but there will always be miscalls. While we may wish to act as if the test is perfect, it is not; our intention is to minimize errors, but they cannot be altogether eliminated.

A cost is associated with each miscall, and this varies by situation. At the time of licensure, the cost of a false negative amounts to giving an incompetent individual a license to practice medicine for the next 40 years; the cost of a false positive is that the individual affected must reapply and likely pass at the next sitting. So for a national certifying body, such as the National Board of Medical Examiners for the Medical Council of Canada, it makes sense to set the pass mark relatively higher and reduce the likelihood of a false negative. Conversely, for a recertification examination, the cost of a false positive is the possibility that physicians, who have performed well for many years, may be coerced into giving up practice, with major adverse effects upon their lives and their patients, when in fact they are still functioning well. Under these circumstances the hurdle must be set lower – the physician must be given the benefit of the doubt. But patient safety is paramount and these debates about the standards for recertification should be aired publicly. The dilemma may be resolved by further testing for those who are at the cut score.

So far this discussion is hypothetical. What empirical evidence is there to support the contention that for recertification a full certifying examination is not required and that a shorter test will suffice? We have no direct evidence that either group deliberately adjusts the cut point higher or lower, but there is at least some circumstantial evidence that such an action may be operative (Cunnington & Norman, 2000). For the Medical Council of Canada the population is drawn largely from recent graduates who tend, by most measures, to be at the peak of their competence. Nevertheless, the Medical Council of Canada fails 4.5% of them. In contrast, data from at least one organization that assesses the performance of physicians in practice give another picture. The College of Physicians and Surgeons of Ontario runs two programs. The peer assessment program does random peer assessed, practice based audits (McAuley et al., 1990). About 10% of primary care physicians are found either to be functioning at an unacceptably low level or their records are so poor that the assessors are unable to determine the level at which they are functioning. Family physicians have a higher rate of being identified as possibly deficient by peer review than specialists (15% versus 2%) we could estimate that about 5% of all physicians are functioning at an unacceptably low level. These physicians are then referred to the Physician Review Program, a one day standardized assessment of the knowledge, skills, and behaviors of family physicians using the tools of multiple choice questions, standardized patient review, and chart stimulated recall (Cunnington, Hanna, Turnbull, Kaigas, & Norman, 1997). Of the referred physicians, only about 10% are rated as unsafe to practice, which is 0.5% of all physicians. Thus, leaving aside the issue that older physicians make up a significant proportion of Physician Review Program candidates and must on average be practicing at a lower level than recent graduates, the College of

Physicians and Surgeons of Ontario still has a failure rate that in some absolute sense is about 1/10 that of the Medical Council of Canada. The roughly 10 fold lower failure rate for physicians taking the recertification examination, as opposed to those taking the certifying examination, suggests that those responsible for recertification are aware of the risk of false positive findings and have deliberately set their "cut points" to minimize such error.

It appears therefore that certification and recertification are not the same thing and that one need not use the same test for recertification as for certification. While standards may reasonably be expected to be the same, the test designed to ensure the maintenance of those standards may on conceptual and psychometric grounds be simpler and less intensive, with a realistic pass-fail mark (cut point).

Test design

The issue of test reliability and validity is central to the responsibility of any organization undertaking to create a competence examination. Simply put, the test has to distinguish between the competent and the incompetent. Given that a physician's ability to make a living may be curtailed as a consequence of such assessment, the test cannot afford to have any false positive results (physicians declared incompetent when they are not). As no test is 100% sensitive and specific, the design of such a test instrument is an onerous responsibility and one in which the default presumption has to be competence unless there is convincing evidence of incompetence. In consequence, an organization undertaking to develop such a test needs to have deep pockets and the support of a large, affluent and powerful organization if it is going to be able to afford adequate numbers of appropriately trained support personnel, a psychometrician experienced in test design, reliability and validity studies, and a supportive cadre of clinicians to draw upon for question material.

The problems start with the test blueprint. How do you define and limit the domain of the field to be assessed? Is the test going to measure what practitioners really do? Is it going to be a knowledge test only or is there going to be a performance element and if so what will it look like? And what do you do with physicians who have limited the breadth of their practices? This raises the dilemma of whether to tailor the test to the individual physician, or whether to insist upon a minimum across the board standard (Southgate & Jolly, 1994).

Once a committee has got through these political minefields it will need to seek out clinicians to write the test materials, which will then have to be tested for reliability. It will also be necessary to show that the test has validity, i.e. that it is really measuring the competence that it purports to measure. And then there is the question of who is going to pay, and how much, and can you make them pay for something they are unenthusiastic about. It's not surprising that organizations have shied away from all these problems in favor of counting continuing medical education hours, nor that only the biggest and most powerful organizations have been willing to take this route.

The tests in practice

In practice, recertifying examinations have assumed different formats for different organizations. In addition, recertification procedures often demand not only passing a recertification examination, but also fulfillment of other non-examination components. The American Board of Internal Medicine recertification program, for example, has three components (Lewis, 1996). The final component is a proctored examination of three modules of 60 questions each focusing on the knowledge necessary to provide quality care to patients. To get to the final exam two other elements are necessary. One is designed to identify physicians whose competence has been called into question by hospitals or licensing boards; it requires verification that the physician holds an unchallenged, unrestricted license to practice. The second component is interesting because it revolves around the concept of self-evaluation, an educational ideal, but one which has been difficult to support by experimental study (Regehr, Hodges, Tiberius, & Lofchy, 1996). It requires the candidate to complete five modular take-home examinations designed to encourage self-study. The anticipated advantage of such open-book testing is that it permits assessment of content that candidates cannot be expected to know routinely, and that it poses its educational challenges in a context where candidates can use the educational resources typically available to them in practice (Norcini & Lipner, 1999). Results of a study on this component of the recertification process found that the modules were difficult to pass on the first attempt, that candidates' scores were comparable to those obtained on proctored certifying exams, that they were about as reproducible as tests of similar length, and that the scores had small but significant correlations with training, previous test performance, and the nature of practice (Norcini, Lipner, & Downing, 1996).

In contrast, the American Board of Emergency Medicine has taken a different direction. In 1988 they introduced four recertification options: the written exam used for initial certification; an oral exam used for initial certification; a written exam for recertification; and an oral exam called chart stimulated recall (CSR) (Munger, 1994). The latter examination consisted of a two part oral exam that focused less on knowledge and more on what physicians do (skills), both in the test situation and in their actual practices (Solomon, Reinhart, Bridgham, Munger, & Starnaman, 1990). The first part involved the examiner evaluating the examinee on the management of 3 simulated clinical cases, with the examiner role-playing the patient, family, and medical support staff. The second component required the examiner to assess an examinee's diagnosis and management of 3 clinical cases from the examinee's own practice (CSR). The analysis of the data from the first 25 candidates of this test showed a reliability coefficient for the three CSR cases of 0.54; for the overall 6 case test of 0.57; a correlation between the CSR and the simulated patient cases of 0.49; and a correlation of 0.37 and 0.45 respectively with the examinee's oral and written certification scores taken approximately 10 years earlier. Over the years 1989-1993, however, only 7% of diplomates undertaking recertification selected the CSR option and, because it was expensive for the board and time-consuming for candidates preparing their charts, the board decided to eliminate the performance-based oral exam.

Other member boards of the American Board of Medical Specialties have followed suit, or are in the process of following suit, in one form or another. The American Board of Orthopedic Surgery initially offered four different routes to recertification: written exam, practice audit, oral exam, and certificate of added qualification (Simon & DeRosa, 1999). Currently it is one of only two boards that offer an oral exam. The exam is structured to evaluate candidates actual practice with their own patients and in 1998 it was taken by one hundred candidates. More recently they have eliminated the practice-audit pathway and have added a computer-administered general clinical examination and a computer-administered practice-profile examination for selected practice areas.

Other jurisdictions have generally rejected recertification by examination. In Canada the organizations that certify family medicine and specialty practice have both chosen to sidestep examinations in favor of time-limited certificates that can be renewed through a process of counting continuing medical education hours. In Australia and New Zealand the Royal Australasian College of Physicians also rejected the idea of examinations, but instead of looking only at continuing medical education hours they also chose to offer as an alternative the option of practice-based assessment.

Outcomes of recertifying examinations

What are the outcomes of recertifying examinations? The first and most obvious is that they set the standards of expectation and performance for the examination and the test committee constructing the exam. However, the additional benefit is the explicit statement by the professional organization of the standards and of the need for them to be maintained. By the expedient of making it clear to the membership what is expected, with clear and unambiguous goals, a large proportion of the target group will make sure that they are able to perform at or above the expected level. To accomplish this goal, physicians will be motivated to keep up to date, possibly through the expedient of effective and focused continuing medical education. The second effect of such a definition of standards is that those who fall short of the standard cannot claim that they were unaware of the expectations or that they were discriminated against by capricious demands or personal vendettas.

Beyond the benefits of standard setting, is there evidence that examinations actually ensure maintenance of competence and reliably identify deficient practitioners? Perhaps some of the best evidence comes not from recertification examinations themselves but from studies of certification exams. Ramsey and colleagues studied the predictive validity of the American Board of Internal Medicine (ABIM) certification process by looking at the performance of 392 physicians who had completed training 5 or 10 years previously and who were, or were not, board certified (Ramsey et al., 1989). The study instruments included a 119 item multiple-choice question (MCQ) test, a self-administered patient questionnaire, evaluations by professional associates (in the areas of clinical skills, communication skills, humanistic qualities and clinical reasoning), and a review of medical records. The results showed that certified physicians received higher scores on the MCQ test and on ratings from professional associates. There was also a high correlation between the score from the MCQ test and the scores from the initial ABIM certification score completed up to 10 years previously (r = 0.73). Certification status was the only variable significantly affecting examination performance and professional associate ratings. But patient satisfaction scores and medical record audit did not reveal significant differences, raising the possibility that tests of knowledge and the judgment of peers do not sample the whole of professional performance. They may be necessary but not sufficient for recertification.

From a different perspective, Tamblyn and colleagues looked at the relationship between licensing examination scores and resource use and quality of care (Tamblyn et al., 1998). They used medical service and prescription claims files in the Province of Quebec health care databases to look at resource use (specialty consultation, symptom relief versus disease-specific prescribing) and quality of care (inappropriate prescribing, mammography screening) in 614 recently licensed primary care physicians. The results showed that physicians with higher licensing examination scores referred more of their patients for consultation (3.8/1000 patients per SD increase in score); prescribed fewer inappropriate medications to older patients (–2.7/1000 patients per SD increase in score) and more disease-specific relative to symptom-relief medications (3.9/1000 patients per SD increase in score); and referred more women for mammography (6.6/1000 patients per SD increase in score).

Ram and colleagues explored a different aspect of the relationship of examinations to clinical practice (Ram, Van der Vleuten, Rethans, Grol, & Aretz, 1999). Rather than looking at written exams, they compared a multiple-station examination (OSCE) using standardized patients (SPs) carried out at the university with video assessment of regular consultations in daily practice in physicians' own offices. For the eight-station OSCE, physicians designed cases and checklists from a blueprint for family practice and SPs were trained to portray the patients for the scenarios. Physicians were allotted 12 minutes for each case, and all physician assessments were videotaped for analysis. The video assessments took place in the participants' own offices. Ten criteria were used to select 16 consultations from each physician's practice. Ninety Dutch physicians completed both parts of the examination. Thirty-five trained peer-observers then scored the videotapes based upon predetermined criteria. The results showed that the reliabilities for the two forms of testing were equivalent (for 2 raters for 8 cases, 0.81 for office assessment and 0.84 for SP assessment) and there was significant correlation between the scores on the two assessment approaches.

The messages of these studies are clear. Testing can reliably measure components of clinical performance (competence). Testing, even as long as 10 years previously, reliably predicts quality of care for years to come. There is a performance difference between those who have, and those who have not, achieved certification status. Certification by testing is a reliable predictor of subsequent clinical performance. Test scores are positively correlated with quality of care. Performance based assessment is as reliable as assessment carried out in physicians' own practices. These results should be reassuring to those organizations that have chosen to recertify by examination as they provide the kind of evidence required to show the public that they are seriously engaged in ensuring that heath care standards are being met.

Recertification by practice-based assessment

One of the main criticisms of recertification by testing is that it assesses competence (can do) and cannot assess all aspects of performance in the workplace (does do). Perhaps this does not matter if the purpose of recertification is to assure the public that a physician has reached a minimum standard. But the high stakes for doctors and patients involved in failing to recertify makes critics of testing uneasy. They say that natural justice demands that a doctor should not be deprived of the right to work unless the wider activities involved in performance in practice are also assessed. Other physicians wish to submit evidence based on practice activity for recertification, arguing that it is closer to patient care than either test results or evidence of continuing medical education hours. Whatever the reasons, assessment of the physician's office and/or hospital practice is an optional part of some recertification programs or can be offered as an exemption. In these situations the problems of reliability and standard setting must be addressed.

Practice based assessment differs from tests of competence in that the material and activities that comprise the assessment derive from the practice of the physician. Every assessment is unique because the clinical practice of each doctor is unique. The assessments may or may not involve a visit to the place of work. The variability of assessments can be reduced by attention to the structure and documentation of the assessment methods, the adequacy of sampling and the training of assessors, but there can never be exact equivalence. The outcomes are based on judgments to which it may be difficult to attach the apparent certainty of numbers. Advocates of testing are in their turn made uneasy.

The American Board of Internal Medicine (ABIM) recertification program provides a good model because it takes into consideration the transformation of competence on beginning practice into performance in actual practice. It addresses, or plans to address, the three principal components of recertification: patient outcomes; medical knowledge and judgment; and professionalism (Norcini, 1999). Patient charts for common conditions (e.g., diabetes, hypertension) and procedures (e.g., flexible sigmoidoscopy) will be reviewed in a structured way (patient history, examination, diagnostic procedures, assessment and management are scored and feedback provided). A clinical preventive services module forms a self-selected part of the program. The heart of the module is an audit of patient records for selected preventive services. After completing the audit the candidate must devise a quality improvement plan. The Board reserves the right to ask for copies of the patient records underlying the audit. The program assesses professionalism by incorporating an assessment of physician behavior by colleagues and patients. It acknowledges that all certified physicians cannot be expected to know everything but can be expected to find out when necessary (an open-book computer-based test) but affirms that there are some things all certified physicians should know whatever the limitations of their practice (a proctored test).

In the United Kingdom, the decision of the General Medical Council to require revalidation for all registered physicians has led to a different emphasis. The purpose of the program is to assure the public that possession of a license implies that a physician is currently fit to practice. The present emphasis throughout the profession is on establishing content validity by elaborating the General Medical Council guidance *Good medical practice* for different disciplines (see Table 1).

Table 1. Criteria for assessing *Clinical Care*[1] for United Kingdom general practitioners as set out in *Good medical practice for general practitioners*

The excellent GP	The unacceptable GP
- Takes time to listen to patients, and allows them to express their own concerns.	- Has limited competence, and is unaware of where his or her limits of competence lie.
- Considers relevant psychological and social factors as well as physical ones.	- Does not listen to patients, and frequently interrupts.
- Uses clear language appropriate for the patient.	- Fails to elicit important parts of the history.
- Is selective but systematic when examining patients.	- Is unable to discuss sensitive and personal matters with patients.
- Performs appropriate skilled examinations with consideration for the patient.	- Fails to use the medical records as a source of further information about past events.
- Has access to necessary equipment and is skilled in its use.	- Fails to examine patients when needed.
- Uses investigations where they will help management of the condition.	- Undertakes inappropriate, cursory or inadequate examinations.
- Knows about the nature and reliability of investigations requested and understands the results.	- Does not explain clearly what he or she is going to do or why.
- Makes sound management decisions which are based on good practice and evidence.	- Does not possess or fails to use diagnostic and treatment equipment.
- Has a structured approach for managing long term health problems and preventive care.	- Undertakes irrelevant investigations.
- Maintains his or her knowledge and skills, and is aware of his or her limits of competence.	- Shows little evidence of a coherent or rational approach to diagnosis.
	- Draws illogical conclusions from the information available.
	- Gives treatments that are inconsistent with best practice or evidence.
	- Has no way of organizing the care for long term problems or for prevention.

Note. [1] *Clinical Care* is one of many headings in *Good medical practice*. Criteria have been developed for each one. They are all included in revalidation

While the present work is directed towards developing criteria, the process is leading to the production of specific criteria and standards for acceptable practice, which will be capable of assessment. The Council has decided that all aspects of the guidance will be considered for revalidation. Relationships with patients, teamwork, participation in accredited professional development and evidence of maintenance of performance are placed alongside the traditional competencies in diagnosis, management and practical skills that make up good clinical care. The nature of the evidence and the choice of methods is not yet determined and is the subject of national consultation. But there is certain to be an assessment of communication skills and teamwork for all doctors, irrespective of discipline, and it is likely that a move to the assessment of patient outcomes will form part of the evidence about good clinical care. Non-medical people will be involved in planning the program and conducting some parts of the assessment such as observing consultations and assessing communication. Another certainty is that the process will not include a major emphasis on traditional tests of competence nor will continuing medical education hours be a basis for demonstrating that a physician is up to date. Open book tests allowing self-assessment and the demonstration of improvement by re-submission are likely to be widely adopted. Local groups, which will be accredited by the General Medical Council, will evaluate the evidence that every doctor must submit. If the evidence is below the standard then a practice visit will follow.

The necessity to agree upon the evidence that will be submitted to the General Medical Council, and to make it equivalent for every doctor, has led to a further debate about standards. Revalidation is at a minimum standard but it covers all aspects of clinical practice. It will therefore require work from every doctor to assemble the evidence to present to the Council. In order to avoid alienating the competent majority there is a debate between the Council and the Medical Colleges about what activities might be said to subsume the minimum standard. In its turn the Council will still require coverage of *Good medical practice* and reliable and valid methods before it will accredit assessments at the higher standard. The overall effect has been to trigger a move to improve the quality of all assessment programs in medicine with attention focused on content validity, reliability, standard setting and training of assessors.

Family physicians in the United Kingdom have an established track record of assessing the quality of individual clinical practice by practice based assessment (Royal College of General Practitioners, 1985). The problems of separating individual performance from those of the outputs of clinical teams are formidable but have been addressed. The most recent program, Membership by Assessment of Performance, introduced in 1999, enables practitioners, who have been in independent practice for 5 years but who are not certified members of the Royal College of General Practitioners, to gain membership by peer review of practice. In the United Kingdom, general practitioners take state examinations to be eligible for independent practice. College membership is optional but usual, and at a higher standard. The development of MAP entailed a widely conducted Delphi exercise to derive the content of the assessment, and work on defining criteria and standards which are published and available to all of those wishing to undertake the program (Holden & Wearne, 2000). The structure of the assessments is similar to those reported from many other PBA programs. There is a visit to the site of practice, verification of pre-submitted material, assessment of medical record keeping, chart stimulated recall, and structured interviews with peer associates and colleagues from other disciplines. The pre-visit assessment includes scrutiny of written reports of audits and critical incident analysis, prescribing data (which is comprehensive in the United Kingdom) and the results of patient satisfaction surveys. But it is striking that there is also a requirement to complete the consulting skills module of the certifying examination before undertaking the PBA. This was introduced in order to moderate the standard between the two assessments. Consulting skills are assessed either through a 10 station simulated patient examination or through assessment of videotaped actual consultations. The assessment is conducted by trained physician and lay assessors, underlining the United Kingdom trend for members of the public to become involved with ensuring professionalism and good communication throughout the medical workforce. This is a new program, implemented in 1999, and data are not yet available about numbers applying or their success.

The Practice Quality Review option within the recertification program for the Royal Australian College of Physicians has been successful (Newble, Paget, & McClaren, 1999). It is offered as an alternative to the standard continuing medical education option, and is positively evaluated by those who have taken it up. The assessment follows a recognized format in that the physician submits information before the visit to give the assessors insight into the style of practice and the doctor's quality assurance and continuing medical education activities. The assessors conduct an extensive review of case records; observe performance with new and revisiting patients; observe technical procedures where relevant and conduct an extensive interview with the physician. The assessor's report is sent to the College, but also provides detailed feedback for the practitioner. Another option, Physician Assessment, has also been introduced based on the approach developed by the ABIM where evaluations are collected from 15 colleagues who rate the physician on 12 dimensions falling into two categories – medical skills and humanistic qualities. It provides a feasible way of obtaining information from peer associates which relates directly to a physician's performance in practice.

Staged programs for relicensure

While there are a plethora of approaches in many countries to ensure that a physician is competent, strategies to anticipate and prevent declining performance of doctors in practice are now a central concern for regulating bodies. They are increasingly adopting proactive or interventional methods. This is resulting in the emergence of national programs that apply to all physicians at all career stages, within which there will be no place to hide. This is, or will be, politically difficult as the medical profession and the public comes to realize the implications. In particular the public will be surprised that these systems have not always been in place.

Canada and the United Kingdom provide good examples of this development. (Southgate & Dauphinee, 1998). In Stage 1 of the Canadian Model for the Monitoring and Enhancement of Physician Performance, the performance of all physicians will be screened via fee for service billing patterns, peer assessment questionnaires and patient satisfaction questionnaires. The vast majority of practitioners will "pass" this first cut without a problem and enhancement steps will be feedback, primarily for reassurance. Revalidation is the equivalent first stage of the United Kingdom program. Patient satisfaction and peer assessment questionnaires are also likely to be adopted.

About 10% of practitioners in the Monitoring and Enhancement of Physician Performance program will be identified from the first screen as at risk or in need and will move to Stage 2 of assessment involving hospital audit, office audit and structured interview of the physician (McAuley et al., 1990). In the United Kingdom, failure to revalidate on the basis of written evidence submitted locally, will trigger a practice visit by a medical and lay person. The assessment will include review and observation of consulting skills, medical record keeping, clinical method including prescribing, teamwork, practice audits, complaints. If a rapid plan for remediation cannot be put in place and seen to be effective, and if patients are at risk, then referral to the General Medical Council, to examine fitness to practice, will follow.

Individually oriented assessment will apply to a very small number (1-2%). In the Monitoring and Enhancement of Physician Performance Stage 3 an objective assessment of need is carried out. This is based on written tests of practice related knowledge, basic clinical skills assessment by objective structured examination or simulated office orals, and detailed interviews in order to set out a specific remedial program for that individual (Cunnington et al., 1997). In the United Kingdom the poorly performing doctor, who is not ill or exhibiting misconduct, is referred to the Performance Procedures. This is in itself a two-stage process involving a nationally organized practice review, by two medical and one lay assessor, followed by tests of competence. All of the doctors assessed so far have entered both stages, which take place within days of each other. Data from the first 6 general practitioners assessed within the full program have confirmed the complex relationship between performance and competence. Early findings are that performance does predict competence, enhancing our confidence in the concurrent validity of the tests of competence. But the United Kingdom view, based on early cases, is that tests of competence are necessary but not sufficient to assess the breadth of performance set out in *Good medical practice* when seeking to identify serious deficiency.

Standards and objectivity in practice based assessments

There is always an attraction to objectivity. Well designed tests of competence can withstand legal challenge and remove some of the more immediate discomfort from those who are judging the professional performance of their colleagues. But where the judgment of peers and the input of the public is about fitness to practice, then a part of the process must involve face-to-face contact. The people conducting the review must take personal responsibility for the evidence they collect, the way they document it and the judgments they make on it. There can be no opportunity to stop a career without being prepared to justify, in court if necessary, why it was necessary to do so. Equally, decisions to find a doctor fit to practise may have to be justified and explained to the public. In the United Kingdom Performance Procedures, peer review supported by (but not overturned by) tests of competence, have already stood such challenges. The approach to maximizing fairness and objectivity during the practice review stage has centered on the use of well designed and documented methods, training of assessors and the collection of evidence from multiple sources. Qualitative research methods have proved very useful here, particularly triangulation of evidence. Each aspect of the review is documented contemporaneously, assigned to a category of *Good medical practice,* categorized by method and assessor, and entered into a computer as the review proceeds. Typically 500-700 independent judgments, supported by evidence, with an audit trail back to the original note, are entered during the two-day visit. Early experience shows that for any heading it becomes obvious to the assessors, as they consider the evidence, whether the weight is accruing to the conclusion that that aspect of practice is acceptable or unacceptable. There are no numerical rules for considering the large amount of information except that a single piece of evidence may not be double counted. Assessors weigh the evidence using the principles of triangulation. They must corroborate evidence from at least three sources before making a judgment. So far all of the panels have been unanimous in their findings and their reports have been accepted despite legal challenge.

PROBLEMS IN RECERTIFICATION

Failure to recertify: the implications

Although much has been written about the desirability and advantages of recertification the issue of what to do with those who fail to recertify has received little attention. And yet it is a critically important issue to the profession and also to the licensing bodies and to the public, whose access to physician services could be affected. To some extent the implications depend upon where the failure lies. The licensing body, which invariably has public members and the press looking over its shoulder, may determine that it has very little flexibility in dealing with failure to relicense. It may conclude that if physicians fail to relicense then indeed they are not licensed to practice. Such a failure could spell economic collapse for the physician. But ultimately public protection from incompetent and dangerous doctors is paramount. This is the basis for the approach taken by the General Medical Council. In the United Kingdom it is clear that doctors who fail to revalidate will be referred into the Fitness to Practise Procedures. There are no exceptions. The screener will determine if the problem is because of health, conduct or performance and the relevant assessments will follow. The doctor's license is at risk. It is not an option to opt out of the system if a physician wishes to remain on the United Kingdom register.

Failure to recertify with a professional body may be different as the organization may feel that it has the responsibility and opportunity to extend a helping hand in terms of educational assistance, extension of deadlines for submission of proof of accomplishment of goals, or opportunities to repeat the recertifying examination or practice based assessment. This might seem benign enough until one considers the response of the licensing body when notified that a physician has failed to recertify. Out of concern for public safety (and public scrutiny) will the licensing body feel obliged to suspend or revoke a physician's license to practice? These issues will undoubtedly be worked out in different ways in different jurisdictions, but the message that failing to recertify has only the benign implications of putting practitioners on notice that they will need to improve their abilities over the next few years will hardly be tenable.

Why do physicians fail to recertify? The temptation is to ascribe it simply to laziness; a lack of commitment and effort to keep up. This intuitive judgment, however, fails to acknowledge the biologic realities inherent in looking at physicians practicing over a lifetime. New physicians undergoing initial certification are a relatively homogeneous group who all share, amongst other things, the advantages of youth. Physicians as they age inevitably suffer the infirmities common to the public at large, including drug and alcohol dependence, medical illness, cognitive decline, mood disorders, divorce, and financial problems. To better understand these problems Turnbull and colleagues undertook a study of the cognitive function of 27 family physicians referred to a 1-day, standardized test of competency because of concerns raised at a peer reviewed practice based assessment (Turnbull et al., 2000). At the end of the day of clinical testing they administered a 1.5 hour screening neuropsychological test using standard instruments for problem solving, learning and memory, attention, and mood. Overall, 7 of 27 physicians showed moderate or severe cognitive difficulty. Mood disturbance was identified in only 3. Of the 8 physicians who scored well on the clinical testing, 7 had no, minimal or mild cognitive impairment. Of the 19 physicians who scored poorly on the clinical assessment, 6 (32%) had moderate or severe cognitive impairment. Of note is the observation that few if any physicians with significant neuropsychological impairment performed well on the clinical assessment. However, only a minority of physicians performing poorly on the clinical test had cognitive difficulty sufficient to explain their lack of competence.

Failure to recertify: remediation

What should be the response of a licensing body when a physician fails the attempt to relicense? Is it delicensure? This drastic step may solve the licensing body's problem but does not do much for the physician or his/her patients. For the professional organizations the answer is likely to be more positive with remediation heading the list. But is remediation effective in this situation; what is the evidence that remediation works in this population?

The effectiveness of remediation is one of those things, like the effectiveness of continuing medical education, which is more a matter of faith than evidence. Few studies have been done. If, as the Turnbull study, noted above, suggests, a third of dyscompetent physicians have moderate or severe cognitive impairment, it would hardly be expected that they would respond positively to even intensive remediation efforts. One of the few published studies on this topic is by Hanna, Premi, and Turnbull (2000). Five severely dyscompetent physicians (aged 50, 55, 69, 72, 72), identified through a provincial quality assurance process, were enrolled in an intensive, remedial continuing medical education program. The facilitator met with the group for two hours twice per month for three years using a problem-based small group format based around cases from the physicians' practices as stimuli to discuss basic and clinical issues. The physicians also discussed evidence-based journals, undertook a self-audit, and during 16 meetings were each required to bring four problem cases and to lead the discussion on the cases. There was extensive use of role-play, and opportunities to interview standardized patients and get feedback about their performance. At the conclusion of the program the physicians undertook a reassessment of their performance using the same standardized one-day assessment that had been used to identify them initially. Of the five only one improved, one remained unchanged, and three deteriorated.

What can be learned from this report? First, it demonstrates that even severely dyscompetent physicians may improve, as was the case for one of the five physicians. Perhaps not surprisingly he was the youngest and most engaged in the educational process. However, three of the four deteriorated, and none of the physicians over age 65 improved. Extensive inferences cannot be drawn from so small a study, but the results do suggest that remediation cannot be considered a panacea for the problem of incompetence (additionally it raises the question of whether there should be a mandatory retirement age for physicians.) The study also suggests that a significant proportion of physicians identified as being dyscompetent may never be able to return to independent practice. For physicians over the age of 65 this may not be a big concern. Given the difficulties inherent in remediation, and the low likelihood of success, they may be best advised (or required?) to retire gracefully before a career-ending tragedy. For physicians in midlife, it may be best for them to undergo formal cognitive testing prior to embarking on remediation efforts. If the results of such testing showed that they have significant cognitive impairment, they might then escape the stigma of incompetence in favor of the label of disabled, and thus be entitled to disability insurance. If they performed well, then there would be a reasonable chance (perhaps 1:2) that, with appropriate motivation, a well designed continuing medical education program, including, where necessary, supervised history taking, clinical examination, and decision making with feedback, the physician could improve to meet the standards required for recertification and relicensure.

Who is going to pay the very significant costs involved in such a program is open for discussion. In North America the cost is likely to be borne by the physicians themselves – a group which presumably has money and would be motivated to invest it in the continuance of their careers. In the United Kingdom the government has agreed to provide some funds to make upgrading of knowledge and skills possible providing that the doctor shows insight and employers agree. Otherwise the physician bears the costs.

Perhaps an even greater obstacle to retraining is finding the required supervisors and programs. The truth is that most of the truly dyscompetent physicians do not have a single problem that can be rectified by a weekend course. One study that identified dyscompetent physicians on a one day standardized test in family practice examined the data for each of eight categories: knowledge, history taking, physical examination, problem solving, management, communication skills, and record keeping (Caulford et al., 1994). They found that for physicians in the highest categories of competence the most prevalent problem was record keeping. In contrast those physicians who were in the lowest categories of competence had major deficiencies in nearly all areas; 60-80% of these physicians had major deficiencies in 6 of the 7 domains and 100% had deficiencies in record keeping. Another problem in arranging retraining is the matter of informed consent from patients. They have a right to know the circumstances of the physician who is to care for them. This is particularly so if high risk and interventional procedures are involved. Many health care organizations are not prepared to risk litigation if things go wrong. The implication is that the problems are multiple and difficult and are unlikely to be easily rectified. These are the kind of problems that turn away experienced and motivated educators. They may see the investment of their time and energy as more likely to be productive when spent with new graduates than in retraining physicians with multiple performance (and possibly behavioral or cognitive) problems.

REFERENCES

Benson, J. A. (1991). Certification and recertification: One approach to professional accountability. *Annals of Internal Medicine, 114,* 238-242.

Caulford, P., Lamb, S., Kaigas, T., Hanna, E., Norman, G. R., & Davis D. A. (1994). Physician incompetence: Specific problems and predictors. *Academic Medicine, 69,* S16-S18.

Charlin, B., Tardiff, J., & Boshuizen, H. (2000). Scripts and medical diagnostic knowledge: theory and applications for clinical reasoning instruction and research. *Academic Medicine, 75*(2), 182-190.

Cunnington, J. P. W., & Norman, G. R. (2000). Certification and recertification: Are they the same? *Academic Medicine, 75*, 617-619.

Cunnington, J. P. W., Hanna, E., Turnbull, J., Kaigas, T. B., & Norman, G. R. (1997). Defensible assessment of the competency of the practicing physician. *Academic Medicine, 72*(1), 9-12.

Davis, D. A., Thomson O'Brien, M. A., Freemantle, N., et al. (1999). Impact of formal continuing medical education. Do conferences, workshops, rounds, and other traditional continuing education activities change physician behavior or health care outcomes? *Journal of the American Medical Association, 282*, 867-874.

Davis, D. A., Thomson, M. A., Oxman, A. D., & Haynes, B. (1995). Changing physician performance. *Journal of the American Medical Association, 274*, 700-705.

General Medical Council (1999). *Good medical Practice.* London: Author. (www.gmc-uk.nl)

General Medical Council (1999). *Performance procedures – A guide to the arrangements.* London: Author.

General Medical Council (1999). *When your professional performance is questioned. The GMC's performance procedures.* London: Author.

Grant, J., & Stanton, F. (1999). *The effectiveness of continuing professional development.* A report for the Chief Medical Officers review of continuing professional development in practice. Edinburgh: Association for the Study of Medical Education.

Hanna, E., Premi, J., & Turnbull, J. (2000). Results of remedial continuing medical education in dyscompetent physicians. *Academic Medicine, 75*, 174-176.

Hewlett, P. O., & Eichelberger, L. W. (1996). The case against mandatory continuing education. *Journal of Continuing Education in Nursing, 27*, 176-181.

Holden J., & Wearne, J. (2000). Membership by assessment of performance: Developing a method for assessing established general practitioners. *British Journal for General Practitioners, 50*, 231-235.

Lewis, R. P. (1996). Recertification: Its time has come. *Journal of the American College of Cardiology, 28*, 260-262.

McAuley, R. G., Paul, W. M., Morrison, G. H., Beckett, R. F., & Goldsmith, C. H. (1990). Five-year results of the peer assessment program of the College of Physicians and Surgeons of Ontario. *Canadian Medical Association Journal, 143*, 1193-1199.

Munger, B. S. (1994). Oral examinations. In E. L. Mancall & P. G. Bashook (Eds.), *Recertification: New evaluation methods and strategies* (pp. 39-47). Evanston: IL: American Board of Medical Specialties.

Newble, D. I. (Ed.) (1994). Guidelines for the development of effective and efficient procedures for the assessment of clinical competence. In D. Newble, B. Jolly, & R. Wakeford (Eds.), *The certification and recertification of doctors. Issues in the assessment of clinical competence* (pp. 69-91). Cambridge: Cambridge University Press.

Newble, D. I., & Paget, N. S. (1996). The maintenance of professional standards programmes of the Royal Australasian College of Physicians. *Journal of the Royal College of Physicians of London, 30*, 252-256.

Newble, D. I., Paget, N. S., & McClaren, B. (1999). Revalidation in Australia and New Zealand: Approach of Royal Australasian College of Physicians. *British Medical Journal, 319*, 1185-1188.

Norcini, J. J. (1999). Recertification in the United States. *British Medical Journal, 319*, 1183-1185.

Norcini, J. J., & Lipner, R. S. (1999). Recertification: Is there a link between take-home and proctored examinations? *Academic Medicine, 74*, S28-S30.

Norcini, J. J., Lipner, R., & Downing, S. M. (1996). How meaningful are scores on a take-home recertification examination? *Academic Medicine, 71*, S71-S73.

Norman, G. R. (1999). The adult learner: A mythical species. *Academic Medicine, 74*, 886-888.

Premi, J., Shannon, S., Hartwick, K., Lamb, S., Wakefield, J., & Williams, J. (1994). Practise based small group continuing medical education. *Academic Medicine, 69*, 800-802.

Ram, P., Van der Vleuten, C. P., Rethans, J. J., Grol, R., & Aretz, K. (1999). Assessment of practicing family physicians: comparison of observation in a multiple-station examination using standardized patients with observation of consultations in daily practice. *Academic Medicine, 74*, 62-69.

Ram, P. G., Van der Vleuten, C. P., Rethans, J. J., Grol, R., & Aretz, K. (1999). Assessment of practicing family physicians: Comparison of observation in a multiple-station examination using standardised patients with observation of consultations in daily practice. *Academic Medicine, 74*, 62-69.

Ramsey, P. G., Carline, J. D., Inui, T. S., Larson, E. B., LoGerfo, J. P., & Wenrich, M. D. (1989). Predictive validity of certification by the American Board of Internal Medicine. *Annals of Internal Medicine, 110*, 719-726.

Regehr, G., Hodges, B., Tiberius, R., & Lofchy, J. (1996). Measuring self-assessment skills: an innovative relative ranking model. *Academic Medicine, 71*, S52-S54.

Royal College of General Practitioners (1985). *Report from general practice. What sort of doctor?* (report 23). London: Royal College of General Practitioners.

Royal College of General Practitioners (1995). *Fellowship by assessment. Occasional paper 50*, 2nd ed. London: Royal College of General Practitioners.

Royal College of General Practitioners (1999). *Membership by assessment of performance. The MAP Handbook.* London: Royal College of General Practitioners.

Secretary of State for Health (1999). *Supporting doctors, protecting patients.* A consultation paper on preventing, recognising and dealing with poor clinical performance of doctors in the NHS in England. Department of Health (doh@prologistics.co.uk).

Sibley, J. C., Sackett, D. L., Neufeld, M. D., Gerrard, B., et al. (1982). A randomized trial of continuing medical education. *New England Journal of Medicine, 306,* 511-515.

Simon, M. A., & DeRosa, G. P. (1999). The value of recertification to orthopedic surgery and to the public. *Journal of Bone and Joint Surgery, 81-A,* 292-294.

Southgate, L., & Dauphinee, D. (1998). Maintaining standards in British and Canadian medicine: the developing role of the regulatory bodies. *British Medical Journal, 316,* 697-700.

Southgate, L., & Jolly, B., (Eds.) (1994). Determining the content of recertification procedures. In D. Newble, B. Jolly, & R. Wakeford (Eds.), *The certification and recertification of doctors. Issues in the assessment of clinical competence* (pp. 178-186). Cambridge: Cambridge University Press.

Southgate, L., & Pringle, M. (1999). Revalidation in the United Kingdom: general principles based on experience in general practice. *British Medical Journal, 319,* 1180-1183.

Solomon, D. J., Reinhart, M. A., Bridgham, R. G., Munger, B. S., & Starnaman, S. (1990). An assessment of an oral examination format for evaluating clinical competence in emergency medicine. *Academic Medicine, 65,* S43-S44.

Tamblyn, R., Abrahamowicz, M., Brailovsky, C., Grand'Maison, P., et al. (1998). Association between licensing examination scores and resource use and quality of care in primary care practice. *Journal of the American Medical Association, 280,* 989-996.

Turnbull, J., Carbotte, R., Hanna, E., Norman, G., Cunnington, J., Ferguson, B., & Kaigas, T. (2000). Cognitive difficulty in physicians. *Academic Medicine, 75,* 177-181.

Section 6: Implementing the Curriculum

Introduction

LYNN CURRY – SECTION EDITOR
CurryCorp

The purpose of this last section is to review evidence on implementing change in medical education curricula and professional curricula in general. This utility of this purpose was considered reasonable given the expected effect of all previous sections in generating a desire in readers to initiate curricular enhancements. Our message, borrowing from current advertising parlance, is "just do it". We offer six chapters of advice on how to make the "doing" more pleasant, more successful and more rewarding to all concerned. Authors in this section review published literature in a range of areas pertinent to curricular change and offer summaries and suggestions intended to be helpful or at least sympathetic in the struggles that are inevitable in managing change of any significant impact. Of course, without that impact, why bother?

Davis and White (Chapter 28) review structure and governance issues in medical schools and curricula. Their argument is that active management of both structure and governance is central to success of curricular change attempts. Illustrations are drawn from a large-scale curricular change at the University of Michigan Medical School. The review concludes with a series of role expectations for all stakeholders involved in curricular governance which will be useful guidance to others contemplating curricular change in professional schools.

In Chapter 29, Jolly addresses the faculty development necessary for implementation of curricular change. Beginning with definitions of faculty development the review then considers how faculty development serves curricular needs. Particular focus is given to new demands on medical curricula: ambulatory teaching, community-based approaches, problem-based learning, move to primary care delivery, and response to national initiatives. This chapter concludes with advice on the choice and design of faculty development.

Bland and Wersal review research on academic leadership in Chapter 30. Leadership behaviors found most effective in guiding organizations through curricular change are identified. Of particular interest are those leadership patterns that accomplish their innovation objectives without incurring negative impact on other valued aspects of the institution such as student preparation, faculty research productivity and school reputation.

Cavanaugh makes an argument in Chapter 31 for re-introducing professional caring in the professional school curricula. Research is reviewed on caring as a core component of professional moral education in relation to the teaching-learning

915

International Handbook of Research in Medical Education, 915–916.
G.R. Norman, C.P.M. Van der Vleuten, D.I. Newble (eds.)
© 2002 *Dordrecht: Kluwer Academic Publishers. Printed in Great Britain.*

environment and related assessments in the health professions. The case is made that large-scale curricular change offers ideal opportunities to model key aspects of professional caring through pedagogical caring. This is an approach to managing curricular change through the innate drive for self-actualization among all members of the professional school community.

Chapter 32 by Chauvin is a review of methods successful in disseminating educational research results with implications for implementing change in professional school environments. The change process is defined variously in four principal change theories, which are then combined in novel integration. Organizational change is considered as a process for both stability and development and models for planned organizational change are presented. A model for facilitating individual change and strategies to utilize evaluation finish the chapter.

The section closes with Chapter 33 by Curry on achieving large-scale change. The thesis is that large-scale change is imminent in medial education and, by extension, in most professional schools. To support that contention a range of evidence is presented: internal and external dissatisfaction, challenges to traditional scopes of practice, significant shifts in primary and secondary stakeholders, successful new models of higher and professional education and the burgeoning role of informatics in education and society. Arguments are advanced about the necessity of professions educators assuming responsibility to manage significant curricular change and previous attempts are examined for lessons to be learned. Change management models are reviewed and illustrated with examples from the published literature on change in medical education. The chapter concludes with a checklist for change agents intended to provide direction to those managing large-scale change in any organizational venue.

28 Managing the Curriculum and Managing Change

WAYNE K. DAVIS AND CASEY B. WHITE

University of Michigan Medical School

SUMMARY

In this chapter we explore the contentious issues related to governance of the medical school curriculum. Within the United States, over more than 50 years, various commissions have issued recommendations regarding curricular governance, while others have attempted to clarify various aspects of curriculum management, including defined roles of students, faculty, and school administrators. We draw heavily from these documents. We also examine the significant external influence that accrediting bodies have exerted on medical school curricular governance structures. We document the methods for, and the importance of, selecting faculty leaders for educational management roles and the necessity of rewards for faculty participating in curricular oversight. The chapter concludes with a synthesis and set of recommendations regarding the principles of curricular governance that are most likely to lead to efficient and effective leadership of the educational program for the M.D. degree.

As with any review of this type, we issue several caveats. Our review of the literature on curriculum governance revealed that most of the information in this area comes from medical schools within the United States and Canada; thus, the chapter has a distinctly "North American bias". Although some if not all of the observations and principles may be applied to other settings, this cannot be assured. Also, even within the medical schools in the United States and Canada, there are vast differences in history, culture, organization and priorities. These differences limit the generalizability of any review of this type. Finally, although it has been recommended on several occasions that, as a part of medical education governance, the medical school should control graduate medical education, this chapter addresses only undergraduate medical education.

International Handbook of Research in Medical Education, 917–944.
G.R. Norman, C.P.M. Van der Vleuten, D.I. Newble (eds.)
© 2002 *Dordrecht: Kluwer Academic Publishers. Printed in Great Britain.*

INTRODUCTION

Business literature abounds with books and articles focused on how to organize and run a business enterprise. Leadership, management expertise, and corporate structures are frequently studied and case studies are written to describe how a particularly successful (or unsuccessful) business has faced challenges. Unlike the literature on business administration, most of the contemporary literature on medical school curriculum management focuses on the need for centralized management in order to bring about curriculum reform. Even the less current commission reports link curriculum management style with the specific goal of bringing about change in medical education; this is most likely the result of a preoccupation with change in medical education that has been evident since the Flexner report of 1910.

Curricular governance in medical education has not been studied apart from the ability of the governance structure to bring about curriculum change. One strong reason for linking governance to curriculum reform is the resistance to change inherent in medical school organizations. Discipline-based departments are reluctant to lose the autonomy they have acquired in the traditional departmental-based structures. The governance structure in most medical schools prior to the 1990s, when the most recent wave of change began, was designed to support the primary and secondary missions of the school: departmentally-based research and patient care. This departmental-based structure was entrenched and prevalent among medical schools.

Recent changes in medical education are primarily the result of changes in medical practice and research. Health care delivery has undergone staggering transformations due to new technology, the introduction of managed care, and the limitation of insurance reimbursements for lengthy hospital stays. At the same time, physicians and researchers have recognized the efficiency and effectiveness of interdisciplinary approaches to research efforts (e.g., ontogenesis and molecular biology) and clinical care problems. These approaches have led to the development of population- and disease-based centers (e.g., geriatrics centers, diabetes centers, cancer centers), which bring together outstanding clinicians and researchers to achieve specific goals. Although these changes have had profound impacts on how medical schools are organized to conduct research and deliver patient care, they have not by themselves produced meaningful change in medical education or its organization.

HISTORY

Historically, medical school courses, the building blocks of the medical school curriculum, have been based in departments. Courses were named for and taught by faculty from these specific disciplines. The departmental structure was organized to support the research mission in the basic science departments and the revenue-earning patient care activities in the clinical departments. In this structure, as history has shown, funding follows successful effort. Evolution of powerful medical school departments occurred after World War II when departments acquired direct access to funding through externally-supported research projects, third-party payers, and Medicare and Medicaid (Hendricson, Payer, Rogers, & Markus, 1993; Bussigel, Baransky, & Grenholm, 1988). This structure was logical and served the research and patient care missions well.

At the time when strong departments were emerging and flexing their proverbial muscles, medical curricula were primarily composed of departmental-based courses and clerkships. The responsible department determined the goals, content and format(s) for teaching each of the courses. Usually there was little intervention or review by the school's curriculum committee, which was composed of department heads or teaching faculty, each representing his/her department's best interests. With healthy funding to underwrite research efforts, medical discoveries proliferated, and teaching hours demanded by the departments swelled. There was more to learn than could possibly be taught in four years, and extension of the time devoted to the curriculum – to meet the combined demands of each of the departments – was not a feasible option.

If one were to examine the curricular governance structure of a typical medical school in the early 1960s one would find a curriculum committee composed of elected or appointed members, each of whom represented the department holding his/her primary appointment. Typically, there were no systematic evaluations of the courses, clerkships or entire curriculum, and in the absence of data, most of the discussion about medical education was opinion-based. Few, if any, meaningful changes resulted from the discussions of the curriculum committee, which was grid-locked by turf protection. Their primary functions seemed to be patrolling the curriculum to make sure no one taught more hours than were assigned, and protecting the curriculum from assault by special interest groups external to the medical school (e.g., those wanting to introduce more behavioral science or those wanting to increase the amount of primary care instruction).

> Departmental governance tends to be more educationally conservative, perhaps because it tends to reinforce departmental identity, exacerbate conflicts over turf, and generate resistance to cross-disciplinary approaches. *(Reynolds et al., 1995, p. 672).*

Bucking this dominant trend, several "new" medical schools such as Maastricht University (the Netherlands) and McMaster University (Hamilton, Ontario, Canada) had the advantage and foresight to put into place unique organizational structures specifically created to support their innovative curricula (Neufield & Barrows, 1974; Bouhuijs, 1990). These structures could best be described as matrix organizations with "department" and "teaching role" as the two orienting forces. These schools were unique and did not serve as a model that was widely copied.

Adding to the barriers faced by the curriculum committee was the lack of administrative structure and what was frequently called "clout" to implement the ideas that did survive the coffee and donuts of the curriculum committee meetings. The chair of the curriculum committee (usually a busy faculty member) was not afforded release time to follow through on the recommendations of the committee. The term of office for most curriculum committee chairs was brief and did not allow continuity of ideas or follow up on innovations. The committee did not collect data on educational activities so there was no basis for decision-making. As assistant and associate dean positions became more prevalent in medical schools, these individuals too were limited in their effectiveness since their roles were not clearly defined and their responsibility to follow through on committee recommendations/actions was neither agreed upon nor enforced. Departmental chairs still held the power to control what was taught by their departmental faculty and the individual teachers were primarily responsible for what was taught. There were instances of entire blocks of content disappearing from the curriculum of many schools if a particular faculty member left the institution, was promoted to an administrative position, or retired.

REPORTS ON MEDICAL EDUCATION

Throughout the twentieth century, medical education was the focus of numerous examinations by commissions and blue-ribbon panels. Christakis (1995) reviewed 19 of 24 reports, dating from 1910 to 1993, that endorsed the reformation of American medical education. Recommendations to centralize curriculum management were first noted in 1940 (Weiskotten, Schwitalia, Cutter, & Anderson, 1940), and were repeated, formulated as recommendations and as warnings, in seven subsequent commissioned reports. Selected portions of individual reports follow:

Medical Education in the United States, 1934-1939 (American Medical Association) 1940

> As a professional institution the medical school considers its curriculum as a unified whole. The organization of the faculty into the various departments and the laying down of a more or less formal curriculum does not imply the independence of the several units. The continued visualization of objectives and the conduct of the educational program as a whole requires frequent departmental, interdepartmental and faculty conferences. *(Weiskotten et al., 1940, p. 81)*

Medical Schools in the United States at Mid-Century (American Medical Association, Amercian Association of Medical Colleges) 1953

... The expanded activities of the modern medical school call for a new type of leadership and a new type of organization *(Deitrick & Berson, 1953, p. 138).*

The Graduate Education of Physicians (American Medical Association) 1966

"The growth of knowledge must lead through specialization and fragmentation to a higher order of organization that will enhance the ability of many kinds of specialists to work together on the problems that are the reason for their existence." *(Millis, 1966, p. 93)*

A Handbook for Change (Student American Medical Association) 1972

Recommendation: That each segment of the curricular program be the responsibility of an interdepartmental teaching committee which will, in consultation with the department of medical education, define the course objectives and evaluate the student's progress *(Graham & Royer, 1972, p. 38).*

Physicians for the Twenty-first Century (American Association of Medical Colleges) 1984 (The GPEP Report)

Medical School deans should identify and designate an interdisciplinary and interdepartmental organization of faculty members to formulate a coherent and comprehensive educational program for medical students and to select the instructional and evaluation methods to be used *(Project Panel on the General Professional Education of the Physician, 1984, p. 20).*

Clinical Education and the Doctor of Tomorrow (N.Y. Academy of Sciences) 1989

The Liaison Committee on Medical Education (LCME), the body responsible for the accreditation of medical schools in the United States and Canada, was challenged to develop a standard that would regard the existence and effective function of an institutionalized authority (committee) for curriculum management as central to medical education. *(Gastel & Rogers, 1989, p. 111)*

Medical Education in Transition (Robert Wood Johnson Foundation) 1992

... A division of effort (departmental autonomy) becomes a barrier to an educational effort like the organ-systems curriculum, which is specifically intended to integrate rather than focus learning on reductionistic scientific thinking. *(Marsten & Jones, 1992, p. 22)*

Educating Medical Students: Assessing Change in Medical Education (Association of American Medical Colleges) 1992

An overarching, transdepartmental administrative structure is required to define educational policies; set institutional goals and objectives; define the concepts, knowledge, skills and behaviors to be learned; and foster the development of educational methods and evaluation strategies. *(Association of American Medical Colleges, 1992, p. 1)*

Enarson and Burg, in an analysis similar to the one performed by Christakis, reviewed the recommendations made in 15 major reports between 1906 and 1992. Among the organizational variables the following recommendation was reported: "*Control of, and responsibility for, the planning, implementation and evaluation of the educational program of each medical school should be given to a central interdisciplinary and interdepartmental group*" (Enarson & Burg, 1992, p. 1142).

It seems clear from the analyses in these commission reports (and based on other literature of the time) that medical school administrators and faculty were beginning to understand the need for a centralized interdepartmental organization for the medical school's teaching mission. However, despite the realization and articulation over decades by those charged with studying medical education that organizational change was desperately needed, there was little progress in this direction. In fact, in the middle 1980s the Association of American Medical Colleges Executive Council was still supportive of department-based management (Hendricson, Katz, & Hoy, 1987). At the same time, the Liaison Committee on Medical Education was strongly recommending curriculum reform but did not challenge department-based management (Kassebaum, Cutler, & Eaglen, 1997). This was in spite of the fact that the 1984 GPEP Report recommended an interdisciplinary and interdepartmental organization of faculty members to manage the curriculum (Project Panel on the General Professional Education of the Physician, 1984).

In meeting the challenge of educating students to be physicians in the 21st century, schools of medicine must develop management systems that promote change and encourage innovation. *(Burg et al., 1992, p. 714)*

Finally, because curriculum change was not coming about despite strong recommendations in the GPEP report, and because change was not going to come about in medical schools with autonomous department-based organizations, the Liaison Committee on Medical Education was challenged to develop a standard "*that would regard the existence and effective function of an institutionalized authority (committee) for curriculum management as central to medical education*" (Gastel & Rogers, 1989, p. 11).

In 1991 the Liaison Committee on Medical Education established a new standard; the most recent wording is as follows: "*There must be integrated institutional responsibility for the design and management of a coherent and coordinated curriculum. The chief academic officer must have sufficient available resources and authority provided by the institution to fulfill this responsibility*" (Kasselbaum, 1997, p. 1130).

This standard was intended as both a carrot and as a stick. Articulating the direction in which educational governance needed to move provided guidance and direction to the school as its faculty worked through the accreditation self study. Since the standard was a "must", there was added incentive to adopt a centralized governance structure for the curriculum for the M.D. degree (at least at the time of accreditation). To date, the development of an accreditation standard seems to be the largest factor in causing schools to reconsider and alter the administration of their curriculum.

LEADERSHIP AND GOVERNANCE FOR CHANGE

Key leadership characteristics

Some medical educators have compared the departmentally-based educational organization of a curriculum to a corporate bureaucracy (Bloom, 1988, 1989, 1995). This comparison is based in part on the fact that the success of medical school departments has been the result of revenues from research endeavors, clinical care or both; thus, these two entities share making money as a common goal. While the similarities and differences between corporate and academic bureaucracies have been documented at length, there is somewhat general agreement that certain leadership attributes may transcend the basic differences between academia and business.

Often, natural leaders within any institution lead by their stature, their charisma, and their accomplishments. *(Kaufman, 1998, p. 511)*

According to Peter Drucker, *"The manager leads by integrity of character. He commands more respect than the most likable man ... he sets high standards"* (Beatty, 1998, p. 105). In the middle 1980s Warren Bennis studied effective leaders and said: *"Leaders [must] have a clear idea of what they want to do"* (Bennis, 1993, p. 89) *"[they] must communicate their vision"* (Bennis, 1993, p. 79) and *"People would much rather follow people they can count on, even if they disagree with their viewpoint"* (Bennis, 1993, p. 82).

These concepts are supported in the literature on medical schools and medical education. In *Social Process and Power in a Medical School* Bucher wrote, *"The assessed stature of a man, whether head or faculty, is very important."* Qualities that might define stature include, *"... the quality of a person's research, whether or not he appears to be clear-thinking, whether he is a decent human being, whether he has good judgment, and whether he 'pulls his load'"* (Bucher, 1970, p. 29). Clearly, successful leadership requires exceptional individuals, whether in business or in education; yet it can be even more complicated than that.

Leadership for change

Any analysis of leadership within a medical school must start with the role of the dean. Unhappiness with the curriculum may originate with the students or the teaching faculty but unless the dean is convinced that change is needed, nothing is likely to occur.

Fundamental leadership characteristics transcend any particular agenda. However, leading a medical school through a major transition such as curriculum reformation requires a different kind of leadership from the dean than managing a medical school during a period when matters are fairly stable. In *Leading Among Leaders: the Dean in Today's Medical School*, Daugherty (1998) concluded, "*A nation at peace and a nation under threat require different types of leaders – as do medical schools*" (p. 649).

The type of leadership described as vital to curriculum change has often been called "entrepreneurial". "*Entrepreneurial leadership is a key feature in the process of change*" (Broomfield & Bligh, 1997, p. 109). Entrepreneurs are defined as risk-takers, and thus by extension the literature on curriculum change supports the notion that a dean who is not afraid to take risks possesses one of the qualities needed to assure successful reform. This quality is essential because curriculum change can be a risky business, especially considering the resistance from departmental chairs, who hold power over their faculty.

In 1991 the Pew Health Professions Commission cautioned,

> Simply breaking down the (departmental) boundaries is not enough, nor is it always appropriate. In creating a new model for health professions education, the more challenging task is to keep all that is valuable within the departmental and disciplinary orientation and simultaneously develop a new model that permits ways of organizing people, knowledge, research, and patient care. (*Shugars, O'Neil, & Bader, 1991, p. 13*)

Samuel Bloom advised: "*Each medical school must plan its own program. It will not succeed, however, unless it addresses the structural problems of organization, the sources of authority and allocation of resources, and the power centers of decision-making*" (Marsten & Jones, 1992, pp. 22-23).

The literature on leadership reveals that the medical school dean who can successfully bring about curriculum change must be decent, clear-thinking, likable and also a respected person who possesses high standards and unquestionable integrity. In addition, this dean must be a risk-taker who is not afraid to shake up the departments, which is something that can only be handled well if handled with great skill. It is also clear that, without the strong support of the dean, any change in the educational program of a school will not occur.

Funding is also fundamental to change. To bring about change, the dean also needs to be willing and able to mobilize sufficient resources, which may mean a re-distribution of funds. In 1993, describing a curriculum revision process at the University of Michigan Medical School, the authors wrote, "*Dean Bole emphasized education from the start. An active chief academic officer, he promised support for teachers and teaching activities, and funding for revitalizing the curriculum. He vowed to return education to a top priority and immediately set about doing so by appointing an associate dean for medical education*" (Davis & White, 1993, p. 334). Successful leaders mobilize resources, human and monetary, to bring about change. At Michigan, Dean Bole collected specific data on departmental teaching effort, compared these data with the distribution of General Funds, and announced changes to the distribution to realign effort with funding, and to fund curriculum leadership and efforts from the dean's office.

Centralizing for change

While the dean must set the tone and create the environment in which change can take place, it is not realistic to believe he/she can provide the hands-on, day-to-day leadership that curriculum change requires. The dean needs a faculty member; one who reports directly to the dean, has intricate knowledge of how the medical school works, is well respected, and has outstanding communication skills. This individual must be well supported financially by the dean and, like the dean, must be chosen based on his/her ability to perform this particular task: curriculum change. This individual will lead the effort, and will chair the faculty committee charged with developing the new curriculum. This must be a thoughtful, careful choice.

Medical education can only be as good as its leaders. *(Deitrick & Berson, 1993, p. 117)*

Daryl R. Conner (1993) describes two types of senior managers and how they deal with change: the first group he labels the *"unconsciously incompetent people who do not implement change effectively in their own lives nor orchestrate it well with others, and they do not know why"* (p. 221). These people simply "don't know that they don't know". According to Conner (1993) their *"change-related failures are often spectacular; therefore, they provide excellent opportunities for cataloging what not to do. When unconsciously incompetent people confront major change, they are usually unable to make the necessary adjustments without displaying dysfunctional behavior. Either they never achieve their change objectives or do so only after expending a great deal more time and money than originally planned"* (p. 221). Conner believes most senior managers are unconsciously incompetent. Could this analysis apply to unsuccessful Associate Deans for Education?

The second groups are the unconsciously competent. These are people who *"tend to do the right things to successfully implement change but do not know what those things are or how they do them"* (Conner, 1993, p. 221). They are "not simply lucky", as many of them thought. They were following specific (though unconscious) guidelines that they had intuitively developed as a result of trial and error. These people were never novices at change. They were always heavily scarred from, and therefore prepared by, many encounters with future shock.

While they are often extremely successful in their execution of change, they also have the capacity to fail miserably. These people can work wonders in some change situations only to fall flat on their faces in others. Without awareness of the behavior that leads to success, it is virtually impossible to reproduce that success consistently. We have concluded that the proficiency these people demonstrate at implementing change depends mostly on whether or not they are having a good day at following their hunches – not exactly the most dependable system on which to rely when dealing with important changes *(Conner, 1993, pp. 221-222)*

During the 1950s and 1960s most United States medical schools realized the need to create an office of curriculum affairs or office of curricular implementation. As the dean's responsibilities continued to grow, many schools also began appointing part time assistant and associate deans for education or curriculum. Currently, these individuals tend to be associate deans with responsibility for the implementation of the undergraduate curriculum. These are the individuals that the dean turns to when it is time for a curriculum review, reform or change.

The leadership characteristics of the dean mentioned above transfer to the associate dean in most instances. However, since the departmental chairs will not accord an associate dean the same power they ascribe the dean, there are special characteristics that are needed. The list is long:

- Consensus-building skills
- Team-building skills
- Ability to inspire and motivate
- Delegation skills
- Mentoring skills
- Ability to say "no"
- Political savvy
- Ability to "hold the line"
- Ability to compromise
- Commands respect from colleagues
- Ability to create a vision
- Understanding power and influence and how to use them.

Communication between the dean and the associate dean is essential. It is vitally important for the dean to share his/her vision for the medical school with the associate dean, and for both to be able to share with the faculty a carefully crafted and thoughtful vision for the future. The associate dean must have the unqualified support and confidence of the dean.

A case-in-point

Dr. Jones had recently been appointed Associate Dean for Education and was eager to implement curricular change. He had been recognized as an excellent clinical teacher and was now in a position to exert his influence over the educational program. He did not know very much about education or administration but was eager to learn. First, he attended a workshop sponsored by the American Association of American Colleges focused on problem-based learning with examples of how it was implemented at three innovative schools.

He returned home and shared what he had learned with the dean, who was even less informed regarding the benefits of problem-based learning or what it would take to change the traditional curriculum in a research-oriented school with strong basic science departments. It was agreed that Dr. Jones would give a report at the next faculty meeting on his experience at the workshop and would use the occasion to announce a curriculum review, the goal of which was to make sweeping changes in the curriculum. The dean was eager to improve the education of the medical students and was supportive of Dr. Jones.

At a faculty meeting the following week Dr. Jones reported with enthusiasm his experiences at the workshop and briefly outlined the components of a problem-based learning curriculum as he saw it. Included in his overview were comments about: interdepartmental teaching, no basic science courses, students working on a paper-based medical problem the first day of medical school, small tutorial groups led by faculty tutors, lots of free time for the students to do independent research on the medical problem, and happy students.

Questions from the faculty included: How do you intend to pay for the increased faculty effort to run this new curriculum? What does the curriculum committee (charged with managing our curriculum) think about this idea? What is the evidence that problem-based learning is better than what we have been doing here very successfully for 150 years? What do the chairs think of this idea? Where is the Executive Committee on this plan? Who will protect the integrity of the information taught to the students if the departments and chairs are not responsible for the content and teaching? How can the students work on a medical problem on the first day of classes when they don't even have a medical vocabulary? How could he assure content coverage with a case-based education? Etc.

Although these questions were quite predictable, Dr. Jones did not have satisfactory answers for any of them. The appropriate committees had not been consulted, and he had not done any groundwork with the chairs, the curriculum committee or the faculty at large. He had no idea how the cases would be developed or how content adequacy would be assured. Clearly, he had no incremental money to satisfy the chairs and faculty that their efforts in this venture would be funded or rewarded.

After 20 minutes of questioning by the faculty, and before the dean could bring any closure to what he considered a disastrous situation, one of the chairs asked to be recognized. He spoke eloquently about the quality of the school's current curriculum. He provided, as evidence, the quality of the faculty who delivered it, the United States Medical Licensure Examination scores of the students, the distinction of the graduating classes, and the quality of residency placements the students received upon graduation. Therefore, he moved that the curriculum should not be changed and that problem-based learning was not acceptable for this school. He allowed that if Dr. Jones could produce convincing evidence that problem-based learning would produce better doctors as graduates and that the graduates would achieve even better residency situations, the matter could be opened again after the proper committees (curriculum, Dean's Advisory and Executive) had been consulted and had approved the plan. The motion passed overwhelmingly.

Dr. Jones was asked to step down as Dean for Education and no changes were made to the curriculum.

Many believe that leaders in medical education are analogous to the sails on a sailboat or, like a snow fence, they cannot change the wind or its direction, but they can redirect the wind for some useful purpose. On a sailboat the wind can be channeled to provide propulsion. Snow fences don't stop the snow from drifting in the wind, they redirect the snow away from the road. The same may be true for leadership. However, it is our belief that leadership can drive change, rather than trying to bring about change by reacting to circumstances and opinions. Successful, meaningful change is unlikely if the leader of the effort merely tries to redirect the opinions and positions of the faculty in the school. The leader must be knowledgeable and willing to express his/her goals and opinions in the process. Most importantly, he/she must be able to articulate a vision that others can embrace.

Committee for change

One of the most important things the dean's appointed leader will do is choose the faculty committee that will work as a team to bring about curriculum change. This group will not be the standing curriculum committee, rather it will be a group hand-selected by the dean and the associate dean with input as deemed necessary from faculty and student advisory groups.

> Committees are the forums through which policy-making for the college as a whole occurs. *(Bucher, 1970, p. 13)*

The membership of the committee that will set curriculum transformation in motion should reflect the particular commitment to change. "De-departmentalizing" the curriculum means a new focus on inter- and multi-disciplinary approaches to education. Thus, committee members should represent a cross-section of disciplines. Early introduction to patients, teaching fundamentals in a clinical context, and sufficient ambulatory experiences will require appropriate clinical membership.

Representation alone, however, does not guarantee an effective committee. In 1997 Broomfield and Bligh wrote about the importance of teams and the features of team roles in bringing about curriculum change. "*Whilst quality of leadership is a major variable in predicting the outcome of team work, other variables should be considered. These variables include the behaviour of members of the team during its work*" (Broomfield & Bligh, 1997, p. 109). The authors believe that if behavior could be predicted, then teams could be constructed to function most effectively.

Although behavior and thus effectiveness may be difficult to predict, the associate dean will not want to choose just those faculty recommended by chairs as having the time to participate in this activity. Rather, some specific qualities will be key. Faculty who teach medical students, who have robust networks and excellent communication skills, and who will work to reach consensus: these are the individuals who can help to bring about change. Perhaps most importantly, "opinion leaders" are needed for this effort. *"The opinion leaders in medical schools vary, depending on the dominant subculture of the organization. They are usually individuals who can use their influence to either advance or impede the implementation of any idea, project, or program"* (Halvorsen, 1998, p. 379).

A case-in-point

Dr. Cooper was recognized as the "hands-down" best teacher in the basic science portion of the curriculum. Rules were actually passed regarding the distribution of teaching awards since Dr. Cooper would win the same award year after year if there were no such distribution rules. In addition to his teaching prowess, he was an articulate, quick, and very savvy faculty politician. One of his habits was to sit in exactly the same chair in the hospital cafeteria each day at lunchtime and conduct dialogue with all who would listen regarding the school and how it was progressing. He was an alum with impressive credentials and clearly a leader among the faculty. His name was mentioned for every committee that was ever appointed to serve the school. He was known to all.

It was no surprise that Dr. Cooper was appointed to the curriculum change committee by the dean. What *was* a surprise was the importance of his informal network in the overall success of the curriculum change effort. If new ideas were to be tried or a controversial proposal to be floated to the faculty, it was Dr. Cooper who would take it to the faculty informally and get feedback. This approach proved to be immensely more effective than "discussions" at faculty meetings. These "discussions" were never very helpful for several reasons: (1) very few faculty showed up to the meetings, (2) the environment (large auditorium with the dean and associate deans in the front, chairs sprinkled throughout in their preferred corners of the room) was not conducive to receiving input from most faculty. They did not feel comfortable presenting opposing views to those of the leadership.

None of these problems was obvious at Dr. Cooper's table in the hospital cafeteria. Junior and senior faculty felt free to listen and argue with whatever was under discussion. Dr. Cooper took the results of his luncheon summits to the planning committee and this input was critical to the successful planning of the new program. Further, since Dr. Cooper floated the ideas to the faculty, in addition to the usual communication channels, there were no surprises when issues were presented for formal discussion at the faculty meetings. Finally, given his excellent communication skills, Dr. Cooper was a powerful force in changing faculty opinions in favor of curriculum change.

Students should also be members of the committee charged with curriculum change. They bring a very important perspective and, in serving on a committee like this, provide evidence that they are willing to put time and energy into an effort that will improve medical education for the classes following them, rather than for themselves.

> The responsibility for curriculum changes in medical schools usually lies almost completely with the faculty, and change, when it occurs at all, is often slow or disruptive. Because medical students are the direct beneficiaries of the curriculum, it is logical to involve them both as barometers of the curriculum status and as active participants in shaping changes. *(Shope, 1989, p. 300)*

In fact, students can be the driving force behind change at some schools. In an article about curriculum change in Great Britain, Lowry (1993) noted that Britain's General Medical Council, while calling for change, did not have a good reputation for implementing or ensuring change in the long term. She wrote:

> Ultimately the strongest driving force for change must be the students and the doctors themselves. They must be empowered to demand excellence in the courses that they attend and realize that their education is not a favour to them but a means of preparing them to be the sort of doctors that we want in the future. *(Lowry, 1993, p. 322)*

At Stanford in 1966 unhappy students made "formal petitions to the dean's office", and according to minutes cited in a 1997 article, "the faculty group concluded that students' concerns were legitimate". Again in 1988, a group of Stanford medical students, like their peers in the 1960s and 1970s, organized Students for an Improved Curriculum. Based on student unhappiness, Stanford "... *then decided to go forward with a curriculum review because such an examination had been mandated five years earlier when the (prior) curriculum had been finally dismantled*" (Cuban, 1997, p. 103).

Whatever the membership, the centralized committee must be appropriately charged and delegated sufficient authority to complete their responsibilities. The very first recommendation of the Josiah Macy, Jr. Foundation report (1989) was: "*Create at each school an appropriate central unit that has authority to plan, organize, monitor, evaluate, and continuously revise the curriculum*" (Gastel & Rogers, 1989, p. 111).

Leadership and governance for long-term stability

If a school is successful in changing its curriculum to a new interdepartmental format, a new governance system for maintenance and continuous improvement is needed. The change process paraphernalia must give way to a structure of leadership focused on long-term implementation. The primary goal is continuous improvement through close monitoring to prevent the necessity for major changes in the program four years hence.

Dean for a change

Today, early in the twenty-first century, there is probably not one medical school dean who feels he/she is leading within a stable environment. Advances in medical discoveries and changes in health care delivery have turned the educational programs upside down, and forced organizational change to accommodate progress. Success as a leader is only partially (albeit essentially) dependent on acute intelligence and other personal qualifications including an ability to achieve compromise and nurture collaboration and integration.

Today, good deans must fight the "good fight", and every fight has opposing sides (read: enemies). The highest-quality medical education is now much more clinically oriented, with more and more activity taking place in the clinics, where attention is focused more on containing costs and generating revenue than on education. It is not inconceivable that the dean who is able to put such a program in place – the salt-of-the-earth, the entrepreneur, the general – might need to walk away when that particular job is done.

> Education consumes time and energy, which interferes with the generation of clinical revenues or grant dollars. *(Arana & McCurdy, 1995, p. 1075)*

Associate dean

The associate dean who leads the team that brings about change may be ready to step down once the faculty approve the new curriculum, but waiting a year or two might better serve the institution. To ensure success, there must be continuity for at least a period of time. The faculty who were on the "change committee" have done their job, and that committee should be recognized, congratulated and excused. The dean and associate dean will want to find administrative roles for at least some who have shown particular skills that will be useful in managing a new curriculum, and continuity will help in this transition. The dean and associate dean should exercise a high level of caution in this task.

However the school decides to organize its centralized governance structure, the new governance model must be presented to the faculty for approval simultaneously with the new curriculum. They both have a new, interdisciplinary approach and thus go hand-in-hand. A model for centralized governance with the associate dean as the school's delegated leader gives the associate dean significant authority, which he shares with the new committee for curriculum governance. Funding for the educational program should also reside with the associate dean.

Centralized committees for curriculum governance

Curriculum leaders

Faculty responsible for the details of the curriculum are needed to lead the program for the school, and should be financially compensated by the dean for these efforts; this further removes any departmental connotation from curriculum management. Organizationally, this can be accomplished best by funding a faculty member to direct each year of the curriculum. At the University of Michigan these individuals are called "component directors". Each one is responsible for a single year of the curriculum, is paid a portion of his salary by the dean's office, and is appointed by the associate dean. Faculty in these roles must truly look beyond their own departments to provide advice, direction and leadership to the faculty leading and teaching the courses. They must ensure appropriate integration and avoid unnecessary redundancy. Daily interactions with students and teachers are essential, as is the ability to interpret the data derived from course and clerkship evaluations. Frequently these component directors are asked to report to the appropriate committees their impressions of curriculum quality derived from internal and external measurements. In 1993, Davis and White wrote:

> The dean and associate dean carefully recruited from among the faculty a director and an assistant director to manage each of the components. These eight faculty members were recruited because they were well-respected scholars and clinicians with tenure who had demonstrated significant commitments to teaching and the ability and willingness to represent the institution rather than their departments. *(p. 334)*

In recruiting faculty to these important positions, mistakes can happen and should be rectified as quickly as possible.

A case-in-point

Dr. Cooper, who was absolutely ideal as a spokesperson/communicator on the dean's committee charged with revising the curriculum, was chosen to lead the second-year curriculum. As a surgical pathologist, a practicing clinician, and an expert teacher, he seemed the logical choice to provide leadership to the second year, which was interdepartmental and viewed as an important preparation of the students for clinical clerkships. In fact, many of the ideas about the content and how it should be taught were actually contributed by Dr. Cooper.

Not long after his appointment things started to go terribly wrong in the second year. Dr. Cooper, who was an excellent communicator while a member of the committee, turned out to be an obstinate tyrant when he had the ability to make decisions such as redirecting teaching effort. He had not learned what most kindergartners learn about working and playing with others. He was an excellent teacher and committee member, but a miserable boss. Even the students rebelled at his stubbornness and lack of interest in their input on issues related to examination scheduling and integration of content. Finally, at the end of his 12-month appointment he concluded, with the assistance of the associate dean, that he was much happier in the classroom and laboratory and that the job of administration was not his cup of tea.

The working committee

Course and clerkship directors, if carefully chosen and well-led by the component directors (year coordinators) and associate dean, will handle the day-to-day management of the curriculum. These individuals should come together as a team, working together with the associate dean to discuss and recommend educational innovations, review and resolve problems, plan for the future, and make changes within courses to ensure educational goals are met and the highest quality is maintained. Issues involving policy should be discussed at length and recommendations brought forward from this committee to the policy committee.

The policy committee

The right people must be involved in curriculum management at the policy level; considering again team roles, the organization of committee membership should be thought about very carefully. At least some members should be appointed based on their intimate involvement in delivering the curriculum, and all of them, as a committee, should have authority to make decisions about curriculum content and educational methods.

Elected members can provide a perspective outside those closely involved in management and delivery of the curriculum, and junior faculty who are interested in or involved in the curriculum can provide a different perspective and learn more about curriculum decision-making and management. Bucher supports the value of involving junior faculty in management, *"Those younger faculty members who have risen most quickly into major committee responsibilities have all been fervently outspoken and highly critical of the status quo. Persons with demonstrated courage and conviction tend to be snapped up quickly"* (Bucher, 1970, p. 43).

Medical students should also be voting members of the curriculum policy committee. Engaging the students in discussion as important decisions are made is key to ensuring all perspectives have been put on the table, and prevents faculty and committees from reacting as problems arise rather than anticipating, discussing, and then making informed decisions. Although important information to be used in management decisions can be obtained by formal student evaluations of the curriculum, engaging students in discussion about issues will provide input at a different, and equally important, level. According to Huppatz:

> Only students are familiar with their needs and capabilities. Students are able to offer a student view on such issues as facilities and resources. For academic issues such as course content and examinations, students can offer feedback from

their current course and identify aspects that worked well and should be retained in the new course. *(Huppatz, 1996, p. 11)*

CURRICULUM AND TEACHING EVALUATION

Our purpose in this chapter is not to detail the components of a successful curricular evaluation system; our purpose is to describe how an evaluation system serves the governance and management of the curriculum.

Valid and reliable evaluation data are essential if the committee(s) and individuals responsible for the curriculum are to succeed in their roles. In the absence of data, anecdotes and "hearsay" evidence will become the default source of decision-making and will not provide a sound basis for guiding the curriculum. Without data it is impossible for the policy committee and working committees to refute statements from students, teachers, course directors and chairs that are either misdirected or self-serving.

A significant component of this chapter has been devoted to curriculum governance designed to guide curriculum change. If a major curriculum change is adopted and implemented, faculty will demand to know, and leaders should know, what the effects of that change are in the longer term. The governance structure must support methods for collecting, analyzing and interpreting data on the program.

Evaluation data can be used to make determinations about the quality of an educational program, and data gathered on individual faculty can be used for promotion, reward and placement of faculty. As medical schools realize the importance of recognizing teaching as a scholarly activity, documentation of faculty teaching efforts has become necessary. *"To address the need for more teaching required in medical schools and to recognize excellence in teaching, several schools have changed their tenure codes to emphasize teaching and to require better records of quality teaching through portfolios or peer review"* (Bland & Halloway, 1995, p. 33). Clearly a well-designed teacher evaluation system serves many purposes in the school.

Curriculum evaluation that relies heavily upon student input will not be popular among students, so it should not be an optional activity for them. There are a number of ways to soothe the sting of the requirement:

- spread it among the class (for example, half of the class evaluates one term, and the other half evaluates the other term);
- make it available on the web, so they are not faced with a series of bubble sheets;
- show them the fruits of their labors (e.g., publicize changes made to the curriculum that resulted from student evaluations).

If the governance structure is new, and if the faculty are not confident of the governance or the role of the dean in the curricular planning/management process, it may be advisable to create a separate faculty-student committee to oversee the evaluation activities. This committee could be responsible for reviewing the raw data and compiling an annual report to the faculty and students. An important consideration would be to ensure that no one believes the dean's office is manipulating the data with some political agenda in mind. Because of the sensitivity of these data, evaluation's place in the organizational structure should be carefully considered.

A case-in-point

The medical school implemented a new curriculum and simultaneously established an ongoing evaluation of the curriculum that included individual teachers and courses. Many faculty were suspicious of the new governance system that centralized (in the dean's office) direction of, and funding for, the curriculum. Therefore, a student-faculty committee was elected to serve as the Committee on Curricular Evaluation (CCE). The CCE was chaired by an elected faculty member and was charged with oversight of all evaluations and the delivery of an annual report to the students and faculty based on the evaluations.

Dr. Brown was a full professor and successful researcher in a basic science department. He was very bright and energetic and considered himself to be a triple threat faculty member since, in addition to his success in the laboratory, he also directed medical student teaching in his discipline and taught in the Ph.D. programs. He liked to stimulate students and did so with a questioning style of teaching that some students considered confrontational. Dr. Brown also contributed unselfishly through administrative service to the school. His popularity and stature with the basic science faculty had resulted in repeated elections to the Executive Committee and appointments to other prestigious university and medical school committees.

Not unexpectedly, Dr. Brown was elected chair of the CCE. The committee had worked successfully for three years prior to Dr. Brown's chairmanship, following the implementation of the new interdepartmental curriculum, and the faculty had grown accustomed to the detailed annual report of the CCE.

This year when the responsible faculty member presented the data to the CCE from the Department of Medical Education, there was a problem. Dr. Brown's teaching had received very poor evaluations from the second year class. In fact, they were so poor that he was rated in the bottom 5% of all teachers in the school. His course was rated at the bottom.

Dr. Brown wasted no time at the CCE meeting using his standing as chair to call into question the validity of all curricular evaluation activities. He changed from being a supporter of the new curriculum and of the evaluation activities to an angry critic. He announced that since there were obviously serious flaws in the evaluation system, there would be no evaluation report to the faculty this year, and the school should cease to waste valuable resources on such a flawed evaluation system. Although other members of the CCE tried to reason with Dr. Brown, he would not be dissuaded. Instead of the annual report from the committee, he submitted a recommendation to the Dean and Executive Committee to stop all evaluation activities.

Although the prior reports were summary documents only, and no detailed evaluation data regarding individual teachers were ever released to the faculty or the students, news traveled quickly throughout the school that the data were not favorable for Dr. Brown. In the end, the Associate Dean for Education was forced to prepare the annual report to the faculty and Dr. Brown resigned as the chair of the CCE. As a result of this unanticipated problem with the teacher evaluation system, from that time on, even the CCE was blinded as to the identity of the teachers who were being evaluated. After much discussion of the issues, the Executive Committee invited an expert in curricular evaluation to consult with the school and ensure the validity of the system and instruments.

Another extremely important task is the selection of the person to direct the actual evaluation efforts. If available, a faculty member from the Department of Medical Education (or equivalent) should be selected for this task. The objectivity and acceptability of this faculty member should be unquestioned. This person should sit ex officio on the Policy level committee to be informed of curriculum planning and to be involved in setting new goals for the evaluation efforts. He/she should also be a member of the faculty-student evaluation advisory committee and should assist the chair of the committee in agenda setting and follow up between meetings. This person should have evaluation expertise and be able to draft the annual report tables and figures to be used by the committee in assembling the annual report to faculty and students.

Funding for the evaluation efforts should be centralized in the dean's office. Undertakings such as a curriculum evaluation on this scale will require sufficient funding, staffing and expertise to make it a success. It is unlikely that the Department of Medical Education will have adequate resources to accomplish a successful evaluation activity of this scope without incremental funding.

FUNDING

In a departmentally based governance model, the dean provides funding to the departments, and the departmental chairs assign faculty to teach. Traditionally, the chairs hold the power over the faculty: to praise, to pay, to promote. They decide who will teach, and, given departmental funding priorities, they do not always choose the most talented or dynamic individuals, and do not always give them the kind of time or credit for the time high-quality teaching requires. Centralized governance and centralized funding, if adopted along with concrete plans for faculty recognition and reward, can give the associate dean leverage to recruit certain faculty to help ensure the quality of teaching in the curriculum, whether new or not.

In a common model for the transition to centralized funding, support for teaching that was previously provided directly to departments is re-deployed within the dean's office. As with centralized governance, many medical schools began to move to a centralized funding model as they adopted a new curriculum. With these changes, a centralized governance structure gives the associate dean authority to work with the faculty to shape and improve the curriculum, and a new centralized funding structure gives him/her money to buy faculty time to serve in leadership roles in the curriculum, to develop new courses or sequences, or to teach.

There have been a number of proposals to link funding to the quality and quantity of medical school faculty teaching efforts. In 1995 the University of Texas at Houston proposed a two-track approach in which one-half of current resources were distributed to the departments and one-half was distributed by the dean's office based on "merit". Reiser said: *"The selection of a department for a merit award should be based on the department's accomplishments in research and teaching in the laboratory, clinical, and policy-making venues of medical work"* (1995, p. 274).

Yale University School of Medicine also adopted a model of funds distribution based on faculty efforts (time) and faculty teaching quality. Using this model, a portion of funds was distributed to faculty (Johnson & Gifford, 1996).

FACULTY

Recognition and rewards

Without tangible rewards, the best faculty will not take the time to teach. As those in charge of assuring the quality of the curriculum, this should be a matter of great concern to the associate dean for education and the curriculum policy committee. In a pressured academic world where faculty are recognized and rewarded for funded research and income from patient care, education may be viewed as important but also as an activity for those who are no longer competitive. Although centralized funding does provide some additional leverage, medical school leadership will encounter difficulty recruiting faculty to an activity with a priority of 3 out of 3. *"Teacher resistance, in innovative as well as stable schools, was uniformly linked to a perceived lack of rewards for teaching and a sense of the importance of research for promotion and tenure"* (Cohen et al., 1994, p. 358).

Even after curriculum reform takes place and historical problems with the curriculum have theoretically been addressed, recruiting faculty to participate in teaching remains difficult, and for the same reasons. In the last few years, eight medical schools have participated in the "Preparing Physicians for the Future: Program in Medical Education" endeavor, sponsored by the Robert Wood Johnson Foundation. Describing the program's outcomes, Kaufman wrote, *"At most of the eight institutions, many faculty members resisted participation in the innovations because they thought added work would be required and because they saw no incentives and rewards for teaching efforts"* (1998, p. S12).

In a study of reforms in medical education, 1369 medical educators were asked about eight specific reforms. Ninety-eight percent of the respondents indicated that they supported or strongly supported a reform to *"... develop a system for evaluating and rewarding faculty for teaching excellence"* (Cantor, Cohen, Barker, Shuster, & Reynolds, 1991, p. 1003). To actually get there, however, medical schools must first accept teaching as a scholarly activity. Allegheny University of the Health Sciences studied this issue at some length and embarked on an interesting process to articulate the characteristics of scholarship. Individuals involved in this study concluded that scholarly activities must have an influence that extends beyond the students and patients interacting directly with the faculty member. They concluded that:

> For an effort to be considered scholarship, it should meet some, if not all, of the following criteria of being public and contributing to the body of knowledge in the field:
>
> Requires a high level of expertise
>
> Breaks new ground or is innovative
>
> Can be documented, and preferably can be archived and retrieved
>
> Can be peer-reviewed
>
> Can be transported to other sites, and replicated or elaborated upon
>
> Has an impact on the discipline or some community of people.
>
> *(Nieman, Donoghue, Ross, & Morahan, 1997, p. 498)*

To successfully recruit and retain the best teachers, rewards must include but do not have to be limited to tenure. Many faculty value highly any recognition by the dean, by colleagues and by students of teaching, particularly outstanding teaching. Awards for excellent teaching can be developed, publicized, and bestowed at major events like the Honors Convocation or Commencement. Letters from the dean to faculty members, with copies to their departmental chairs, recognizing teaching contributions and thanking faculty for their time and effort, are highly regarded. Nominal cash bonuses or access to funding for travel to a professional meeting might not be great recruitment tools, but they are effective ways to convey appreciation for the time and quality of teaching.

As noted in the GPEP report, *"The willingness of faculty members to devote significant time and energy to an integrated program for the general professional education of medical students will depend on whether or not their contributions to this basic institutional mission are accorded academic recognition"* (Project Panel on the General Professional Education of the Physician, 1984, p. 24).

Development

Properly trained faculty members are vital to the quality of the curriculum, and yet access to faculty development programs has varied widely from medical school to medical school. The good news is that curriculum revision has given medical schools and faculty an opportunity to think about teaching skills and approaches, and the importance of these to the educational program.

Many revisions have occurred in the last ten years. Some changes are as sweeping as adopting a problem-based approach to medical education, while some are smaller-scale changes such as reducing time spent in lecture and replacing it with small-group or independent learning activities. If faculty are not trained to teach in the newly adopted formats, it is unlikely they will teach successfully. In adopting a new pathology curriculum at the University of California, Davis, Lanphear noted, *"… a faculty member could not be expected to develop the new skills to perform in a new educational context without suitable training"* (Lanphear & Cardiff, 1987, p. 49).

Writing about reform adopted at SUNY Buffalo, Rollins said: *"Implementation of [General Physician Initiative] reforms may be hampered if faculty are not convinced of the importance of new instructional strategies or are not skilled in using them"* (Rollins et al., 1999, S108). A student questionnaire evaluating the curriculum change at SUNY revealed: *"the new approach challenged instructors to change their classroom management styles, but few shifts in teaching practices occurred. What was intended to be small group discussions turned into lectures"* (Rollins et al., 1999, pp. S108-109).

Medical school leaders and departmental chairs must embrace education as a priority, and demonstrate their commitment through formal, institutional recognition and rewards for teaching. In 1986, reporting at the Research in Medical Education Annual Conference, Hunt expressed:

> The need for expanded faculty development and the institution of a reward system for excellence in teaching. Medical faculty members are faced with the challenge of serving in a number of roles including patient care provider, researcher, scholar and teacher. Hence, successful curriculum reform efforts must institute strong support mechanisms and rewards for faculty members who devote time and energy to excellence in teaching. *(Hunt, Grover, & Holtzapple, 1986, p. 81)*

The curriculum policy committee, charged with using evaluation data to support and recommend curriculum changes, needs to concern itself with faculty development to assure the quality of teaching in the curriculum. This committee can recommend that specific faculty or all faculty participate in development activities.

It is important to keep in mind that the need for faculty development extends beyond the context of major curricular reform or innovation, and faculty need to understand fully the personal benefits of these programs. For example, developing or sharpening teaching skills in ambulatory settings not only increases the quality and effectiveness of faculty teaching, but also helps to relieve some of the time pressures inherent in teaching in the busy clinic settings.

Regardless of the scope of the development activities, they are primarily designed with two goals: (1) to provide faculty with an opportunity to teach as effectively as possible, and (2) to assure the high quality of the educational program.

CONCLUSION

Information in book chapters like this can only offer perspectives based on experience. This chapter and most of the literature cited here are just that; they are not conclusions drawn from research.

As we stated at the start of the chapter, there is a sizeable body of literature on centralized medical school governance directly related to curricular change. How that centralized governance structure actually works in the longer run should start appearing soon in publications and as presentations at meetings.

Given the authors' experiences, the relative shorter-term success of centralized governance, and the probable staying power of interdisciplinary approaches to issues and problems in health care and research, it is likely that centralized governance will be in place in medical education for some time to come.

The following summarizes in a succinct manner the recommendations of the authors.

GUIDELINES FOR PRACTICE

Roles in centralized curricular governance

It is essential for individuals involved in curricular governance to understand their roles so they can meet their responsibilities appropriately. Table 1 shows a list of those roles, and responsibilities within each role.

COMMON CHARACTERISTICS OF CENTRALIZED GOVERNANCE

The following are characteristics of a centralized governance structure that is in place and functioning well.

1. Educational experiences are organized according to the content and teaching methods, not according to departmental structure.
2. Faculty who participate in the educational program are compensated for their teaching, administrative and evaluation efforts.

Table 1. Roles in curricular development

Students	Participate in a systematic evaluation of courses and teachers.
	Provide student input to curriculum committees regarding student experiences with the curriculum.
	Disseminate information from curriculum committees to student body.
Teaching Faculty	Responsibility for content expertise to be taught/integrated per medical school goals.
	Provide direct instruction and guidance to students.
	Ensure their teaching is in agreement with overall curriculum plan.
	Work to improve their teaching skills.
	Cooperate with other faculty with regard to content and sequencing.
	Participate in evaluation of courses and peer teachers.
Course Director	Oversee planning and implementation of their course.
	Ensure their course achieves its goals and is coordinated appropriately within and across the curriculum.
	Observe teaching faculty and provide feedback.
	Review relevant evaluation data and make recommendations for changes.
Departmental Chair	Support and reward faculty involved in teaching.
	Review evaluation data and anticipate changes (in teachers) that may be recommended.
	Work with Associate Dean on appropriate teaching assignments.
Year Coordinators	Guide all teaching efforts in their year.
	Coordinate with other Year Coordinators to ensure continuity of curriculum.
	Solve problems among/between courses.
	Report regularly to the Associate Dean for Medical Education and the faculty.
	Review evaluation data; recommend and implement changes.
Associate Dean for Medical Education	Chair the Curriculum Policy Committee.
	Recruit and supervise the Year Coordinators.
	Review evaluation data, make and consider recommendations for changes, ensure implementation of approved changes.
	Manage the medical education budget.
	Work with chairs, course directors, and faculty to resolve educational problems.
	Organize and arrange for periodic renewal workshops/retreats.
	Plan, guide and fund new curricular innovations.
	Implement major curriculum changes (e.g., new required clerkship).
	Ensure compliance with LCME educational standards.
Curriculum Policy Committee	Establish and monitor educational policies for the school.
	Approve major curriculum changes.
	Review/approve recommendations from the Year Coordinators and the Associate Dean.
	Review evaluation data and make decisions accordingly.
	Ensure adequacy of content of the courses and the overall curriculum.
	Provide feedback to faculty regarding educational program.
Dean	Establish and maintain the school's priority for education of medical students.
	Articulate the mission of the school's educational program.
	Create and protect the educational budget.
	Provide rewards for teaching efforts.
	Implement methods to reward faculty excellence in teaching.

3. Curricular governance occurs at several levels (course, clerkship, year, entire program). At each level, appropriate faculty are selected to lead the efforts and these individuals are compensated from the centralized educational budget.
4. At each level, faculty committees composed of teaching faculty from that level meet as an organized committee to plan, deliver and evaluate the curriculum within their purview. Faculty compensated for their administrative efforts should chair these committees.
5. At the highest level of governance (the school level) a faculty/student committee, chaired by the Associate Dean for Medical Education, is delegated responsibility for the management and operation of the curriculum.
6. This curriculum policy committee must have the ability to change course content, delete courses no longer relevant, and reassign curriculum time. The committee reports only to the dean and the faculty.
7. Membership of the central educational committee is not elected in a way that would force the members to represent departmental interests above the interests of students or the school.
8. The Associate Dean, as the chief academic officer for the Dean, has control of the funding for the educational program as delegated from the dean.

While several medical schools have achieved many of these criteria, to our current knowledge no school has achieved all of them.

RECOMMENDATIONS FOR FUTURE RESEARCH

1. Examine the linkage between funding and educational effort and quality.
2. Document successful culture changes and curriculum innovations (with data on specific successes of particular methods) that grew out of reform and centralization of curricular governance.
3. Design and study models of faculty reward systems and the relationship to educational outcomes.
4. Examine the links between governance structure (centralized, interdepartmental, departmental, etc.) and the content and organization of the curriculum they produce.
5. Conduct detailed cost of medical education studies (format and outcomes) and document changes based on these studies.

REFERENCES

Arana, G. W., & McCurdy, L. (1995). Realigning the values of academic health centers: the role of innovative faculty management. *Academic Medicine, 70(12)*, 1073-1078.

Association of American Medical Colleges. (1992). *ACME-TRI Report: Educating medical students.* Washington, D.C.

Beatty, J. (1998). *The world according to Peter Drucker.* New York: Free Press.

Bennis, W. (1993). *An invented life.* Reading, MA: Addison-Wesley.

Bland, C. J., & Halloway, R. L. (1995). A crisis of mission: faculty roles and rewards in an era of health-care reform. *Change, September/October 1995*, 30-35.

Bloom, S. W. (1988). Structure and ideology in medical education: an analysis of resistance to change. *Journal of Health and Social Behavior, 29*, 294-306.

Bloom S. W. (1989). The medical school as a social organization: the sources of resistance to change. *Medical Education, 23(3)*, 228-241.

Bloom, S. W. (1995). The place of science of the health professions. *Medical Education, 29 (Supplement 1)*, 76-78.

Bouhuijs, P. (1990). Organization and educational innovation. In C. Van der Vleuten & W. Wijnen (Eds.), *Problem-based learning: perspectives from the Maastricht experience* (pp. 9-15). Amsterdam: Thesis Publication.

Broomfield, D., & Bligh, J. (1997). Curriculum change: the importance of team role. *Medical Education, 31(2)*, 109-114.

Bucher, R. (1970). Social process and power in a medical school. In M. N. Zold (Ed.), *Power in organization* (pp. 3-47). Nashville, TN: Vanderbilt Press.

Burg, F. D., McMichael, H., & Stemmler, E. J. (1986). Managing medical education at the University of Pennsylvania. *Journal of Medical Education, 61(9)*, 714-720.

Bussigel, M. N., Baransky, B. M., & Grenholm, G. G. (1988). *Innovative processes in medical education.* New York: Praeger.

Cantor, J. C., Cohen, A. B., Barker, D. C., Shuster, A. L., & Reynolds, R. C. (1991). Medical educators' views on medical education reform. *Journal of the American Medical Association, 265(8)*, 1002-1006.

Christakis, N. A. (1995). The similarity and frequency of proposals to reform US medical education: constant concerns. *Journal of the American Medical Association, 274(9)*, 706-711.

Cohen, J., Dannefer, E. F., Seidel, H. M., Weisman, C. S., Wexler, P., Brown, T. M., Brieger, G. H., Margolis, S., Ross, L. R., & Kunitz, S. J. (1994). Medical education change: a detailed study of six medical schools. *Medical Education, 28(5)*, 350-360.

Conner, D. R. (1993). *Managing at the speed of change: how resilient managers succeed and prosper where others fail.* New York: Villard Books.

Cuban, L. (1997). Change without reform: The case of Stanford University School of Medicine, 1908-1990. *American Educational Research Journal, 34(1)*, 83-122.

Davis, W. K., & White, B. A. (1993). Centralized decision making in management of the curriculum at the University of Michigan Medical School. *Academic Medicine, 68(5)*, 333-335.

Daugherty, R. M., Jr. (1998). Leading among leaders: the dean in today's medical school. *Academic Medicine, 73(6)*, 649-653.

Deitrick, J. E., & Berson, R. (1953). *Medical schools in the United States at mid-century.* New York: McGraw-Hill.

Enarson, C., & Burg, F. D. (1992). An overview of reform initiatives in medical education, 1906 through 1992. *Journal of the American Medical Association, 268(9)*, 1141-1143.

Gastel, B., & Rogers, D. (1989). *Clinical education and the doctor of tomorrow.* New York: Josiah Macy Foundation.

Graham, R., & Royer, J. (Eds.) (1972). *A handbook for change.* Philadelphia, PA: W. M. Fell Co.

Halvorsen, J. G. (1998). Motivating change: a missiological model [editorial]. *Family Medicine, 30(5)*, 378-382.

Hendricson, W. D., Katz, M. S., & Hoy, L. J. (1987). Question on philosophy, organization and function of medical school curriculum committees. *Proceedings of the Annual Conference on Research in Medical Education, 26*, 185-190.

Hendricson, W. D., Payer, A. F., Rogers, L. P., & Markus, J. F. (1993). The medical school curriculum committee revisited. *Academic Medicine. 68(3)*, 183-189.

Hunt, B. J., Grover, P. L., & Holtzapple, P. G. (1986). New directions for organizing structural curriculum reform. *Proceedings of the Annual Conference on Research in Medical Education, 25*, 77-82.

Huppatz, C. (1996). The essential role of the student in curriculum planning. *Medical Education, 30(1)*, 9-13.

Kassebaum, D. G., Cutler, E. R., & Eaglen, R. H. (1997). The influence of accreditation on educational change in U.S. medical schools. *Academic Medicine, 72(12)*, 1127-1133.

Kassebaum, D. G., Eaglen, R. H., & Cutler, E. R. (1997). The meaning and application of medical accreditation standards. *Academic Medicine, 72(9)*, 808-818.

Kaufman, A. (1998). Leadership and governance. *Academic Medicine, 73(9 supplement)*, S11-S15.

Lanphear, J. H., & Cardiff, R. D. (1987). Faculty development: an essential consideration in curriculum change. *Archives of Pathology and Laboratory Medicine, 111(5)*, 487-491.

Liaison Committee on Medical Education. (1997). *Functions and structure of a medical school.* Washington, DC: Association of American Medical Colleges and Chicago, IL: American Medical Association.

Lowry, S. (1993). Making change happen. *British Medical Journal, 306(6873)*, 320-322.

Marston, R. Q., & Jones, R. M. (Eds.) (1992). *Medical education in transition.* Princeton, NJ: Robert Wood Johnson Foundation.

Millis, J. S. (1966). *The graduate education of physicians.* Chicago, IL: American Medical Association.

Neufeld, V., & Barrows, H. (1974). The McMaster philosophy: an approach to medical education. *Journal of Medical Education, 49*, 1040-1050.

Nieman, L., Donoghue, G., Ross, L., & Morahan, P. (1997). Implementing a comprehensive approach to managing faculty roles, rewards, and development in an era of change. *Academic Medicine, 72(6)*, 496-504.

Project Panel on the General Professional Education of the Physician (1984). *Physicians for the Twenty-First Century: the GPEP Report.* Washington, D.C.: Association of American Medical Colleges.

Reiser, S. J. (1995). Linking excellence in teaching to departments' budgets. *Academic Medicine, 70(4)*, 272-275.

Reynolds, C. F., Adler, S., Kanter, S. L., Horn, J. P., Harvey, J., & Bernier, G. M. (1995). The undergraduate medical curriculum: centralized versus departmentalized. *Academic Medicine, 70(8)*, 671-675.

Rollins, L. K., Lynch, D. C., Owen, J. A., Shipengrover, J. A., Peel, M. E., & Chakravarthi, S. (1999). Moving from policy to practice in curriculum change at the University of Virginia School of Medicine, the East Carolina University School of Medicine, and SUNY – Buffalo School of Medicine. *Academic Medicine, 74(1)*, S104-S111.

Shope, T. (1989). Student-initiated analysis and change of a medical school curriculum. *Academic Medicine, 64(6)*, 300-301.

Shugars, D. A., O'Neil, E. H., & Bader, J. D. (1991). *Healthy America: Practitioners for 2005: an agenda for action for U.S. health professional schools.* Durham, NC: Pew Health Professions Commission, 1991.

Weiskotten, H. G., Schwitalia, A. M., Cutter, W. D., & Anderson, H. H. (1940). *Medical education in the United States, 1934-1939.* Chicago, IL: American Medical Association.

29 Faculty Development for Curricular Implementation

BRIAN C. JOLLY
University of Sheffield

SUMMARY

This chapter looks at how faculty development has assisted in implementing new curricula. It starts by elucidating the concept of faculty development. Essential features include both individual and corporate responsibility for anticipating personal and professional needs, the delivery of activities to meet these needs and the necessity for continuation of and reflection on this process.

Then, using a narrative approach, it reviews research on the benefits of faculty development in three sections. First, faculty development that addresses the needs of institutions' current curricula and teachers. Second, it describes research that centers on the role of faculty development in the birth and maturation of radically new curricular approaches, including problem-based learning, community-based medical education and the extended use of ambulatory settings. Third, guidelines for the appropriate choice of faculty development strategies are discussed.

Finally potential research issues are outlined. These include the need for an eclectic methodology for such studies, and for continued, but better, research on short courses, sabbaticals and workshops, and particularly on curriculum enhancement programs. Two issues that need further work are the influence of context on development programs, and the need for focused long-term evaluation of the impact of faculty development initiatives.

INTRODUCTION

Modifying a curriculum is likely to be difficult. Without faculty development it may well be impossible. At least, that is the conventional view and one giving rise to numerous papers and articles about institutional approaches to curriculum renewal and educator preparation, or simple descriptions of faculty development programs (e.g. McLeod et al., 1997; Rubeck & Witzke, 1998; Nieman, 1999). However, even assuming the efficacy of the intervention, the vexing questions on this issue are what type of faculty development will be appropriate and how much is enough?

International Handbook of Research in Medical Education, 945–967.
G.R. Norman, C.P.M. Van der Vleuten, D.I. Newble (eds.)
© 2002 *Dordrecht: Kluwer Academic Publishers. Printed in Great Britain.*

This review will include evidence that addresses these questions. Such evidence is sparse. Research, especially in controlled or evaluative modes, has not been extensive. Nor has it been particularly programmatic. Moreover, unfortunately, it has not been underpinned by unified theoretical perspectives.

The conceptual frameworks and models of faculty development in western professional/educational settings derive from a broadly based and eclectic philosophical foundation borrowed from numerous fields (Brew, 1995). The existence of activities in faculty development as diverse as lectures, seminars, action groups, mountaineering, survival courses, psychotherapy, and co-counseling testifies to the almost limitless boundaries of what has become known as faculty development. This rubric has included, in general terms, personal development, as in the sabbatical or elective; professional development, such as study for a higher degree or specialist qualification; and workforce tuning, such as the need to train a workforce to deal with unforeseen acute medical problems, e.g. HIV.

Nevertheless there has been a recent explosion of interest in faculty development in academic medicine (Towle, 1998). This has taken place, particularly in Europe, against a background of rapid change and development in other sectors of higher education where we have witnessed the growth of specific University departments devoted to faculty development, and its inculcation into the rubric of quality assurance procedures (Elton, 1998).

In medicine the predominant need in faculty development has concerned the teaching skills of clinical educators (Lowry, 1993). However the pace of change has been such that, in some institutions, faculty are just getting to grips with basic teaching skills for "old" curricula, when new sweeping changes take place. How difficult might it be for a clinician to operate as an effective problem-based learning tutor, when they have yet to be proficient in the basic attributes of clinical teaching as defined, for example, by Mattern et al. (1983)? In North America such problems have been addressed by workshop programs quickly moving from basic skills to advanced preparation (e.g. Grand'Maison & Des Marchais, 1991).

This review will start with some definitions of the concept of faculty development. Then we will look at research addressing curriculum development along three dimensions. First, because of the general dearth of research in all areas, it seems sensible to glean as much as possible from any studies that *have* been done. Thus we will look at studies that address the needs of institutions' current curricula and their medical teachers. This is also partly because some institutions are still struggling with inculcating a basic educational approach, or with ensuring the quality of their current curriculum provision, through faculty development. Second we will examine studies that have attempted to track the role of faculty development in the birth and maturation of new curricular approaches. Finally, pointers to providing a rationale for the appropriate choice of faculty development strategies, and research issues, will be discussed.

As research in this area is not often constructed around randomized-control studies, or even quasi-experimental ones, a meta-analysis approach is not appropriate. This review will take a traditional narrative approach. It is based on a background paper prepared for the Cambridge Conference on Community Based Medical Education in Ann Arbor, Michigan in 1995. Initially, we included all studies we could find on Medline and Psychlit databases concerning any reference to faculty (or "staff" – the United Kingdom term) development aimed at curriculum change towards community-based and ambulatory education between 1970 and 1994. In early 2000 we supplemented this with a repeat search, targeting any major curriculum change, including, e.g. problem-based learning. Non-Medline indexed medical education journals were searched by direct reference. This resulted in approximately 150 references. Dentistry was included, but papers from nursing and allied professions were excluded.

DEFINITIONS

The term faculty development implies that activities are being undertaken by academic staff in educational institutions and that some progress or growth will occur as a result, both for the individual and, crucially, for the institution. The link with the notion of growth is significant as it introduces a network of values and assumptions about the nature of the human condition and its moral and ethical attributes (Perry, 1968). While individual growth is undoubtedly important, it is sometimes assumed that it should be subservient to institutional growth. Hence, in reality, faculty development frequently means making personnel more fit for the purpose of the institution. This has been a challenging concept in medical institutions of learning and research. Here, traditionally, personal and professional qualities, e.g. intellect and productivity, especially in research capacity, have often been valued above institutional ones (Handy, 1976) and, more importantly, above humanistic and educational ones. This is less common in industry or commerce, where much more emphasis is given to the need to develop the whole workforce (e.g. see Department of Employment United Kingdom, 1992).

The contrast between individual and institutional needs, and the role of the institution in provision of faculty development activities, are reflected in the following definitions of faculty development.

- a continuous process in which opportunities are provided for professional growth of the individual within the academic environment (Allen, 1990)
- employer sponsored activities, or provisions such as release time and tuition grants, through which existing personnel review or acquire skills, knowledge and attitudes related to job or personal development (ERIC, 1995)
- a process whereby the ability of faculty to perform their work roles is enhanced. The process is structured according to the objectives which it is designed to meet (Millard, 1993)
- enhancement of educational knowledge and skill of faculty members so that their educational contributions can extend to advancing the educational program rather than just teaching within it (Rubeck & Witzke, 1998)

- a broad concept which covers the systematic identification of the present and anticipated needs of an organization and its members, and the development of programs and activities to satisfy these needs. It is concerned with all aspects of a person's work (Elton, 1987)
- any planned activity designed to improve an individual's knowledge and skills in areas considered essential to ... performance ... in a department or residency program ... (Sheets & Schwenk, 1988)
- a tool for improving the educational vitality of our institutions through attention to competencies needed by individual teachers and to the institutional policies required to promote academic excellence (Wilkerson & Irby, 1998).

Such variable definitions are common. Hitchcock et al. (1993) suggest that the definition of faculty development in medical education has broadened over the last 15 years. This is particularly so for relatively prolific writers in the field. For example, Stritter and Hain (1977) first construed faculty development simply as workshops on teaching skills, while by 1983 (Stritter, 1983) this had expanded to strategies to improve teaching performance of faculty, and later others (Bland & Schmidtz, 1986) broadened the concept to include research skills.

Important common features of the definitions of faculty development are:

- the existence of individual as well as corporate responsibility to anticipate personal and professional needs
- the delivery of activities to meet these needs
- the necessity for continuation of and reflection on this process.

WHAT ARE CURRENT CURRICULAR NEEDS AND HOW ARE THEY ADDRESSED THROUGH FACULTY DEVELOPMENT?

The literature exhibits variation in ways of defining needs for faculty development, each predisposing towards certain outcomes. Observational studies or meta-analyses tend to identify what is good practice (for adoption) or undesirable activity (for elimination). Surveys of faculty tend to identify current self-perceived needs. Evaluation of specific faculty development activities can throw limited light on what works. Finally armchair speculations, despite an obvious lack of evidence or data, have been one, possibly the only, way of predicting the likely faculty development needs for the future.

General academic needs

Recent trends in health care and medical education have been taking place against a rapidly developing general academic environment. Post 1960, in the United Kingdom, 3 separate reports identified the need for increased faculty development (Robbins, 1963; Hale, 1964; UGC, 1984). University teachers in the USA, United Kingdom and Australia have more recently been urged to increase accountability, become more responsive to national needs and goals, less insular and bound by ivory tower mentality, and more productive (DoE, 1989; DEET, 1990; Curry & Wergin, 1993; Bok, 1982). In the early 1990s United Kingdom universities were asked, as the result of an extensive review (Jarratt, 1985), to strategically develop their staff development activities. Subsequently, in the United Kingdom, a number of strands involving faculty and institutional development have been woven into place including appraisal, research output, subject review (a process of peer review of the quality of education provided – see http://www.qaa.ac.uk/, accessed 30/07/2000) and educational audit (ratification of institutional quality control procedures).

In the USA a comprehensive survey of 756 colleges and universities (Centra, 1976) identified four types of faculty development, subsequently modified by Stritter (1983) for use in medicine – traditional practices (e.g. sabbaticals), instructional assistant practices (help with teaching), evaluation of teaching (student ratings, etc.) and faculty improvement activities. These activities have subsequently been expanded to include fellowships, short courses and workshops, and "train the trainer" courses at both national and regional level in the United Kingdom and USA (Skeff et al., 1997a; Towle, 1998).

Current faculty development needs in medicine

Observational studies address issues associated with the delivery of current curricula or the "here and now" of teaching practice. However, it is apparent that different contexts give rise to different criteria of "good" teaching (e.g. Mattern et al., 1983; Ullian et al., 1994; Jolly, 1994; Weinholtz, 1986; Irby 1994). Hence being overprescriptive in defining what a clinical teacher, in a certain setting, needs to be able to do, may be inadvisable.

Irby (1992) attempted to identify what academic physicians need to know, by analyzing the teaching of six distinguished clinical teachers. The results suggested that clinical teachers could benefit from learning about a variety of teaching methods and models, that novice teachers should study those more experienced and that faculty development should be content (i.e. case or discipline) based. In a further refinement (Irby, 1994), using the paradigm of craft knowledge (Calderhead, 1987), experienced teachers related in 2-hour interviews and think-aloud exercises what they employed as their knowledge base in their teaching rounds. Irby also undertook observations of the ward team. He identified 6 types of knowledge: knowledge about medicine, patients, patients' contexts, learners, general principles of teaching, and content-specific instruction. By "content-specific" Irby meant the way that teachers used case-based ("illness") teaching scripts or lesson plans to guide the learning of others. The last two are quite complex areas and reflect previous conclusions by Jolly and Macdonald (1989, 1986) that, to be effective, clinical teachers need expertise in clinical teaching, learning theory and educational evaluation. Slater and Cohn (1991) conducted similar observation studies for occupational therapy, with clinicians analyzing videotapes of their own and their colleagues' practice using the Dreyfus (1986) five-stage model of skill acquisition. Although their results were ill defined in the paper, they highlighted the need to have professionals reflect more on their own practice using expert-novice dialogue.

Surveys have been used to identify teachers' self perceived faculty development needs. Occasionally such surveys may be instrumental in achieving a curriculum change or may be a necessary step to embedding the transformation. Baldwin et al. (1995) used multiple one-hour focus group interviews to isolate perceived faculty development needs in pediatric, internal and family medicine generalists, and a checklist to ascertain a cross section of faculty needs. In interviews generalists felt undervalued by specialist colleagues. As a result they felt they needed more support through institutional recognition, more networking and more control over their time. In the checklist, however, two of the most frequently ticked items identified perennial problems in medical curricula: the need to teach individuals and small groups in clinic and the need to evaluate the teaching program.

In Canada, Harrison and Forgay (1990) surveyed faculty of all dental schools to identify needs from 32 prespecified items which they also subjected to factor analysis. From a 46% response rate they identified 6 major areas: conducting courses, clinical evaluation and clinical guidelines, interpersonal teaching skills, educational theory, the management of time and stress, and research and writing skills. However, the importance of each area varied according to faculty characteristics. For example women identified interpersonal skills and running courses as most important, and were also interested in educational theory, whereas men were not particularly enthusiastic about any of the areas. Provision of faculty development courses was rated much higher by didactic (basic-science) teachers than by clinical teachers. Also, those with some training already in education were very much more interested in most of the other topics. The authors concluded that there is a threshold of knowledge about a topic which, when traversed, unlocks awareness of the need for more successful or rewarding teaching methods.

Having discussed the needs for faculty development identified by research, we now turn to descriptions of faculty development programs designed to underpin curricular changes. Such programs have often been developed under an explicit claim to be tuning the workforce, either locally or nationally, or implementing specific new programs such as PBL or teaching in ambulatory or community settings.

Faculty development and new curricula

Many curriculum changes have been implemented at the end of the 20th century. These changes include the move to ambulatory and community settings for medical education and the adoption by many schools of problem-based learning as the main educational methodology. Many schools have undertaken parallel initiatives on all three fronts. Faculty development programs have been widely adopted at the same time. Hence it is not always possible to treat each of these three main trends in isolation although, below, we classify them largely for ease of presentation. Also the impact of staff development has been differentially managed in different countries, due to prevailing local conditions. In addition some investigations have been directed towards identifying the characteristics of a planned change in order to frame and facilitate appropriate faculty development, rather than to evaluate its impact, and these are also included here.

Moving towards ambulatory teaching

A number of studies address the nature of ambulatory (outpatient) teaching, with a view to its implications for, or the impact of, faculty development (Lawson & Moss, 1993; Irby et al., 1991; Packman & Krackov, 1993; Warren & Coke, 1993; Kovach, 1993; Fincher & Albritton, 1993; Steward, 1993; Perkoff, 1986; Gruppen et al., 1993). Ambulatory teaching is characterized by extensive variation in prevalence of case types within a pre-existing heterogeneous casemix, variable (dependent on case) degrees of responsibility assigned to individual students for patient care, more case presentations and a generally higher number of student-patient interactions than in ward-based teaching, together with a relatively high turnover of teachers per student. These attributes define the major goals for faculty development, for example the need to focus on 1-1 teaching, on coping with uncertainty and on the diversity of disease presentation. However, the stable frequency of some disease patterns or clinical conditions in North American clinics has been confirmed by two separate studies – hypertension, diabetes, rheumatological problems, and back pain or other muscular discomfort occurred most often (Fincher & Albritton, 1993; Gruppen et al., 1993).

In the 1960s–1990s, in the United Kingdom, ambulatory teaching was already part of medical education, as ambulatory clinics, ward work and other interventions were traditionally part of most hospital clinicians' responsibilities, although the availability of sub-specialty expertise in the family medicine setting was limited. Hence it is probable that the move to such settings in the United Kingdom has not engendered such an interest in faculty development issues. For example recent utilization of day surgery programs for teaching has not entailed extensive faculty development activities (Seabrook et al., 1997).

In the USA Woolliscroft and Schwenk (1989) have identified a number of features of ambulatory teaching that aid program planning. They include the fact that patients generally are not as ill as those in hospital, and that the ambulatory setting is perhaps the only place to learn about daily patient care and chronic illness. However, in their view the major characteristic of ambulatory care is that the locus of control lies with the patient and not the hospital "system". They point out that *"this fundamental difference underlies all aspects of developing educational programs ... most educational issues flow from this basic difference"* (p. 645).

In a summary of some of the studies cited above, Steward (1993) also highlights other implications for educational strategy which stem from moving to an ambulatory setting. He suggests abandoning the "complete history and physical" as an objective of courses taught in ambulatory settings. He also suggests that there are things that students might learn better in hospital, and these need identification (see also O'Sullivan, 2000). Both of these radical issues had to be addressed in staff development activities underpinning a move to teaching beginning clinical students in community settings (Murray et al., 1999). However, in that study it was the primary care generalists who had to change to adopt the "complete history and physical" as an objective, rather than it being relinquished by the hospital clinicians.

Anderson et al. (1997) performed a qualitative study of 14 peer-nominated faculty developers working in ambulatory education. They concluded that these educators' activities needed to engender more outcome-based evaluation. Also that the short workshops that they run might more usefully include: emphasis on educational planning rather than teaching skills; more about post-educational event analysis, such as reflection, integration and self direction; and attempts to train more learners and teachers to achieve learning objectives consistently in the clinical setting.

Community-based approaches

Folse, Da Rosa, and Wood (1991) surveyed departments of surgery from 21 community-based and 17 traditional schools to acquire information on practice and policy of faculty development. They found that neither the community nor traditional schools are necessarily uniform in their needs. Both types reported the same amount of effort in medical student teaching, but community schools were relatively (but not statistically significantly due to small Ns), more focused on patient care and traditional schools on postgraduate teaching and research. Traditional schools were more departmentalized and had more surgeons, but they were less committed voluntarily to teaching programs than their community counterparts.

DeWitt et al. (1993) describe an approach to community faculty development for training pediatric residents in practice settings. The approach included input on educational planning, teaching styles, learning styles, assessment and feedback as they related to the typical one-to-one clinical supervision or small group tutorial. Adult learning theory and logistic planning of activities in community settings were also identified. DeWitt involved community and full time academic physicians in a "spiral curriculum" programme of 1-3 days on clinical precepting, consisting of short (but initially 1 hour) didactic inputs followed by seminars, workshops, discussions, role-plays and small group presentations. Course tutors attempted to model, in the course process, the concepts they were introducing. Sessions considered for example, "What makes a teacher good?". Participants showed gains in knowledge of concepts and use of techniques and welcomed more role play and the shorter didactic inputs. Interruptions of a medical nature (bleeps) were intrusive, and the issue of location (on- vs off-campus accommodation) was never satisfactorily resolved. The authors concluded that "such programs should focus on developing skills in the two main methods ... clinical precepting and brief presentations". Another study looked at a program designed to increase formal mentoring skills (Morzinsky et al., 1994). This was an action research project – faculty skills were enhanced by actually creating and using a mentoring program; participants learnt on the job aided by a summer picnic, a mid program luncheon, a participant recognition ceremony and some workshops.

It is reasonable to assume that, in the move towards community settings, utilization of scant teaching resources is part of the issue as well as what precisely is done with them. It is therefore surprising to note continued resistance to the movement of training to non-ward-based sites. Krackov et al. (1993) identify a number of barriers including institutional resistance, finance and lack of incentives. Institutional resistance stems largely from apparent loss of control and the assumption that quality of education will suffer. There is frequently difficulty in finding sites for teaching because clinicians are overburdened by service commitments, sites are remote, transport is difficult, etc. The authors suggest that both incentives and recognition for clinical teachers are essential, and that relevant faculty development is mandatory.

Problem-based learning

Probably the most self-contained, focused and extensive faculty development has occurred where schools have adopted problem-based learning as their main educational strategy, particularly where they were not "green field" schools or where they previously had a long tradition of orthodoxy. A number of schools undertaking problem-based (PBL) revisions to curricula have introduced training for faculty (Neufeld et al., 1989; Kaufman et al., 1989; Evans & Taylor, 1996; Stern, 1998). Although there are few published reports of such courses, the format, from personal experience and communications, is remarkably uniform. It usually includes theoretical explanations of PBL (at some stage), small group discussion, individual reading, construction of PBL problems and experience of the PBL method initially with a non-medical problem.

One of the most comprehensive approaches has been at Sherbrooke, (Grand'Maison & Des Marchais, 1991). Here, the program consisted of four complementary but stand-alone elements offered from 1984 to 1990; a 2-day introductory workshop on educational principles, a 1-year, 100-hour course, on "medical pedagogy", an introductory workshop on PBL and a 3-day course followed by a 1-day refresher course on PBL tutoring. The take-up from faculty was 60%, 33%, 75% and 82% of full time teachers respectively for the four components. Evaluation was reported only on attrition rates and participant satisfaction, which were low and high, respectively. Nevertheless, curriculum leaders regarded the PBL workshop as the main contributor to the shift to PBL in the school. The workshops also focused on attitudinal as well as academic aspects of the changes implemented. Grand'Maison and Des Marchais (1991) highlight a number of other lessons learnt from such work:

- development must be tightly based on needs
- it must be continuous
- activities to change attitudes must be initiated a long time before curriculum change is started
- there must be a small core of motivated faculty
- outside experts must be very well briefed.

Nayer (1995) has comprehensively reviewed faculty development initiatives in PBL. As well as Sherbrooke, she cites Maastricht University (Bouhuijs, 1990), Ben Gurion Medical School (Benor & Mahler, 1990), Toronto, Hawaii, Harvard (Wilkerson & Hundert, 1991) and Auckland. She notes that few faculty development programs have been evaluated to gauge the impact on faculty, but that those that have indicate that faculty improves attitude, knowledge and teaching performance.

The move to primary care

There have been a number of approaches to faculty development for primary care. Evaluations of a family medicine fellowship program (McGahie et al., 1990; Bland et al., 1987) suggested that physicians completing the course simply have a more all-round academic orientation than a matched control group of non-attenders; they had more research interests, were more likely to have addressed a national meeting; belonged more frequently to a national society and published more. However, they were equally interested in teaching and administration. Most other family medicine programs address the skills of generalists in observing, analyzing, discussing and giving feedback on students' activity in the clinical encounter. Two studies (Anderson et al., 1991; Bird et al., 1993) concentrated on developing faculty's abilities to review videotapes of students' consultations with patients and give feedback appropriately, while a third (Preston-Whyte et al., 1993) also measured the effect of the course on faculty's ability to write objective learning contracts with a student. In this study three quarters of respondents said they also foresaw improvements in their own consultation skills as a result of learning about teaching them to students. The American College of Physicians and Pew Foundation sponsored a university and community-based faculty development program, based on the Stanford model, aimed at 6 goals, 3 of which entailed enhancing the teaching capabilities of general physician-educators (Skeff et al., 1999). Outcomes, which were only self-report based, indicated achievement of most of the goals. However, community-based faculty increased their ratings of general teaching ability and their sense of integration into the affiliated institution after the program more than hospital-based teachers. The authors concluded that such joint ventures were important to achieve diversification of the teaching settings.

Biddle et al. (1994) studied a 1/2 day per week primary care course for 1 year and interviewed 22 faculty. He found that providing good role models, skills of observation and feedback and the management of the 1-1 tutorial situation were important. Fenton and Povar (1993) suggested that in primary care situations the educational goals are different, focusing on the doctor-patient relationship, epidemiology and the natural history of disease, amongst others. Higgins (1989) concurs, describing students in primary care as more likely to see acute, but non-hospitalizable conditions, being more challenged, and needing a close working relationship between teacher and student.

A follow-up of Canadian family medicine faculty development programs (Steinert, 1993) found that 81% (13/16) offered in-house schemes. The principles of family medicine were not prominent, but clinical supervision and teaching skills were. Compared to 1983 (Steinert et al., 1988) departments had a person responsible for faculty development, had conducted a systematic needs assessment, had more structured courses and paid more attention to rural and community issues.

National programs/surveys

Several papers have addressed the need to link faculty development to teaching skills and curriculum design activities for new curricula geared to the General Professional Education of the Physician (GPEP, 1984) and General Medical Council (GMC, 1993) requirements (Lanphear & Cardiff, 1987; Towle, 1991; Lowry, 1993). In fact Lanphear describes a process of curriculum change as the focus for a faculty development program, in which attendance at an overarching curriculum committee itself promoted development of faculty charged with decision making. He also highlights the need for personal development in such a challenging environment, but the solutions proposed – "supportive and therapeutic counseling" were in his paper delivered by curriculum change agents themselves. Rubeck and Witzke (1998) monitored the use of faculty development in the eight schools participating in the Robert Wood Johnson Foundation (RWJ) curriculum change program. Despite signing up to common goals and receiving funding from the Foundation, schools were varied in their visions, and in their profile, utilization and evaluation of faculty development activity. There was no systematic evaluation of faculty development across the 8 schools, although participants' and observers' perceptions suggested there had been shifts towards more appropriate use of educational terminology, improved skills of individuals, and more diverse management strategies. A further paper on two of the RWJ institutions (Grayson et al., 1999) isolates faculty development as a small part of one of seven elements common to both in the success of the initiative. These were: using national priorities to promote the need for change, establishing top-up financial support in addition to the RWJ, redesigning the vision and organizational structure, establishing a monitoring and evaluation strategy, sustaining a positive attitude towards primary care through careful conference and locum arrangements, integrating the primary care physicians through positive management support, and sustaining interest in the generalist agenda through joint local and national faculty development workshops.

McLeod (1987) surveyed all Canadian medical schools for the incidence and effectiveness of faculty development activities in teaching skills, using methods previously devised by Centra (1976). Seventy-five percent of schools (12/16) indicated that they had faculty development programs. Interestingly all of these had sabbaticals with at least half salary, as well as workshops, seminars and programs. The most common topics included by those running workshops were instructional methods, curriculum evaluation, assessment methods, and educational trends. All schools had rating of instruction by students as the primary method of diagnosing inadequacies. Faculty rated the effectiveness of various development techniques; sabbaticals and workshops were highest rated, and awards for excellence in teaching and circulation of newsletters were ranked 29th and 34th respectively. Also, although assessment of instructional skill was highly rated it was rare for teachers to receive feedback, and schools did not in general have a committee devoted to faculty development. A 10 year follow-up (McLeod et al., 1997) indicated a significant change in faculty development emphasis on a wide front. Sabbaticals and conference funding were still evident, but systematic rating of and rewards for teaching excellence, peer review of teaching, grants for instructional development and the existence of a faculty development committee had increased across the board. The programs that were rated as most effective were instruction on lecturing and small group work, information technology, sabbaticals, awards for teaching, and cheap/no-cost faculty development. However, it was not clear whether faculty development initiatives had contributed towards or been prompted by new programmatic curriculum change.

Recruitment and retention of ethnic minority faculty with appropriate academic skills has been the goal of two faculty development programs (Rust et al., 1998; Freeman et al., 1998). These respectively 8 and 5 week workshops include targeted experience of working with minorities and teaching from minority faculty. Both have shown increased skills in participants and improved retention of ethnic minority faculty. However Rust (pp. 166-167) highlights that faculty development can only be partially effective when combating demonstrated large scale economic, social and educational barriers to participation of ethnic minorities as both faculty and students in medical education.

There have been a number of state-wide, national or international faculty development programs emanating from the USA including Advanced Trauma Life Support and the Stanford Faculty Development Programme. Skeff (Skeff et al., 1992a, 1992b, 1988) has been most prolific in the design and evaluation of such schemes. The basic premise is that a cascade system, of training trainers who then train other faculty, is an efficient way of improving the general level of teaching competence. This comes from diffusion theories of innovation which suggest that change agents with characteristics similar to their target audience are more effective. In Skeff's program facilitators engage in 7 seminars aimed at essential components of good teaching:

- establishing a positive learning climate
- control of teaching sessions
- goals

- promoting comprehension and retention
- assessment of the learner
- providing feedback
- promoting self-directed learning.

Methodologies included brief lectures, review and discussion of videotapes, role-play with videofeedback, specification of personal (participant) learning goals and reading. The most salient evaluation data collected were junior faculty's ratings of participants' teaching activity before and after the course. Increases were seen in all areas except learning climate and promoting self-directed learning, but ratings were initially high in these areas anyway.

Skeff makes a number of observations, anticipated by other investigators (Stritter, 1983), from these developments:

- Institutions may need to deliberately promote, even coerce, participation for faculty to appreciate benefits of faculty development activities
- As a result of training, self awareness about teaching ability increases and subjective rating of skill may be depressed, reducing self-reported effectiveness of courses, but increasing actual skill
- Short (14 hour) courses are unlikely, by themselves, to bring teachers to the highest levels of ability.

Leadership

The insufficiency of using merely the "teaching skills" approach to faculty development is described in several reviews of the anticipated needs of clinical teachers in new curricula (Lowry, 1993; Calman, 1994; Irby, 1992; Plamping & Towle, 1994).

The necessity for strong leadership and for its sustenance and support in new curricular strategies have been identified as common characteristics of institutional strategies for faculty development (Ullian & Stritter, 1997). This has been echoed by reviewers of the Robert Wood Johnson (RWJ) Initiative (Mennin & Krackov, 1998). In their analysis it is plain that such faculty development as existed was unilaterally directed towards the goals of the leaders, and supported their authority. The faculty development was largely institution focused, rather than individually oriented. Faculty development was a tool to broker understanding and ownership of changes. Kaufman (1998) suggests that the role of leadership in the RJW, and its use in governance and curriculum management structures, might be at least as important, if not more important than, faculty development.

Evans (1995) in a comprehensive and insightful paper describes the need for a new model for faculty development to accommodate the rapid changes impacting on health care and education. Although Evans tends to equate "faculty development" to "career progression", he typifies the existing model of advancement as involving substantial engagement in research, high scientific productivity, interaction with colleagues, and the ability to act as a mentor and peer reviewer. The major changes making the continuation of the old model untenable are (pp. 15-17):

Contraction of resources for health care and education

Limited money for research and more competition

Increasing patient care loadings on faculty

Fewer physicians with the skills for a scholarly career

Academic departments losing the capacity to subsidize academic activity by clinical care

A reduction in the public's automatic regard for "the Doctor" leading to increased scrutiny.

Evans then goes on to identify a number of factors for which academic clinicians will need to prepare themselves in the very near future (pp. 17-18):

Co-operation not competition

Reduced departmental and individual autonomy

More heterogeneous roles for all health professionals

Over zealous adherence to the previous model of advancement will hinder individuals' development

Academic centers will need to act as institutions not as collections of departments, hence more explicitly addressing institutional (society's?) goals through faculty development.

As a result a new model of faculty (career) development is proposed. The major additions to what is currently on the agenda include: greater emphasis on health promotion and disease prevention, attention to managed care, a greater role of patients, families and community in decision making and a shift towards humanistic and away from biomedical models of care. Another less strong implication is that faculty development has the potential to encourage major career changes, but also can become ineffective if those trained decide on reorientation to another interest. Hence, for institutions, maximizing payoff from faculty development is an important issue.

In the final section of this report we review very briefly generalized lessons from, and the theoretical approaches to, faculty development.

THE CHOICE OF APPROACHES TO FACULTY DEVELOPMENT

There is one remaining question about faculty development in this review: What are the characteristics of effective programs?

It is very poorly answered by the literature. Attempts to link activities precisely with outcomes have not been very frequent or fruitful. Most theoretical approaches are borrowed from adult education or are cobbled together for expediency to enable a rationale for a course or program to be developed, e.g. see Carroll (1993).

The earliest report of faculty development in a medical education context relates to the workshops designed and run by Frank Stritter at North Carolina and Alabama focusing on teaching skills (Stritter & Hain, 1977). The methods were active, involving brainstorming, consensus generation, didactic presentations, group (10-20) discussion, videotape review and critique and role play or small group microteaching activities. Stritter's work in this area has burgeoned (Stritter et al., 1994), culminating with the development, based on earlier work by Des Marchais et al. (1990), of a 2-year teaching scholars program. This consists of 10-12 3-hour seminars, reflection or activity aimed at application of principles in daily teaching practice and a 1-year research project with a plenary presentation. The program has been successful both in raising the profile of teaching and in training faculty.

Andriole et al. (1998) evaluated a 1-day workshop comprising 5 topics (adult learning, learning needs assessment, questioning, feedback and performance evaluation (assessment)) designed to enhance the teaching skills of practicing surgeons, that involved small group role-play, with feedback and discussions on application to specific clinical settings. The participants were surveyed 4-6 months after the event. All 62 participants reported changing their approach to teaching. Most changed in all topic areas but, specifically, very few had utilized citations given them, accessed additional resources or referred to handout material.

In a comprehensive review of strategies for improving teaching through faculty development, Wilkerson and Irby (1998) classify faculty development developments as having usually developed from one of three conceptual frameworks: behavioral, cognitive and social learning theories. Acknowledging that many of the studies on which the review is based are generally confounded or flawed (as experimental studies), and that some were not in medical education, the authors identify a few useful and apparently enduring outcomes. Longer (more than 2 days) rather than shorter workshops, the use of student ratings coupled with individual feedback from a peer, and fellowships, have all been associated with demonstrable effects on teachers' knowledge, skills and attitudes towards teaching. In the case of feedback, in one non-medical study effects could be detected 14 years later. The impact on teaching of longer workshops and their continuity over 18 months has recently been confirmed (Elliot et al., 1999). However, in a study of graduates of fellowship programs, Anderson et al. (1997b) found that, although 76% remained in academic medicine, their scholarly productivity was limited. Less than 35% had published one article or book chapter. Hitchcock et al. (1993) identify 3 areas for development in medical schools: teaching skills, research skills and what they termed "multiple skills": writing, decision making, administration and grant acquisition. However Reid et al. (1997), in a structured review of outcomes of faculty development programs, showed that participants in different types of activity (full time and part time fellowships, workshops, seminars) all benefit in teaching skills. However, they confirm that the impact of faculty development activities centered on research has not been as easy to demonstrate as that on teaching.

Nayer (1995) reviewed the impact of different PBL faculty development programs. She identified that PBL tutoring usually requires longer workshops than traditional "teaching" skills – not less than 4 and up to 10 days – perhaps because tutors need to unlearn some skills. Question construction was a skill that was difficult to learn. She also reviewed studies of PBL tutor performance and concluded that some tutors may need content updating to be effective if the problem construction is weak or the students are junior.

Skeff et al. (1998) investigated the transferability of workshops designed for clinicians to basic scientists' needs – a potentially important issue in schools moving from traditional to PBL curricula. He used a one group pre-post test design, with follow-up as much as five months later. Although only 8 faculty participated, he found substantial, although not always statistically significant, changes in participants' knowledge of teaching principles, ability to prepare for, undertake and analyze teaching, and their enthusiasm.

Although many of the studies reviewed attempt evaluation, few have looked at replicable cause-effect linkages. This is understandable as such investigations would be difficult. Faculty development is as much ad-hoc as programmatic and usually of finite length but with the potential to deliver infinite effects. Institutions generally do not fund faculty development to provide subjects for inevitably lengthy and costly research projects. Much of the scant research in this area was done in the 1980s, when resources were more generous.

Bland and Stritter (1988) conducted an illuminative/naturalistic site review and interview study of 5 family medicine faculty development programs to isolate the critical elements of their success, and to guide further funding. They isolated 30 characteristics, the most important of which are:

1. A faculty development program must have a clearly stated and readily perceived mission
2. It should be systematically designed and targeted to specific sub-groups
3. A range of skills, not just teaching, should be covered
4. Theory and practice should be taught
5. Practice must be a feature of the course
6. Program personnel should maintain contact with participants
7. Faculty must be committed to the program, and knowledgeable about content areas relating to the discipline from which the participants come
8. Participants should attend in groups from the same institution
9. Support should be available to participants "back home".

Hitchcock et al.'s (1993) review identified three further issues:
• involve faculty in designing their own program
• use faculty assessment as an initial step

- change the institutional environment.

Jolly (Jolly 1993), using experience from 11 years of teaching a 5-day more effective teaching course, has identified aspects of those courses which seemed to lead to happy participants. He argues that although happiness in a program does not guarantee appropriate academic outcome it is nevertheless an important ingredient for a memorable experience. These aspects were:

- For the course; devise group or individual activity which is challenging; the course must practice what it preaches; there must be adequate time for reflection and discussion; it must move fast; it should include mini-didactic presentations from experts; it may include some elements of coercion and competition; knowledge about teaching can be embedded in academic content (cf. Advanced Trauma life Support Instructors' courses ATLS (1994)
- For participants; define groups carefully; do not create groups with only 1 minority member; make courses residential
- For faculty: all faculty must be present at all plenary sessions; share teaching loads equitably, even if you have "star" teachers.

Ten years ago, Bland et al. (1990) made a valiant attempt to coalesce findings from available literature. The result resembles a recipe book of faculty development approaches, but is nevertheless far too comprehensive and scholarly to summarize here. Carroll's (1986) review of adult education theories is patchy in its use of theory and imprecise in its linkage of theory to practice and outcome. Others have tried to look at faculty development in terms of personal development or teaching theory (Riley, 1993; Ramsden, 1994). This looks the most fruitful avenue to explore. Riley traces her own development as a lecturer as a reflection of the evolution of faculty development activities. She has moved from "expert" – the tutor knows things that the learner does not, through "entertainer" – keeping audiences happy by use of techniques (teaching skills), to "engineer" – devising problems and activities for her students to solve and on to "equal" – to create a safe, friendly but challenging environment in which learning from each other can take place. This accords with Ramsden's "Theory 3 of Teaching" (p. 114) in which teaching is construed as allowing learners to apply and modify their own ideas and hence learning "*is something the student does rather than something that is done to the student*" (p. 114). For Ramsden the solution to designing appropriate educational development activities for faculty is akin to their provision for students; what is needed is for the institution and its faculty to be steeped in a model of teaching and learning that is congruent across all levels of activity from undergraduate to principal. This model should support, nourish and sustain all members of the learning community. In this argument he also rejects the "recognition of teaching as a rewardable activity" lobby as naive and energy consuming because of confusion over what is understood by "teaching". He sees faculty development as legitimately operating at a political and strategic level.

It is difficult to summarize such a diverse, but frequently repetitive and confusing, chunk of literature. The theoretical evolution of faculty development has been a patchwork quilt of half-used acknowledgements to various authors and frameworks. The practical issues have been led by immediate need and expediency – in fact one of the most interesting aspects of the literature is the extent to which personal growth theory (see pp. 2-3) has been excluded from practice. Perhaps this is a function of the pressures educationalists experience in the clinical settings. Such high tension activity is bound to affect the delivery of courses. Yet it is interesting (especially in relation to what Ramsden says above) that, in a climate in which we are urging students to become self-motivated, self-educating, reflective practitioners, the overwhelming burden of faculty development is seen as providing courses (institutionalized programs) on finite topics for the immediate digestion and use of clinicians.

RESEARCH ISSUES

This brief review of faculty development in action has prompted a number of observations.

1. There are very few papers describing faculty development programs in medical education, and there is no conventional framework for doing so. Many faculty development programs are not fully described; fewer than 30% include any details of local needs assessment, leadership and resource support, participant attendance and cost (Meurer & Morzinski, 1997). Even if they did, the conventional research paradigm sits uneasily with the detail and complexity required to effectively describe and evaluate faculty development. Hence, it is difficult to attribute change directly to the faculty development program (Reid et al., 1997; Irby & Hekelman, 1997). Also many programs depend on self ratings/reports. Skeff et al. (1997b) point out that faculty may not perceive their own skills accurately. This may lead sometimes to self-ratings decreasing after programs, possibly because participants are made more aware of their deficiencies. Some programs may succeed because of selection bias: participants already have a strong aptitude for and commitment to teaching (Reid et al., 1997). Also, Reid points out that, although student ratings and peer observation may provide good external sources of evidence for faculty development success, the observers may have little insight into whether these changes are due to the program. In fact the author has experienced situations where students have down-rated faculty, as a result of them adopting more problem-based or student-centered approaches, even when these have been fully explained to students. Students do not always accept or interpret curriculum change in same way that faculty may have prepared for.

2. The range of activities in medical teaching make it unlikely that the mainstream higher education (HE) faculty development literature will be very enlightening.

3. Sabbaticals, short 1-2 day workshops and seminars are the most popular means of faculty development in medical education, but all are under-researched.

4. Even in institutional faculty development aimed at curriculum development many courses cover basic skills such as presentation skills and specific capacities like problem-based tutoring. There were no reports of faculty development covering curriculum design or evaluation in the USA between 1990 and 1997 (Simpson & Ullian, 1997).

5. It is the context of faculty development that governs its content, but this is frequently underdescribed in research.

6. Most faculty developers in medicine agree that courses should generally try, in their delivery, to incoporate the principles they are advocating. A small core of motivated faculty can achieve much in faculty development terms.

7. More and better-directed evaluation of the effects of such courses is needed, to include the long term effects and perceptions of all stakeholders (e.g. the students, administrators, see Spencer et al., 2000; Murray et al., 2000).

REFERENCES

Allen, D. L. (1990). Faculty development. *Journal of Dental Education, 54,* 266-267.

Anderson, J., Hess, G., Rody, N., & Smith, W. (1991). Improving a community preceptorship through a clinical faculty development program. *Family Medicine, 23,* 387-388.

Anderson, W. A., Carline, J. D., Ambrozy, D. M., & Irby, D. M. (1997). Faculty development for ambulatory care education. *Academic Medicine, 72,* 1073-1075.

Anderson, W. A., Stritter, F., Mygdal, W. K., Arndt, J. E., & Reid, A. (1997). Outcomes of three part-time faculty development fellowship programs. *Family Medicine, 29,* 204-208.

Andriole, D. A., Evans, S. R., Foy, H. M., Atnip, R. G., & Mancino, A. T. (1998). Can a one-day workshop alter surgeons' teaching practices? *American Journal of Surgery, 175,* 518-520.

ATLS – Advanced Trauma Life Support (1994). *Instructors manual.* Chicago: American College of Surgeons.

Baldwin, C. D., Levine, H. G., & McCormick, D. P. (1995). Meeting the faculty development needs of generalist physicians in academia. *Academic Medicine, 70,* S97-S103.

Benor, D. E., & Mahler, S. (1990). Training medical teachers: rationale and outcomes. In H. Schmidt, M. Lipkin, M. W. de Vries, & J. Greep (Eds.), *New directions for medical education; problem-based and community oriented medical education* (pp. 248-259). New York: Springer Verlag.

Biddle, B., Siska, K., & Erney, S. (1994). A description of ambulatory teaching in a longitudinal primary care program. *Teaching and Learning in Medicine, 6,* 185-190.

Bird, J., Hall, A., Maguire, P., & Heavy, A. (1993). Workshops for consultants on the teaching of communication skills. *Medical Education, 27,* 181-185.

Bland, C. J., & Schmidtz, C. C. (1986). Characteristics of the successful researcher and implications for faculty development. *Journal of Medical Education, 61,* 22-31.

Bland, C. J., & Stritter, F. T. (1988). Characteristics of effective family medicine faculty development programs. *Family Medicine, 20,* 282-288.

Bland, C. J., Hitchcock, M. A., Anderson, W. A., & Stritter, F. T. (1987). Faculty development fellowship programs in family medicine. *Journal of Medical Education, 62,* 632-641.

Bland, C. J., Schmidtz, C. C., Stritter, F. T., Henry, R. C., & Aluise, J. J. (1990). *Successful faculty in academic medicine: essential skills and how to acquire them.* New York: Springer.

Bok, D. (1982). *Beyond the ivory tower: social responsibilities of the modern universities.* Cambridge, MA: Harvard University Press.

Bouhuijs, P. (1990). Faculty development. In C. Van der Vleuten & W. Wijnen (Eds.), *Problem-based learning: perspectives from the Maastricht experience* (pp. 63-68). Amsterdam: Thesis Publications.

Brew, A. (1995). *Directions in staff development.* Buckingham: Society for Research in Higher Education and Open University Press.

Calderhead, J. (Ed.). (1987). *Exploring teachers thinking.* London: Cassell.

Calman, K. (1994). The profession of medicine. *British Medical Journal, 309*, 1140-1143.

Carroll, R. G. (1993). Implications of adult education theories for medical school faculty development programmes. *Medical Teacher, 15*, 163-170.

Centra, J. (1976). *Faculty development practices in US Colleges and Universities*. Princeton: Educational Testing Service.

Curry, L., & Wergin, J. F. (1993). *Educating professionals: responding to new expectations for competence and accountability*. San Francisco: Jossey Bass.

DEET (Department of Employment, Education and Training). (1990). Australian Commonwealth Government. Research Paper No. 7. A Guide to Development of Competency Standards for Professions.

Department of Employment. (1989). *Enterprise in higher education, briefing document*. Sheffield: Department of Employment.

Department of Employment. (1992). *Investors in people*. United Kingdom: HMSO.

Des Marchais, J. E., Jean, P., & Delorme, P. (1990). Basic training program in medical pedagogy: a 1-year program for medical faculty. *Canadian Medical Association Journal, 142*, 734-740.

DeWitt, T. G., Goldberg, R. L., & Roberts, K. B. (1993). Developing community faculty: principles, practice and evaluation. *American Journal of Diseases of Children, 147*, 49-54.

Dreyfus, H. L., & Dreyfus, S. E. (1986). *Mind over machines*. New York: Macmillan.

Elliot, D., Skeff, K. M., & Stratos, G. A. (1999). How do you get to the improvement of teaching? A longitudinal faculty development program for medical educators. *Teaching & Learning in Medicine, 1999, 11*, 52-57.

Elton, L. (1987). *Teaching in higher education: appraisal and training*. London: Kogan Page.

Elton, L. (1998). Staff development and the quality of teaching. In B. C. Jolly & L. H. Rees (Eds.), *Medical education in the millennium* (pp. 199-204). Oxford: Oxford University Press.

ERIC, Educational Resources Information Consortium, Database definition (1995).

Evans, C. H. (1995). Faculty development in a changing academic environment. *Academic Medicine, 70*, 14-20.

Evans, P. A., & Taylor, D. C. M. (1996). Staff development of tutor skills for problem-based learning. *Medical Education, 30*, 365-366.

Fenton, B. A., & Povar, G. J. (1993). An alternative clerkship model for ambulatory training: an interdisciplinary primary care experience. *Teaching and Learning in Medicine, 5*, 197-201.

Fincher, R-M. E., & Albritton, T. A. (1993). The ambulatory experience of junior medical students at the Medical College of Georgia. *Teaching and Learning in Medicine, 5*, 210-213.

Folse, J. R., DaRosa, D. A., & Wood, M. (1991). An evaluation of surgery departments in community-based medical schools. *Archives of Surgery, 126*, 1122-1127.

Freeman, J., Loewe, R., & Benson, J. (1998). Training family medicine faculty to teach in underserved settings. *Family Medicine, 30*, 168-172.

General Medical Council. (1993). *Tomorrow's doctors*. London: General Medical Council.

GPEP. (1984). Physicians for the twenty-first century. Report of the Project Panel on the General Professional Education of the Physician and College Preparation for Medicine. *Journal of Medical Education, 59*, 1-208.

Grand'maison, P., & Des Marchais, J. (1991). Preparing faculty to teach in a problem-based learning curriculum: the Sherbrooke experience. *Canadian Medical Association Journal, 144*, 557-562.

Grayson, M. S., Newton, D. A., Klein, M., & Irons, T. (1999) Promoting institutional change to encourage primary care: experiences at New York Medical College and East Carolina University Medical School. *Academic Medicine, 74 (Suppl)*, S9-S15.

Gruppen, L. D., Wisdom, K., Anderson, D. S., & Wooliscroft, J. O. (1993). Assessing the consistency and educational benefits of students' clinical experiences during an ambulatory care internal medicine rotation. *Academic Medicine, 68*, 674-680.

Hale, E. (1964). *Report of the Committee on University Teaching Methods*. London: HMSO.

Handy, C. (1976). *Understanding organisations* (Chapter 7). Harmondsworth: Penguin Books.

Harrison, R. L., & Forgay, M. G. (1990). Self-perceived needs for faculty development at Canadian dental schools. *Journal of Dental Education, 54*, 240-243.

Higgins, P. M. (1989). Teaching medicine in general practice: the Guy's experience. *Medical Education, 23*, 504-511.

Hitchcock, M. A., Stritter, F. T., & Bland, C. (1993). Faculty development in the health professions. *Medical Teacher, 14*, 295-309.

Irby, D. M. (1992). How attending physicians make instructional decisions when conducting teaching rounds. *Academic Medicine, 67*, 630-638.

Irby, D. M. (1994). What clinical teachers in medicine need to know. *Academic Medicine, 69*, 333-342.

Irby, D. M., & Hekelman, F. P. (1997). Future directions for research on faculty development. *Family Medicine, 29*, 287-289.

Irby, D. M., Ramsey, P. G., Gillmore, G. M., & Schaad, D. (1991). Characteristics of effective teachers of ambulatory care medicine. *Academic Medicine, 66*, 54-55.

Jarratt, Sir A. (1985). *Report of the Steering Committee for Efficiency Studies in Universities.* London: Committee of Vice-Chancellors and Principals of the Universities of the United Kingdom.

Jolly, B. C. (1993). Having a good time. In A. Towle (Ed.), *Effecting change through staff development* (pp. 15-17). London: Kings Fund.

Jolly, B. C. (1994). *Bedside manners: teaching and learning in the hospital setting* (Chapter 1). Maastricht: University of Limburg Press.

Jolly, B. C., & Macdonald, M. M. (1986). More effective evaluation of clinical teaching. *Assessment and Evaluation in Higher Education, 12*, 175-190.

Jolly, B. C., & Macdonald, M. M. (1989). Education for practice: the role of practical experience in undergraduate and general clinical training. *Medical Education, 23*, 189-195.

Kaufman, A. (1998). Leadership and governance. *Academic Medicine,, 73*(Suppl), S11-S15.

Kaufman, A., Mennin, S., & Waterman, R. (1989). The New Mexico experiment: educational innovation and institutional change. *Academic Medicine, 64*, 290-294.

Kovach, R. (1993). Ambulatory education in the internal medicine clerkship at Southern Illinois University School of Medicine. *Teaching and Learning in Medicine, 5*, 205-209.

Krackov, S. K., Packman, C. H., Regan-Smith, M. G., Birskovich, L., Seward, S. J., & Baker, F. D. (1993). Perspectives on ambulatory programs: barriers and implementation strategies. *Teaching and Learning in Medicine, 5*, 243-250.

Lanphear, J., & Cardiff, R. D. (1987). Faculty development: an essential consideration in curriculum change. *Archives of Pathology & Laboratory Medicine, 111*, 487-491.

Lawson, M., & Moss, F. (1993). The move from inpatient teaching. In A. Towle (Ed.), *Innovative learning and Assessment* (pp. 46-49). London: Kings Fund.

Lowry, S. (1993). Teaching the teachers. *British Medical Journal, 306*, 127-130.

Mattern, W. D., Weinholtz, D., & Friedman, C. (1983). The attending physician as teacher. *New England Journal of Medicine, 308*, 1129-1132.

McGahie, W. C., Bogdewic, S., Reid, A., Arndt, J. E., Stritter, F. T., & Frey, J. J. Outcomes of a faculty development fellowship in family medicine. *Family Medicine, 22*, 196-200.

McLeod, P. J., Steinert, Y., Nasmith, L., & Conochie, L. (1997). Faculty development in Canadian medical schools: a 10 year update. *Canadian Medical Association Journal, 156*, 1419-1423.

McLeod, P. J. (1987). Faculty development practices in Canadian medical schools. *Canadian Medical Association Journal, 136*, 709-712.

Mennin, S. P., & Krackov, S. K. (1998). Reflections on relevance, resistance and reform in medical education. *Academic Medicine, 73* Suppl, S60-64.

Meurer, L. N., & Morzinski, J. A. (1997). Published literature on faculty development programs. *Family Medicine, 29*, 248-250.

Millard, L. (1993). Staff development for a new communication and learning course. In A. Towle (Ed.), *Effecting change through staff development* . London: Kings Fund.

Morzinsky, J. A., Simpson, D. E., Bower, D. J., & Diehr, S. (1994). Faculty development through formal mentoring. *Academic Medicine, 69*, 267-269.

Murray, E., Gruppen, L., Catton, P., Hays, R., & Woolliscroft, J. O. (2000). The accountability of clinical education: its definition and assessment. *Medical Education, 34*, 871-879.

Murray, E., Jolly, B. C., & Modell, M. (1999). A comparison of the educational opportunities on junior medical attachments in general practice and in a teaching hospital. *Medical Education, 33*, 170-176.

Nayer, M. (1995). Faculty development for problem-based learning programs. *Teaching and Learning in Medicine, 7*, 138-148.

Neufeld, V. R., Woodward, C. A., & MacLeod, S. M. (1989). The McMaster MD program: a case study of renewal in medical education. *Academic Medicine, 64*, 423-427.

Niemann, L. Z. (1999). Combining educational process and medical content during preceptor faculty development. *Family Medicine, 31*, 310-312.

O'Sullivan, M., Martin, J., & Murray, E. (2000). Students' perceptions of the relative advantages and disadvantages of community-based and hospital-based teaching. *Medical Education, 34,* 648-655.

Packman, C. H., & Krackov, S. K. (1993). Practice-based education for medical students: the doctor's office as classroom. *Teaching and Learning in Medicine, 5,* 193-196.

Perkoff, G. T. (1986). Teaching clinical medicine in the ambulatory setting: an idea whose time has come. *New England Journal of Medicine, 314,* 27-31.

Perry, W. G. (1968). *Forms of intellectual and ethical development in the college years.* New York: Holt Reinhart & Winston.

Plamping, D., & Towle, A. (1994). Service increment for teaching, *British Medical Journal, 309,* 197-198.

Preston-Whyte, M. E., Fraser, R., & McKinley, R. K. (1993). Teaching and assessment in the consultation. A workshop for general practice clinical teachers. *Medical Teacher, 15,* 141-146.

Ramsden, P. (1992). *Learning to teach in higher education.* London: Routledge.

Reid, A., Stritter, F. T., & Arndt, J. E. (1997). Assessment of faculty development program outcome. *Family Medicine, 29,* 242-247.

Riley, J. (1993). The process of developing as an educator. In A. Towle (Ed.), *Effecting change through staff development* (pp. 8-14). London: Kings Fund.

Robbins, Lord. (1963). *Higher education: Government statement on the report of the Committee under Lord Robbins.* London: HMSO.

Rubeck, R. F., & Witzke, D. B. (1998). Faculty development: a field of dreams. *Academic Medicine, 73*(suppl), S32-37.

Rust, G., Taylor, V., Morrow, R., & Everett, J. (1998). The Morehouse faculty development program: methods and 3 year outcomes. *Family Medicine, 30,* 162-167.

Seabrook, M. A., Lawson, M., & Baskerville, P. A. (1997). Teaching and learning in day surgery units: a UK survey. *Medical Education, 31,* 105-108.

Sheets, K. J., & Schwenk, T. L. (1988). Faculty development for family medicine educators: an agenda for future activities. *Teaching and Learning in Medicine, 2,* 141-148.

Simpson, D. E., & Ullian, J. A. (1997). Curriculum design and evaluation in faculty development. *Family Medicine, 29,* 251.

Skeff, K. M. (1988). Enhancing teaching effectiveness and vitality in the ambulatory clinic. *Journal of General Internal Medicine, 3*(Suppl), 26-33.

Skeff, K., Stratos, G., Berman, J., & Bergen, M. (1992). Improving clinical teaching: evaluation of a national dissemination program. *Archives of Internal Medicine, 152,* 1156-1161.

Skeff, K. M., Stratos, G., Bergen, M., & Albright, C. L. (1992). The Stanford Faculty Development Program: a dissemination approach to faculty development for medical teachers. *Teaching and Learning in Medicine, 4,* 180-187.

Skeff, K. M., Stratos, G. A., Bergen, M. R., & Regula, D. P. (1998). A pilot study of faculty development for basic science teachers. *Academic Medicine, 73,* 701-704.

Skeff, K. M., Stratos, G. A., Bergen, M. R., Sampson, K., & Deutsch, S. L. (1999). Regional teaching improvement programs for community-based teachers. *American Journal of Medicine, 106,* 76-80.

Skeff, K. M., Stratos, G. A., Mygdal, W., Dewitt, T. A., Manfred, L., Quirk, M., Roberts, K., Greenberg, L., & Bland, C. M. (1997). Faculty development a resource for clinical teachers. *Journal of General Internal Medicine, 12*(suppl), S56-63.

Skeff, K. M., Stratos, G. A., Mygdal, W., Dewitt, T. A., Manfred, L., Quirk, M., Roberts, K., & Greenberg, L. (1997). Clinical teaching improvement: past and future for faculty development. *Family Medicine, 29,* 252-257.

Slater, D. Y., & Cohn, E. S. (1991). Staff development through analysis of practice. *American Journal of Occupational Therapy, 45,* 1038-1044.

Spencer, J., Blackmore, D., Heard, S., McCrorie, P., McHaffie, D., Scherpbier, A., Sen Gupta, T., Singh, K., & Southgate, L. (2000). Patient-oriented learning: a review of the role of the patient in the education of medical students. *Medical Education, 34,* 851-857.

Steinert, Y. (1993). Faculty development in family medicine. *Canadian Family Physician, 39,* 1917-1922.

Steinert, Y., Levitt, C., & Lawn, N. R. (1988). Faculty development in Canada: a national survey of family medicine departments. *Canadian Family Physician, 34,* 2163-2166.

Stern, P. (1998). Skills for teaching: a problem-based learning faculty development workshop. *American Journal of Occupational Therapy, 52,* 230-233.

Steward, D. E. (1993). Moving medical education out of the hospital. *Teaching and Learning in Medicine, 5,* 214-216.

Stritter, F. T. (1983). Faculty evaluation and development. In C. H. McGuire, R. Foley, A. Gorr, & R. W. Richards (Eds.), *Handbook of health professions education* (pp. 294-318). San Francisco: Jossey Bass.

Stritter, F. T., & Hain, J. H. (1977). A workshop in clinical teaching. *Journal of Medical Education, 52,* 155-157.

Stritter, F. T., Herbert, W. N. P., & Harward, D. H. (1994). The teaching scholars program: promoting teaching as scholarship. *Teaching and Learning in Medicine, 6,* 207-209.

Towle, A. (1991). *Critical thinking: the future of undergraduate medical education.* London: Kings Fund.

Towle, A. (1998). Staff development in UK medical schools. In B. C. Jolly & L. H. Rees (Eds.), *Medical education in the millennium* (pp. 205-210). Oxford: Oxford University Press.

UGC. (1984). *A strategy for higher education into the 1990s.* London: HMSO.

Ullian, J. A., & Stritter, F. T. (1997). Types of faculty development programs. *Family Medicine, 29,* 237-241.

Ullian, J. A., Bland, C. J., & Simpson, D. E. (1994). An alternative approach to defining the role of the clinical teacher. *Academic Medicine, 10,* 832-838.

Universities and Colleges Staff Development Agency (UCoSDA). (1994). Occasional Paper No. 10: Continuing Professional Development for Staff in Higher Education: Informing Strategic Thinking. Sheffield: CVCP.

Warren, C. P. W., & Coke, W. (1993). Ambulatory care teaching in internal medicine at the University of Manitoba. *Teaching and Learning in Medicine, 5,* 202-204.

Weinholtz, D. (1986). Effective attending physician teaching. *Proceedings, Research in Medical Education Conference (RIME) 24th Ann Conf American Association of American Colleges* (pp. 151-156). Washington: AAMC.

Wilkerson, L., & Hundert, E. (1991). Becoming a problem-based tutor: increasing self-awareness through faculty development. In D. Boud & G. Feletti (Eds.), *The challenge of problem-based learning* (pp. 159-172). New York: St Martins Press.

Wilkerson, L., & Irby, D. M. (1998). Strategies for improving teaching practices: a comprehensive approach to faculty development. *Academic Medicine, 73,* 387-396.

Wooliscroft, J. O., & Schwenk, T. L. (1989). Teaching and learning in the ambulatory setting. *Academic Medicine, 64,* 644-648.

30 Effective Leadership for Curricular Change

CAROLE J. BLAND AND LISA WERSAL
University of Minnesota Medical School

SUMMARY

Educational institutions are increasingly expected to make larger and quicker changes in their curricula to address expanding knowledge, advances in technology, and the needs of their graduates to succeed in a changing world. Thus, it is important to understand how leaders can best lead or facilitate curricular change. This chapter reviews the dominant approaches for understanding and studying leadership, and then focuses on recent research on academic leadership, and specifically, leadership for curricular change. Leadership behaviors found most effective in guiding educational organizations through curricular change include being "flexible", developing and communicating a shared vision, viewing the organization through more than one perceptual "frame", utilizing "assertive participative governance", building and maintaining a common organizational culture and set of values, and actively engaging in goal setting.

INTRODUCTION

What constitutes effective leadership for curriculum change? This is the question addressed in this chapter. While considerable research has investigated leadership in specific organizations or settings, few studies are available to guide one wishing to understand the leadership abilities specifically associated with successful curriculum change. Today, educational institutions are increasingly expected to make larger and quicker changes in their curricula to address expanding knowledge, advances in technology, and the needs of their graduates to succeed in a changing world. Thus, it is important to understand how leaders can best lead or facilitate curricular changes.

In this chapter we begin with a brief overview of the dominant approaches for understanding leadership, in order to give the reader a substantive backdrop for the more specific studies that follow. We then describe how the concept of academic leadership is related to faculty morale and academic organization productivity,

International Handbook of Research in Medical Education, 969–979.
G.R. Norman, C.P.M. Van der Vleuten, D.I. Newble (eds.)
© 2002 *Dordrecht: Kluwer Academic Publishers. Printed in Great Britain.*

citing relevant research. Finally, we describe the studies that specifically relate to academic productivity and curricular change.

This chapter is based on foundational leadership theories and then focuses on recent scholarly research that has been conducted in curricular change. However, we want to alert the reader to the fact that there is also an abundance of guidance on leadership available in textbooks, reports of personal experiences, and opinion papers. These types of sources are also worthwhile, as they often reflect and amplify ideas found in the research literature. Texts based on personal reflection and experience can provide added dimensions that research may lack, such as the leader's inner thoughts and interpretations of experiences, or precisely what was said or done in interpersonal interactions.

FOUNDATIONAL LEADERSHIP THEORIES

We begin by reviewing the dominant approaches to understanding leadership. These leadership theories can be clustered into six major categories (Bensimon, Neumann, & Birnbaum, 1989):

1. Trait theories focus on the personal characteristics (e.g., physical, personality) of the leader. While one may still find references in current studies to personal qualities that are thought to enhance leaders' effectiveness, "*trait theories are no longer a major focus of organizational research*" (Bensimon et al., 1989, p. 8). After analyses of hundreds of leadership studies (Bass, 1981; Fiedler & Garcia, 1987; Gibb, 1968), researchers argue convincingly "*no traits have proven to be essential for successful leadership*" (Bensimon et al., 1989, p. 8).
2. Power and influence theories attempt to explain the impact of leadership in terms of how much power or influence the leader possesses, the source of that power (i.e., referent, expert, legitimate, reward, or coercive) (French & Raven, 1959), and how it is used. Early research focused on the top down use of influence. Later research using social exchange theory (i.e., leader-member exchange theory), addressed influence as a reciprocal process between leaders and followers (Dansereau, Graen, & Haga, 1975).
3. Behavioral theories study what the leader actually does. Early research focused on classifying leader behaviors (i.e., autocratic, participative, or laissez faire) and linking them to leader effectiveness (i.e., productivity vs. subordinate satisfaction) (Lewin, Lippitt, & White, 1939). Later research expanded on this by asking whether those defined as effective leaders emphasized task or intergroup relations (Stodgill, 1959) or both (high supportive and high task) (Blake & Mouton, 1994).
4. Contingency theories went one step further to suggest that both the nature of the task (e.g., well-defined or ambiguous) and the environment in which the leader resides affect the type of leadership approach likely to be most effective. Effective leadership behavior from a contingency approach is viewed as either something that must be modified to suit the situation (House, 1971; Vroom &

Yetton, 1973) or a stable characteristic to be matched to a particular situation (Fiedler, 1967).

5. Cultural and symbolic theories stress the idea that *"organizational structures and processes are invented, not discovered"* (Bensimon et al., 1989, p. 21). In other words, structures are the product of the definitions, norms, values, and rules that are negotiated by the organization's members. As a consequence, a leader's effectiveness is based on his/her influence on or maintenance of a common structure of values and beliefs.

6. Cognitive theories suggest that leadership is a social attribution. It is based on the members' perceptions of an organization and its tasks. They attribute leadership qualities to a named leader as a way to define the organization and to legitimize the role of the leader (Bensimon et al., 1989; Fiedler & Garcia, 1987; Sergiovanni & Corbally, 1984; Sims, Gioia, & Associates, 1986).

Another schema for understanding leadership has to do with the perceptual frames through which leaders view and conceptualize their organization (Bolman & Deal, 1991). Perceptual frames theorists suggest that people view situations through cognitive "frames" or "lenses", which determine how they interpret and respond to circumstances. These theorists delineate four perceptual frame categories:

1. the structural frame, emphasizing formal roles and relationships,
2. the human resource frame, focusing on the needs of people,
3. the political frame, in which conflict over scarce resources is the focus, and
4. the symbolic frame, through which organizations are viewed as cultures with shared values.

Research suggests that having the capacity to view their environment through more than one frame advantages leaders. This skill expands their repertoire of creative responses to any given situation, because they are not locked into a particular way of seeing and interpreting the circumstances. Also, because they can more readily view a given situation through someone else's preferred "frame", they have greater capacity to empathize with others. Leaders who view their organization through only one frame are more vulnerable to changes in their environment and less able to deal constructively in boundary spanning situations (Bolman & Deal, 1992). However, since perceptual frames are an internal construct, they may or may not match the actions that a leader takes.

All of the above theories are useful in understanding organizational leadership in general, and they provide substantive background for our next task. Having reviewed the foundational theories on leadership, let us now consult current research on academic leaders that draws on these theories, in order to better understand academic leadership and leadership of curricular change projects in particular.

ACADEMIC LEADERSHIP

Most of today's research on leadership is spawned from behavioral theories. This focus on leadership behaviors reflects current beliefs that skillful leadership can be learned; leadership skills are not necessarily inborn traits tied to personality. We will therefore direct our attention primarily to leadership behaviors in the discussion that follows. The astute reader will note that one of the behaviors discussed dovetails with the ideas of the cultural and symbolic theorists discussed above, in that the preferred leadership behavior is to build and maintain a shared culture and common value set among organization members. But before examining leadership behaviors in depth, let us first say a few words about the centrality of leadership to faculty morale, organizational productivity, and curricular change.

An overarching finding in the research on academic leadership is that leadership is a major determinant of faculty morale and organizational productivity (Blackburn, 1979; Bland & Ruffin, 1992; Bland & Schmitz, 1986; Seldin, 1990), and leadership is one of the most often cited determinants of effective curricular change. In many studies that examine curricular change, effective leadership is found to be vital to successful innovation. In fact, leadership shows up *"even in studies that did not deliberately attempt to investigate it"* (Louis, 1992, p. 945). In their review of the literature on curricular change, Bland, Starnaman, Wersal, Moorhead-Rosenberg, Zonia, and Henry (2000b) found leadership to be the factor most often cited in association with successful curricular change. Other key factors include: on-going training support, tailored to the specific needs of faculty and staff; successful negotiation of external and internal political structures; a cooperative and collaborative work environment; broad-based investment by organizational members in the change effort; and formative evaluation, coupled with corrective action to improve the change process. Because the role of the leader is so central to successful change, studies also reveal that stable leadership, that is, having the same person or persons remaining at the helm throughout the change process, is positively associated with successful innovation (Bland, Starnaman, Hembroff, Perlstadt, Henry, & Richards, 1999; Miles & Louis, 1987). Bland et al. (2000b) further conclude that leadership takes on such import in the change process because the leader largely makes possible the other elements essential for successful change.

LEADERSHIP BEHAVIORS FOR CURRICULAR CHANGE

Certain leadership behaviors or clusters of behaviors are found so often in the literature on effective academic leaders and specifically on leaders of curricular change, which is the focus of this chapter, that they deserve special attention. These include abilities to be "flexible", to develop and communicate a shared vision, to view the organization through more than one perceptual "frame", to utilize "assertive participative governance", to build and maintain a common organizational culture and set of values, and to actively engage in goal setting

(Bland & Schmitz, 1988; Bland et al., 2000b). We will discuss each of these behaviors or behavior clusters, citing relevant supportive studies from the literature.

Flexibility and communication of a shared vision

An effective leader invites broad-based participation and collaboration in the formation of a shared organizational vision, remaining flexible enough to acknowledge the multiple views that various participants contribute to the process. At the same time, the leader must not allow the vision to become too diffuse or obscured, such that the integrity of the vision is compromised. A careful balance is required (Eastwood & Louis, 1992; Fullan & Stiegelbauer, 1991; Richards, 1996). The leader has a primary responsibility to clearly and repeatedly articulate the vision for change through multiple means of communication (Brooks, Orgren, & Wallace, 1999; Bussigel, Barzansky, & Grenholm, 1988; Cohen et al., 1994; Firestone & Corbett, 1988; Fullan, 1985; Glaser, Abelson, & Garrison, 1983; Hendricson, Payer, Rogers, & Markus, 1993; Kaufman, 1998; Lindberg, 1998; Miles & Louis, 1987; Richards, 1996; Rollins, Lynch, Owen, & Shipengrover, 1999; Ross, Appel, & Kelliher, 1999). An effective leader must guide the group through the process of unfreezing old perceptions of their organization or procedures and then *"refreezing"* the new reality (Eastwood & Louis, 1992; Fullan & Stiegelbauer, 1991; Richards, 1996).

Multiple perceptual frames

One way that flexibility is demonstrated is through the ability to utilize multiple perceptual frames (structural, human resource, political, or symbolic), as noted earlier. In a study of 28 health professions schools in seven sites across the United States, participating in the Community Partnerships for Health Professions Education (CPHPE), a W. K. Kellogg Foundation Initiative in Health Professions Education, Bland et al. (1999) found that the most successful change leaders utilized at least two perceptual frames when viewing their organizations, with the human resource frame always being one of the two. Addressing human resource concerns includes providing appropriate training, allowing for participative governance, and creating an atmosphere conducive to open, honest, and frequent communication.

Assertive participative governance and a common organizational culture and value set

One of the most noteworthy clusters of successful leadership behaviors is to engage in "assertive participative governance", that is, actively and consistently seeking input from others, and providing structural mechanisms for organization members to accomplish the organization's mission. This set of behaviors has consistently been found to correlate with positive academic outcomes, such as research productivity and faculty morale. When Rice and Austin (1988) began their study of high-morale colleges, for example, they hypothesized that effective leadership contributes to high morale. They assumed that a variety of leadership approaches could contribute to high morale, and that what mattered most was that the leader was competent and effective in his or her chosen leadership style. What they found through their research was strikingly unexpected. From their surveys of more than 1000 colleges and in-depth studies of the ten colleges with the highest morale, they found that leaders of successful institutions consistently used the same leadership style, rather than a variety of styles. *"Every one of the ten colleges with high morale and satisfaction had a leadership that was aggressively participatory in both individual style and organizational structure"* (p. 54).

A participative leadership style is also found to correlate with positive academic outcomes and research productivity. In their study of 155 laboratories in the Paris area, Pineau and Levy-Leboyer (1983) concluded *"[T]he best laboratories were characterized by 'participatory' working relations: more meetings, the technicians were personally involved in the results, and more interpersonal relations between the researchers and the heads"* (p. 154). Kerr (1984) puts it bluntly: *"[L]iterally hundreds of studies have incontestably demonstrated the superiority of participative leadership and group decision-making"* (p. 234). Although he points out that there are certainly times when participative leadership is not the best governance approach, in academic organizations it is usually preferred.

Specific participative leadership behaviors that facilitate high morale and productivity include holding frequent meetings with clear objectives, building and maintaining common values, maintaining good leader-member relationships, facilitating open communication, allowing expressions of all points of view, sharing information completely, and vesting ownership of projects with all group members (Birnbaum, 1983; Bland & Ruffin, 1992; Dill, 1986a, 1986b; Epton, Payne, & Pearson, 1983; Hoyt & Spangler, 1979; Locke, Fitzpatrick, & White, 1983; Pelz & Andrews, 1966; Pineau & Levy-Leboyer, 1983). The importance of building and maintaining a shared set of values and a common organizational culture while utilizing participative governance also shows up in a recent study by Bland et al. (1999). This study was part of a larger evaluation of the W. K. Kellogg Foundation project (CPHPE), a five-year initiative involving projects at seven sites.

The goal of the initiative was to produce more primary care health providers by making enduring curricular change. In the study, researchers specifically identified the leadership behaviors that correlated with enduring curricular change and desired changes in students. To study the leaders of the seven sites, data were collected from participants via telephone interviews, mailed surveys, and focus groups, on predictors of project success and leaders' use of 16 key leadership behaviors. Focus groups also gathered project leaders' views of skills and knowledge necessary for effective leadership.

The study found that the primary individual leading a project was more influential in achieving positive outcomes than was a leadership team. Using a leadership team was helpful in certain circumstances, especially in building coalitions, but the importance of the primary leader's behavior to project outcomes was striking. Leadership strategies associated with positive outcomes were: having a consistent leader; use of multiple cognitive frames, especially a human resource frame; use of a broad range of leadership behaviors, particularly participative governance and cultural/value influence; and having a majority of community representatives on the partnership board. (Cultural/value influencing behaviors refer to practices of articulating the stories or symbols that represent the meaning and values of the institution.) The authors concluded that while effective leaders use a broad array of behaviors, they particularly emphasize the use of participative governance and cultural/value influencing behaviors. In addition, they use these behaviors with greater frequency than organizational power behaviors (e.g., using organizational authority; providing rewards or allocating resources).

Goal setting

Another leadership behavior consistently found in productive organizations is goal setting. Nearly all studies on effective leaders or effective organizations find that productive groups have clear organizational goals, and that the people within them have articulated personal goals that are compatible with the organizational goals (Locke & Latham, 1984). This finding is echoed in studies specific to education. For example, Bland and Schmitz (1988, 1990) reviewed the last 20 years of research on faculty and institutional vitality across all of higher education and found that a vital organization is characterized by clear, coordinating goals.

This profile of the effective academic leader – one who facilitates group productivity through the pairing of common goals and structure with highly participative governance – is echoed in the research on effective university department chairs (Creswell, Wheeler, Seagren, Egly, & Beyer, 1990). For example, Knight and Holen (1985) investigated whether there was a significant relationship between department chair behaviors (defined as faculty perception of the chair's "initiating structure" activities and "consideration" behaviors) and faculty members' perceptions of the chair's accomplishment of typical responsibilities, such as overseeing curricular design of academic programs and facilitating teaching and research. The term "initiating structure" is widely used to refer to *"the leader's behavior in delineating the relationship between himself and members of the workgroup, and in endeavoring to establish well-defined patterns of organization, channels of communication, and methods of procedure"* (Halpin, 1966, p. 86). "Consideration" refers to *"behavior indicative of friendship, mutual trust, respect, and warmth in the relationship between the leader and the members of his staff'* (Halpin, 1966, p. 86).

Knight and Holen (1985) included the ratings of 458 chairs by 5830 faculty members in 65 colleges and universities across the United States, and results across these sites were strikingly consistent. Chairpersons rated high on both initiating structure and consideration behaviors were also rated highest in effectively accomplishing and performing the common responsibilities of a chair. Conversely, chairpersons rated low on both dimensions received the lowest ratings on performing their responsibilities. Skipper (1976) also conducted several studies investigating higher-education administrators' use of initiating structure and consideration behaviors. He consistently found that, at the dean's level and above, high scores on both dimensions characterized the most effective administrators.

CONCLUSION

Even though curricular change is a difficult process, there is useful guidance in the literature as to the kinds of leadership behaviors that will have a positive impact toward accomplishing successful and enduring curricular change. Furthermore, a recent study by Bland, Starnaman, Harris, Henry, and Hembroff (2000) begins to allay the commonly held fears that successful curricular change comes only at the price of negative impacts on other important outcomes, such as student preparation, faculty research productivity, or school reputation. In their study, CPHPE, Bland and colleagues tracked twelve factors thought to contribute to successful curricular change, including leadership behaviors. They found, as previous studies have elucidated, that participative leadership behaviors were positively correlated with desired outcomes. They also found that the institutions studied accomplished their innovation objectives without incurring negative impact on other valued aspects of the institution, or its students, faculty, or other educational or research outcomes.

So, in terms of effective leadership for curricular change, the literature guides us to know what "works" and we have also begun to experience and report that practicing the behaviors and strategies that promote curricular change need not have negative ramifications on other institutional objectives. Still, in practice, there remains a gap between knowing what to do and having the skills to do it, or, even with the skills, to actually do it. Moreover, practical experience reveals that there can also be a gap between *thinking* one is "doing it" (one's own perception of one's leadership abilities) and *actually* doing it (this includes others' perceptions of leaders' actions and whether those actions are truly effective). The challenge of bridging these gaps remains. Thus, these "gaps" are where future research must be done if we are to take advantage of the knowledge we have acquired from past research in this area.

RECOMMENDATIONS FOR FUTURE RESEARCH

1. What are the most effective methods of teaching leaders the necessary skills to guide their organizations through periods of curricular innovation?
2. In what ways do leaders' personal characteristics play a role in their ability to learn and apply effective leadership behaviors?
3. Is there a hierarchical ordering to the leadership behaviors identified as being conducive to curricular change? That is, are certain behaviors more crucial than others?
4. Are certain leadership behaviors more effective when used in conjunction with other behaviors? For example, is goalsetting more effective when accompanied by flexibility?

GUIDELINES FOR PRACTITIONERS

1. Be open to honest feedback from persons close to you and employ formative evaluation as a tool to find out how skillful you are at the desired leadership behaviors: being flexible, communicating a shared vision, utilizing multiple perceptual frames, practicing participative governance, building and maintaining a common organizational culture, and engaging in goal setting.
2. Know that change requires investment of organizational resources over a long period. Innovation projects usually take more time and effort than initial projections estimate. Be prepared to invest for the "long haul".
3. Cultivate individuals to share in project leadership.
4. Make the effort to see situations from other points of view.
5. Develop a shared vision and use every opportunity to reinforce it.
6. Be confident in setting goals and measuring your progress toward them. Celebrate each achievement – even the "small" ones.

REFERENCES

Bass, B. M. (Ed.). (1981). *Stodgill's handbook of leadership: a survey of theory and research*. New York: Free Press.
Bensimon, E. M., Neumann, A., & Birnbaum, R. (1989). *Making sense of administrative leadership: The "L" word in higher education*. Washington, D.C.: Association for the Study of Higher Education.
Birnbaum, P. H. (1983). Predictors of long-term research performance. In S. R. Epton, R. L. Payne, & A. W. Pearson (Eds.), *Managing interdisciplinary research* (pp. 47-59). New York: John Wiley & Sons.
Blackburn, R. T. (1979). Academic careers: Patterns and possibilities. *Current Issues in Higher Education, 2*, 25-27.
Blake, R. R., & Mouton, J. S. (1994). *The managerial grid*. Houston, TX: Gulf Publishing Company.
Bland, C. J., & Ruffin, M. T., IV. (1992). Characteristics of a productive research environment: Literature review. *Academic Medicine, 67*, 385-397.
Bland, C. J., & Schmitz, C. C. (1986). Characteristics of the successful researcher and implications for faculty development. *Journal of Medical Education, 61*(January), 22-31.

Bland, C. J., & Schmitz, C. C. (1988). Faculty vitality on review: Retrospect and prospect. *Journal of Higher Education, 59*(2), 190-224.

Bland, C. J., & Schmitz, C. C. (1990). An overview of research on faculty and institutional vitality. In J. H. Schuster & D. W. Wheeler (Eds.), *Enhancing faculty careers: Strategies for development and renewal* (pp. 41-61). San Francisco: Jossey-Bass.

Bland, C. J., Starnaman, S. M., Harris, D. L., Henry, R. C., & Hembroff, L. (2000a). "No Fear" curriculum change: monitoring curriculum change in the W.K. Kellogg Foundation's National Initiative on Community Partnerships and Health Professions education program. *Academic Medicine, 75*, 623-633.

Bland, C. J., Starnaman, S. M., Hembroff, L., Perlstadt H., Henry, R., & Richards, R. (1999). Leadership behaviors for successful university-community collaborations to change curricula. *Academic Medicine, 74*(11), 1227-1237.

Bland, C. J., Starnaman, S. M., Wersal, L., Moorhead-Rosenberg, L., Zonia, S., & Henry, R. (2000b). Curricular change in medical schools: How to succeed. *Academic Medicine, 75*, 575-594.

Bolman, L. G., & Deal, T. E. (1991). *Reframing organizations: artistry, choice, and leadership*. San Francisco: Jossey-Bass.

Bolman, L. G., & Deal, T. E. (1992). Leading and managing: Effects of context, culture, and gender. *Educational Administration Quarterly, 28*(3), 314-329.

Brooks, W. B., Orgren, R., & Wallace, A. G. (1999). Institutional change: Embracing the initiative to train more generalists. *Academic Medicine, 74*(1 suppl), S3-S8.

Bussigel, M., Barzansky, B. M., & Grenholm, G. G. (1988). *Innovation processes in medical education*. New York: Praeger.

Cohen, J., Dannefer, E. F., Seidel, H. M., Weisman, C. S., Wexler, P., Brown, T. M., Brieger, G. H., Margolis, S., Ross, L. R., & Kunitz, S. J. (1994). Medical education change: A detailed study of six medical schools. *Medical Education, 28*, 350-360.

Collins, J. C., & Porras, J. I. (1994). *Built to last: successful habits of visionary companies*. New York: HarperBusiness.

Creswell, J. W., Wheeler, D. W., Seagren, A. T., Egly, N. J., & Beyer, K. D. (1990). *The ccademic chairperson's handbook*. Lincoln, NB: University of Nebraska Press.

Dansereau, R., Jr., Gaen, G., & Haga, W. J. (1975). A vertical dyad linkage approach to leadership within formal organizations: A longitudinal investigation of the role-making process. *Organizational Behavior and Human Performance, 13*, 46-78.

Dill, D. D. (1986a). Research as a scholarly activity: Context and culture. In J. W. Creswell (Ed.), *Measuring faculty research performance* (pp. 1-23). New York: Jossey-Bass.

Dill, D. D. (1986b, April). Local barriers and facilitators of research. Paper presented at the Annual Meeting of the American Education Research Association, San Francisco.

Eastwood, K. W., & Louis, K. S. (1992). Restructuring that lasts: Managing the performance dip. *Journal of School Leadership, 2*, 212-224.

Epton, S. R., Payne, R. L., & Pearson, A. W. (Eds.). (1983). *Managing interdisciplinary research*. New York: John Wiley & Sons.

Fiedler, F. E. (1967). *A theory of leadership effectiveness*. New York: McGraw-Hill.

Fiedler, F. E., & Garcia, J. E. (1987). *New approaches to effective leadership: Cognitive resources and organizational performance*. New York: John Wiley & Sons.

Firestone, W. A., & Corbett, H. D. (1988). Planned organizational change. In N. Boyan (Ed.), *Handbook of research on educational administration* (pp. 321-340). New York: Longman.

French, J. R. P., & Raven, B. (1959). The bases of social power. In D. I. Cartwright (Ed.), *Studies in social power* (pp. 150-167). Ann Arbor, MI: Research Center for Group Dynamics – Institute for Social Research, University of Michigan.

Fullan, M. (1985). Change processes and strategies at the local level. *Elementary School Journal, 85*(3), 391-420.

Fullan, M., & Stiegelbauer, S. (1991). *The new meaning of educational change*. (2nd ed.) New York: Teachers College Press.

Gibb, C. A. (1968). Leadership. In G. Lindzey & E. Aronson (Eds.), *The handbook of social psychology* (2nd ed.). Reading, MA: Addison-Wesley.

Glaser, E. M., Abelson, H. H., & Garrison, K. N. (1983). *Putting knowledge to use: Facilitating the diffusion of knowledge and the implementation of planned change*. San Francisco: Jossey Bass.

Halpin, A. W. (1966). *Theory and research in administration*. New York: Macmillan.

Hendricson, W. D., Payer, A. F., Rogers, L. P., & Markus, J. F. (1993). The medical school curriculum committee revisited. *Academic Medicine, 68*(3), 183-189.

House, R. J. (1971). A pathgoal theory of leader effectiveness. *Administrative Science Quarterly, 16,* 321-338.

Hoyt, D. P., & Spangler, R. K. (1979). The measurement of administrative effectiveness of the academic department head. *Research in Higher Education, 10*(4), 291-304.

Kakabadse, A., Nortier, F., & Abramovici, N-B. (1998). *Success in sight: visioning.* London: International Thomson Business Press.

Kaufman, A. (1998). Leadership and governance. *Academic Medicine, 73*(9 suppl), S11-S15.

Kerr, S. (1984). Leadership and participation. In A. P. Brief (Ed.), *Productivity research in the behavioral and social sciences* (pp. 229-251). New York: Praeger.

Knight, W. H., & Holen, M. C. (1985). Leadership and the perceived effectiveness of department chairpersons. *Journal of Higher Education, 56*(6), 677-690.

Lewin, K., Lippitt, R., & White, R. K. (1939). Patterns of aggressive behavior in experimentally created "social climates". *Journal of Social Psychology, 10,* 271-299.

Lindberg, M. A. (1998). The process of change: stories of the journey. *Academic Medicine, 73* (9 suppl), S4-S10.

Locke, E. A., & Latham, G. P. (1984). *Goal setting: a motivational technique that works!* Englewood Cliffs, NJ: Prentice Hall.

Locke, E. A., Fitzpatrick, N. W., & White, F. M. (1983). Job satisfaction and role clarity among university and college faculty. *Review of Higher Education, 6*(4), 343-365.

Louis, K. (1992). Organizational change. In M. C. Alkin (Ed.), *Encyclopedia of Educational Research* (6th ed., pp. 941-947). New York: Macmillan: Maxwell Macmillan International.

Miles, M., & Louis, K. (1987). Research on institutionalization: a reflective review. In M. Miles, M. Ekholm, & R. Vandenberghe (Eds.), *Lasting school improvement: Exploring the process of institutionalization* (pp. 25-44). Leuven, Belgium: ACCO (Academic Publishing Company).

Pelz, D. C., & Andrews, F. M. (1966). *Scientists in organizations: Productive climates for research and development.* New York: John Wiley & Sons.

Pineau, C., & Levy-Leboyer, C. (1983). Managerial and organizational determinants of efficiency in biomedical research teams. In S. R. Epton, R. L. Payne, & A. W. Pearson (Eds.), *Managing interdisciplinary research* (pp. 141-163). New York: John Wiley & Sons.

Rice, R. E., & Austin, A. K. (1988). High faculty morale: What exemplary colleges do right. *Change, 20*(2), 50-58.

Richards, R. W. (Ed.). (1996). *Building partnerships: Educating health professionals for the communities they serve.* San Francisco: Jossey-Bass.

Robert, M. (1991). *The essence of leadership: Strategy, innovation, and decisiveness.* New York: Quorum Books.

Rollins, L. K., Lynch, D. C., Owen, J. A., Shipengrover, J. A., Peel, M. E., & Chakravarthi, S. (1999). Moving from policy to practice in curriculum change at the University of Virginia School of Medicine, East Carolina University School of Medicine, and SUNY-Buffalo School of Medicine. *Academic Medicine, 74*(1 Suppl), S104-S111.

Ross, L. L., Appel, M. H., & Kelliher, G. J. (1999). The role of the generalist physician initiative in the merger of Hahnemann University and the Medical College of Pennsylvania. *Academic Medicine, 74*(1 Suppl), S16-S23.

Seldin, P. and Associates. (1990). *How administrators can improve teaching: moving from talk to action in higher education.* San Francisco: Jossey-Bass.

Senge, P. M. (1994). *The Fifth discipline field book: Strategies and tools for building a learning organization.* New York: Currency, Doubleday.

Sergiovanni, T. J., & Corbally, J. E. (Eds.). (1984). *Leadership and organizational culture: New perspectives on administrative theory and practice.* Urbana: University of Illinois Press.

Sims, H. P. Jr., Gioia, D. A. and Associates. (1986). *The thinking organization: Dynamics of organizational social cognition.* San Francisco: Jossey-Bass.

Skipper, C. E. (1976). Personal characteristics of effective and ineffective university leaders. *College and University, 51*(2), 138-141.

Stodgill, R. M. (1959). *Individual behavior and group achievement.* New York: Oxford University Press.

Vroom, V. H., & Yetton, P. W. (1973). *Leadership and decision making.* Pittsburgh: University of Pittsburgh Press.

PERSPECTIVES ON PROFESSIONAL AND PEDAGOGICAL CARING

In common word usage, caring fails to fit well within a single definition. Caring is better considered by a *family of meanings* in the manner described by Kaplan (1964). When used as a verb, caring denotes doing or action and Gaut (1983) itemizes three shared features for its family of meanings: (1) attention to or concern for; (2) responsibility for or providing for; and (3) regard, fondness or attachment. It is notable that these shared features indicate an interaction of affect, cognition and behavior.

In the health professions literature, the concept of caring is intertwined with several attitudinal and behavioral qualities such as humanism, altruism, compassion, empathy and integrity. Moreover, reference to caring is uniformly present as a core component of any itemized listing or description of professionalism, whether couched affectively, cognitively or behaviorally. Leininger (1981) offered the following definition of professional caring, that spans affective, cognitive and behavioral components and emphasizes that professional caring is intentionally directed toward welfare of the recipient:

> The cognitive and deliberate goals, processes, and acts of professional persons or groups providing assistance to others, and expressing attitudes and actions of concern for them, in order to support their well-being, alleviate undue discomforts, and meet obvious or anticipated needs. (*p. 46*)

Caring and moral education

Professional and pedagogical caring are commonly considered within the rubric of moral education (see for example, Branch, 2000; Noddings, 1992). Definitional imprecision poses measurement difficulties in empirical research such that the scholarly study of caring is subject to pitfalls similar to those cited in reviews of research on moral education. That is, the complex interplay of affect, cognition and behavior makes variables difficult to define precisely enough to measure. The resulting definitions are often unsuitable, particularly if the result reflects an attempt to "chop up morality into cognitions, affects and behaviors". This result is unsuitable because "*there are no pure feelings completely devoid of cognitions, no cognitions completely devoid of affects, and all behavior is the result of cognitive-affective processes*" (Bebeau, Rest, & Narvaez, 1999, p. 22).

There are two conceptualizations proposed in the literature, one addressing moral education and the other professional caring, which provide a congruent framework for considering the interactional processes involved in caring and moral behavior in a similar manner. Moreover, these conceptual frameworks facilitate consideration of caring as moral behavior with the attendant interplay of affect and cognition.

Bebeau et al. (1999) propose a comprehensive morality model of four component processes to guide research and moral education which may be viewed as congruent with the explicative analysis results of Gaut's (1983) set of conditions for intentional caring. Gaut's first condition is awareness – that the individual must recognize and attend to the other's need for caring; similarly the first component of the Bebeau et al. morality model is moral sensitivity involving awareness and interpreting the situation. Gaut's second condition is knowledge – *"to know that certain things could be done to improve the situation"* (p. 318) with due regard for respect of the person as an individual with rights, values and choices; similarly, the second component of the proposed morality model is moral judgment involving knowledge and judging which action is right or wrong. Lastly, Gaut's *"positive change condition"* (p. 321) involves choosing an action intended to bring about a positive change in the other wherein this change must be judged solely on the basis of what is good for the other's welfare in the particular situation (i.e., welfare of other criterion). This compares to the moral motivation component of the proposed morality model (prioritizing moral values over personal values).

The fourth component of the Bebeau et al. (1999) morality model goes beyond Gaut's (1983) conditions of caring framework. This component is moral character, described as *"having the strength of your convictions, having courage, persisting, overcoming distractions and obstacles, having implementing skills, having ego strength"* (Bebeau et al., 1999, p. 22). Additional literature relating the concept of caring to virtue and self-actualization is pertinent here.

Caring, virtue and self-actualization

A bioethical perspective of caring is offered by van Hooft (1996) which he derives from virtue theory and argues that *"what we do in situations of moral difficulty or practical quandary is an expression of what we care about most deeply"* (p. 83). An international medical specialty society has also connected caring with virtue by specifying a set of ten core virtues required to be a moral professional who cares for and about patients: prudence (knowing the right action), courage (fortitude to do what is right in the face of aversive conditions), temperance (grace under pressure), justice (fairness and consistency), unconditional positive regard (respect and human acceptance), charity (effacement of self-interest), compassion, trustworthiness, vigilance and agility (adroitness, resilience) (SAEM Ethics Committee, 1996).

In a similar vein, Milton Mayeroff's seminal work *On caring* (1971) explored philosophical underpinnings within an overall formulation of caring as "helping the other to grow" and identified knowing, patience, honesty, trust, humility, hope and courage as "major ingredients of caring". Mayeroff conceives caring as a self-actualization process in which the needs of the other are placed before self, and by focusing on and being responsive to the other, one's self-growth is actualized. He notes, therefore, that teachers need students just as students need teachers. In this view physicians need patients just as patients need physicians.

Professional and pedagogical caring

In the context of helping relationships (e.g., teacher-learner, physician-patient), caring can be viewed as an interactive process involving attitudes, behaviors and actions grounded in the moral value of respect for self and others. At least two individuals are required for a caring interaction and importantly, actions of the "carer" must be directed to benefit the other rather than self (Gaut, 1983). Noddings (1992) further describes this interaction by a relational definition in which a caring relation is an encounter between two human beings – a carer and recipient of care (cared-for) – wherein each party must contribute in respective characteristic ways. For the carer, this includes "engrossment" (open, non-selective receptivity) in which dialogue forms the basis for responses in caring, and "motivational displacement" (responding in a manner that furthers the other's purpose). In return, the cared-for must receive, recognize and respond to complete the caring encounter. Noddings claims that caring teachers listen and respond differentially to students; she emphasizes that modeling is vital in helping students develop the "capacity to care" and holds teachers responsible for creating caring teacher-learner relationships to facilitate student development of the attitudes and skills required for caregiving in the world of work, parenting and civic responsibility.

In addressing pedagogical caring specifically, Hult (1979) typifies roles and contexts in which teacher caring is demonstrated. For example, teachers demonstrate "caring about" things and people by the attention, concern, skill and due regard with which their duties are fulfilled, as well as demonstrating "caring for" students in purposeful ways that recognize student needs, expectations and rights for pedagogical services (including critical appraisal as well as praising). The published literature regarding teaching and learning caring in the health professions points to the presence of caring behaviors and attitudes in the professional school learning environment as an important pedagogical component in the development of professional caring ability.

RESEARCH ON CARING, LEARNING ENVIRONMENT AND ASSESSMENT

Electronic searching of the health professional literature by the key word "caring" reveals a large volume of nursing publications in which professional and/or pedagogical caring is the central theme and the term caring appears in nearly every title. Medical education literature is less directly accessible by this keyword; most medical education publications pertaining to caring in this regard are indexed and titled by more general terms such as professionalism and humanism, or specifically address particular attributes of caring such as empathy and compassion. It is unclear whether this difference reflects definitional difficulties with the term caring discussed earlier in this chapter or perspectives that may differ based on discipline.

In contrast, nursing education has been engaged in a widespread "caring curriculum movement" involving an educative-caring curriculum in which caring is translated and transmitted in the practices of nurse education (Bevis & Murray, 1990). The dominant theme of the caring curriculum in nursing education holds caring to be the core value of educator-student relationships. The underlying premise is that pedagogical caring in teacher-learner relationships is essential to nursing education for two reasons: (a) students must experience caring in their educational environment to develop professional caring ability, and (b) a trusting and caring educational environment is required to empower students to think critically (Paterson & Crawford, 1994).

Research in nursing education

There is a large, rapidly expanding, international nursing literature addressing teaching, learning and measuring caring ability, with research on caring involving quantitative as well as qualitative approaches to inquiry. A common finding is that modeling is important in the pedagogy of caring. For example, Kosowski (1995) found role modeling to be the most frequent learning mode based on phenomenological study of student perceptions regarding how professional nurse caring is taught and learned. Hughes (1992) also found that teacher modeling of caring behaviors during interactions with students was fundamental to the teaching-learning caring process. As noted by Paterson and Crawford (1994), caring is not something that is "done to" students but rather is the context in which teaching-learning interactions take place.

A longitudinal study designed to measure the effects of childhood home and nursing school learning environment on caring was undertaken involving a nationwide sample of U.S. female baccalaureate nursing students in the 1990s. The study was conceived according to an educational socialization model described by Good and Brophy (1986) in which learning environment is viewed as an intervening variable between school inputs (e.g., attitudes and beliefs which students bring to school from home life experiences) and student outcomes; the model proposes that teachers and students are affected by school structures, processes and beliefs embodied in the learning environment.

In the first phase of the study, 67% of those randomly sampled from a national student nurse database returned a completed questionnaire booklet incorporating instruments for which previous evidence of reliability and validity were available (Cavanaugh & Simmons, 1997). The *Parental Bonding Instrument* provided a measure of student perceptions regarding parental caring experienced prior to entry to nursing school via a 12 item subscale representing the bipolar "caring vs. indifference/rejection" behaviors and actions of parent figures (Parker, Tupling, & Brown, 1979). A measure of student perception of caring in the learning environment of their professional school was derived from 16 items comprising four scales (Respect, Trust, Morale, Caring) of the *CFK School Climate Profile* (Johnson & Johnson, 1992). Three scales of the *Caring Ability Inventory* congruent with Mayeroff's (1971) conception of caring components (Knowing, Patience,

Courage) provided a 37 item measure of the students' ability to care for others as developed and previously validated in studies involving college undergraduates and professional nurses (Nkongho, 1990). The design of this study permitted exploration of relationships between student inputs to nursing school with respect to caring experiences in the home environment during childhood and adolescence, as well as caring behavior influences during nursing school in terms of the learning environment, and student outcomes in terms of caring ability.

Initial analyses based on 350 senior nursing students revealed mean Caring Ability Inventory scores higher than those previously found for a sample of college undergraduates but not as high as those observed for a sample of professional nurses. Multiple regression analysis revealed school climate ratings to be a modest but statistically significant predictor of student caring ability scores, while the parental bonding variable failed to achieve statistical significance (Simmons & Cavanaugh, 1996). This evidence indicated that caring behaviors and modeling in the learning environment influenced student caring ability deterministically irrespective of ratings of home life experience prior to entry into nursing school.

In the second phase of the study, both junior and senior level nursing students who had participated in phase one were reassessed. Successful longitudinal follow-up of about 200 student nurses after graduation and 1-2 years of professional practice revealed continued caring ability growth in that caring ability scores significantly increased by nearly one standard deviation as compared to their matched scores as students ($p < 0.001$). Moreover, caring ability scores as a student were significantly correlated with those as postgraduates ($r = 0.59$, $p < 0.001$), and the postgraduate scores demonstrated a low but statistically significant correlation with student school climate ratings (Simmons & Cavanaugh, 2000). Considered collectively, findings from nursing research on learning environment and caring tend to support Noddings' (1992) theoretical proposition that student educational experiences in being cared for influence their ability to develop the "capacity to care".

Research in medical education

There is evidence that the medical education learning environment may adversely affect students in developing or maintaining caring as a professional practice ethic. Studies of medical students via anonymous self-report surveys have revealed widespread perceptions of psychological mistreatment such as being frequently shouted or yelled at, humiliated or belittled by residents, interns, clinical faculty and by nurses (Baldwin, Daugherty, & Eckenfels, 1991; Wolf, Randall, On Almen, & Tynes, 1991). In a study of 665 students from several U.S. medical schools, 98% reported witnessing physicians refer derogatorily to patients, and 80% reported having misled a patient or done something they believed constituted unethical behavior with many attributing this behavior to fear of poor evaluation or "to fit in with the team" (Feudtner, Christakis, & Christakis, 1994). There is further evidence that attributes of professional caring may be undervalued in physician practice, especially as regards promotion for teaching physicians. A study of 214 physicians employed by a large teaching hospital in Israel consistently rank ordered the following quality statement as the *most* important for being "a good physician" and the *least* importantly for being promoted in the hospital: human relation to patients and ability to understand patients' problems and emotions (Carmel & Glick, 1996).

Following implementation of a new curriculum model in the early 1990s, a U.S. medical school implemented an annual student survey on learning climate; aims of this initiative included creating a model of student satisfaction with the learning environment which offers *"practical and educational significance and that could serve as a catalyst for educational intervention"* (Robins, Gruppen, Alexander, Fantone, & Davis, 1997, p. 135). The reported model is derived from regression analysis of seven predictor items addressing predominantly humanistic aspects of the learning environment on a rating of satisfaction with the overall learning environment. Interestingly, the strongest predictor for the total group of 430 students was an item reflective of pedagogical caring (i.e. medical student education is a high priority for faculty) with a standardized regression weight of 0.41, and this was consistently the strongest predictor for each of the gender and ethnicity subgroups as well (regression weights vary between 0.34 and 0.47). All subgroups provided similar ratings for the extent to which the educational program promotes critical thinking, but men tended to report greater satisfaction than women on predictor items and white students reported greater overall satisfaction with the learning environment than minorities. As noted by the authors, the inclusion of predictor items in addition to the single global learning environment rating permits monitoring of environmental reforms more closely (Robins et al., 1997); thus this initiative holds promise for facilitating awareness and improvement of caring behaviors and attitudes by faculty in the medical school learning environment.

There are further examples of research in medical education that incorporate measures of learning environment related to professional and pedagogical caring. Similar to that described above, however, the instrumentation and item content are not termed as measures of caring *per se*. For example, Arnold, Blank, Race, and Cipparrone (1998) proposed an instrument designed to measure professional attitudes and behaviors within the environment of medical education and residency training. In this 14-item questionnaire, students and residents based ratings on their observations and experiences in clinical education with regard to resident and attending physician teachers. Factor analysis of 529 respondents from five institutions in the northeast region of the United States identified three subscales: excellence (e.g., role models, placing needs of patients first), honor/integrity and altruism/respect. To a large extent the content of items as well as the factors identified are clearly related to components of professional caring, but the authors describe the instrument as yielding measures of "professionalism". As another example, Testerman, Morton, Loo, Worthley, and Lamberton (1996) have proposed and studied the psychometric properties of a 14 item instrument called the Cynicism in Medicine Questionnaire, in which two of four subscales (faculty cynicism, institutional cynicism) clearly relate negatively to learning environment factors reflective of caring.

With the contemporary interest in continuous quality improvement in education, medical student and resident perceptions of the learning environment may be readily obtained and used in a practical manner to monitor and improve pedagogical caring, regardless of the particular instrument title. Instruments cited in the preceding examples of nursing and medical education research are published in the literature in full, tend to be brief and easy to administer and score; moreover most may be suitable for sizable subgroup analysis (e.g., gender, ethnicity). Systematic evaluation of the medical learning environment provides an opportunity to monitor relevant aspects of the learning environment and guide improvements to facilitate desirable affective and behavioral student outcomes such as humanism and caring ability.

Learning environment vs. individual assessment

The American Board of Internal Medicine (ABIM) has further developed a method of assessment of the "humanistic qualities" of individual physicians. ABIM's Project Professionalism has defined humanistic qualities as a formal component of clinical competence and as a requirement for certification (Stobo & Blank, 1994). This initiative considers attitudes and behaviors that maintain patient interest above physician self-interest as the core of professionalism; notably, this is the core value of professional caring in moral education.

The ABIM has developed and distributed widely its standards to promote professionalism within the medical education environment and has identified professionalism as a separate category on the certification examination blueprint (American Board of Internal Medicine, 1992). Currently ABIM recertification also includes standardized scoring of professional associate ratings and patient satisfaction questionnaires for each candidate. This involves 20 peer physicians and 40 patients providing confidential ratings on each candidate's professionalism and humanistic qualities (e.g., responsiveness to patients, respect, compassion); ABIM analyzes these ratings and provides each candidate a score report for self-evaluation (ABIM, 1999).

An interesting study of an internal medicine residency program reports a similar multifocal approach to the assessment of humanistic attributes in individual physicians (Klessig, Robbins, Wieland, & Rubinstein, 1989). Caring attributes (e.g., respect, integrity, empathy, compassion) were self-assessed by residents as well as faculty rating each resident and patients doing the same. Each group provided ratings on a previously validated patient satisfaction questionnaire, while residents and faculty also each completed an additional "Faculty Evaluation Form" endorsed by the ABIM for use in residency programs. However, results reveal faculty and resident ratings significantly inversely related, and patient ratings did not significantly correlate with either faculty or resident ratings, suggesting that these groups may differentially view or place differing values on humanistic behavior.

Present evidence suggests that assessment of pedagogical and professional caring which is observable or perceived within the learning environment may be more interpretable and useful for medical education, especially as regards curricular concerns. However, increasing efforts are being directed to the development of measures with suitable psychometric integrity for the individual assessment of physician caring behaviors and actions as a component of standardized assessments of professionalism.

IMPROVING CARE FACILITATION IN THE CURRICULUM

Care facilitation refers to the forces or conditions that facilitate discovery of the meaning and uses of caring in intellectual and professional activities (Leininger, 1986). In education, we bring an implicit emphasis to all things that are the focus of assessment. Therefore by incorporating any of the above described assessment strategies we are likely to facilitate the transmission of care throughout the curriculum, both formal and informal.

However, educational methods used in the teaching-learning process can also effectively incorporate caring principles and practices to facilitate the transmission of caring attitudes and behaviors. Even in the setting of traditional didactic instruction to large student groups, teachers can transmit professional standards of "caring about" by the attention, concern and regard demonstrated in fulfilling lecturer duties and providing meaningful assessments that ensure the likelihood of realizing student learning outcomes (Hult, 1979). Teachers can effectively demonstrate caring by open, non-selective receptivity in all teaching-learning settings; students should feel welcome to ask questions or offer comments as caring teachers will listen and respond differentially to their students and concerns (Noddings, 1992). In this way teachers may care for students in the collective sense and demonstrate professionalism in pedagogical caring.

Role modeling

Other medical education teaching-learning settings offer additional opportunities to transmit caring at an interpersonal level. For example, small group methods such as problem-based learning groups, clerkship rotations and preceptor methods used in clinical training permit teaching-learning interactions to occur on a closer, more individual basis. In these settings, teacher-learner encounters span somewhat formal interactions involving structured learning tasks and responses (e.g., attending rounds) to the quite informal interchanges and continuous student observation that accompanies the student simply being present in the clinical setting for clerkships and rotations.

All formal and informal teachers (classroom and clinical faculty as well as supervising residents) must be attentive and committed to their role as a model for facilitating moral development in aspiring professionals, and the enactment of professional role modeling must be consistent throughout all settings of teacher-learner interactions and instances in which students observe teachers. It must be recognized that, in pursuing their role as students, aspiring professionals are continuously learning from their teachers through the behaviors and actions that are both casually observed as well as more overtly directed to them. In considering moral education from the perspective of an ethic of caring, modeling is the fundamental component; *"modeling is important in most schemes of moral education, but in caring it is vital"* (Noddings, 1992, p. 22).

Role modeling may be viewed as a central component of the "informal curriculum". It should be recognized in curricular planning, documentation and assessment. Assessment strategies discussed earlier can be utilized to monitor individual faculty and group performance as role models for the development of caring beliefs, attitudes and behaviors as well as related affective competencies such as professionalism, humanism and altruism.

Mentoring

Each opportunity for a caring relationship is to some extent structured by time and purpose in teaching-learning contexts (Hult, 1979). Teacher role modeling serves as an exemplar but may be considered a somewhat indirect teaching-learning method in the transmission of caring; the intention is to demonstrate consistency in modeling professional values and behaviors without necessarily explicating such to an individual or group. Alternatively, mentoring provides the opportunity for pedagogical caring to operate more overtly and actively, on an individual or interpersonal basis. In the mentoring context, the teacher-learner role relationship is not merely that the student belongs to a group of students, but rather that the teacher pursues an in-depth and comprehensive knowledge of the student as a unique individual; this provides the basis for pedagogical caring on an interpersonal (as opposed to purely intellectual) level.

The term mentor comes from Homer's *Odyssey* in which Mentor has the role relationship of nurturing and educating Odysseus' son. Mentoring provides extensive opportunity for professional socialization as a whole and transmission of caring in particular. It is a longitudinal relationship between teacher and student permitting pedagogical caring in the complete sense of Mayeroff's (1971) "helping the other grow".

Mentoring appears to be the tacit methodology involved in the historical apprenticeship model of medical training. The mentoring relationship extends beyond teaching specific skills by encompassing personal, professional and civic development to facilitate student integration into the professional community through socialization to its norms and expectations (Reynolds, 1994). Importantly, mentoring relationships permit teachers to demonstrate professional caring at an interpersonal level and allow for the dialogue, practice and confirmation components of Noddings (1992) "ethic of care" model to occur.

Faculty development may be useful in facilitating teacher awareness and ability to utilize mentoring as a method and context for student moral development. Importantly mentoring must be recognized in faculty reward and promotion methods because mentoring requires longitudinal teacher-learner relationships, which necessitate the devotion of teacher time. Whereas class size and curricular structure may limit opportunities for longitudinal mentoring relationships in some medical school environments, such should be an integral part of residency and fellowship training programs (for example, see Markakis, Bekcman, Suchman, & Frankel, 2000).

Coaching

Anderson (1999) has argued *"concerns about ensuring the widest opportunity to the largest number of our young people have led us to distort and dilute the meaning of being a mentor"* (p. 4). He argues that every member of a medical school class cannot be mentored in the deeper sense of true mentor relationships, but students can be provided guidance, role models and career advice. Schon (1987) offers an alternative (or perhaps complementary) approach via a pedagogical method of coaching.

Schon (1987) juxtaposes "knowing-in-action" based on propositional knowledge conveyed in traditional teaching-learning methods (e.g., lecture, reading, objective testing) with the need for practitioners to learn how to professionally function in "indeterminate zones of practice" characterized by uniqueness, uncertainty and values conflict. He cites the practicum portion of the educational process, in which students do not simply attend but rather live in the experience, as the educational context in which coaching for "reflection-in-action" allows aspiring professionals to learn by exposure and immersion. In practicums, such as medical student clerkships and resident rotations, the learner is supervised by a senior practitioner who may at times teach in the conventional sense (explaining, conveying information), but Schon stresses that the main activities of a coach are demonstrating, advising, questioning and criticizing. The nature, direction and purpose of dialogue between coach and student embody the effectiveness of coaching.

Considering the extent to which it is typical to rely on aspiring and young physicians for the bulk of clinical education (e.g. residents supervising medical students), coaching skills should be emphasized to promote effective learning in this context as well as the importance of the "informal curriculum" for learning opportunities facilitating moral development. Many of these informal teachers need to be aided in understanding that their teaching role and educational impact greatly exceed simply expanding or reinforcing the scientific and technical knowledge of students. Teacher knowledge of perspectives on professional and pedagogical caring, salient characteristics of an educative-caring curriculum, and assessment of care facilitation in the learning environment can be helpful in explicitly enabling teachers to foster learner development of professional caring ability.

CONCLUSION

Professional caring is a complex phenomenon operationalized through interactions between teachers and learners as well as between health care providers and patients. Research indicates a connection between the learning environment and development of caring attitudes and behaviors in aspiring health professionals. The medical education community tends to consider attributes of professional caring as subcomponents of broader physician competencies and qualities such as humanism and professionalism. However, it is important for medical educators to purposely identify and exemplify professional caring in the curriculum, both in formal and informal teacher-learner interactions, as well as attend to cognitive, affective and behavioral perspectives. Role modeling, mentoring and coaching can effectively incorporate caring principles and practices to facilitate the transmission of caring attitudes and behaviors in aspiring physicians.

RECOMMENDATIONS FOR FUTURE RESEARCH

Clarify professional caring as a component of clinical competence

Further research is needed in the health professions to more clearly delineate professional caring as a construct and to explore relationships with related components of clinical competence, which are variously termed professionalism, humanism, altruism, etc. Caring has been described as an "elusive and imprecise concept" defined and made operational for research in a variety of ways, but commonly considered to consist of a set of behaviors and activities in the context of the health professions (Kyle, 1995). Noddings' (1992) notion of an "ethic of care" places caring firmly within the framework of moral education, while others have delineated caring by the attitudinal and behavioral qualities underpinning and giving rise to caring, most notably Mayeroff's (1971) seminal thesis on the "ingredients of caring". The four-component model proposed by Bebeau et al. (1999) might be useful for further articulation of professional caring within the rubric of moral education and development. This model offers the advantage of situational specific exploration as a function of attending to each component process – moral sensitivity, moral judgment, moral motivation and moral character. Perhaps a starting point for thinking about methodology is provided by Valentine (1989) wherein a structured conceptualization method involving the development of separate concept maps for different groups (e.g., health professionals vs. patients) was employed to develop concrete representations of professional caring, thus permitting exploration of construct validity through pattern analysis. Research of this nature may also help explain reported discrepancies between self, peer and patient ratings of physician caring attributes (for example, see Klessig et al., 1989).

Socio-cultural research on professional caring

Gilligan (1982) asserted a socio-cultural basis for differences between caring in men and women and there is some health professional literature to support this theory. For example, in a study of moral orientation it was observed that a predominantly female sample of nurses used care considerations more often than a predominantly male sample of physicians, lending support to Gilligan's claim that Kohlberg's (1976) justice-based theory reflects the moral reasoning of males while her care-based theory reflects the moral reasoning of females (Peter & Gallop, 1994). However, the researchers acknowledged that the relationship between gender and care-based versus justice-based moral orientation is complex and requires considerable further exploratory study.

Leininger (1984) has also noted that, although human caring is a universal phenomenon, there is cultural variation in expressions, processes and patterns of caring; therefore health professionals need culturally-based knowledge and skills to be transculturally effective in humanistic caring. Multicultural awareness and research are receiving greater attention in medical education, providing the opportunity to incorporate professional caring in this area of inquiry and further our understanding of socio-cultural implications.

Influence of professional caring on patient outcomes

It is not uncommon for health care providers to believe that non-technical elements of professional caring (for example, respect, trust, concern, compassion) facilitate favorable patient responses. Indeed, Leininger (1986) expresses strong conviction that the professional caring ability of health professionals influences patient outcomes, but she acknowledges that the problem of identifying and verifying human care attributes by empirical methods makes exploration difficult. Further research is needed to develop psychometrically useful tools for measuring patient perception and responsiveness to the non-technical professional caring they receive which will enable scientific inquiry regarding the relationship between humanistic caring by health professionals and patient outcomes.

GUIDELINES FOR PRACTITIONERS

Formalize the teaching and learning of professional caring in the medical education curriculum

Although scholars continue to struggle with definitional frameworks and debate theoretical perspectives of moral development, it is both possible and proper to identify professional caring as a core competency for aspiring physicians, as well as to incorporate teaching-learning activities that facilitate and exemplify caring in the curriculum.

Promote faculty development of pedagogical and professional caring knowledge, skills and behavior. Recognize and reward exemplary performance

Provide both formal and informal teachers with development opportunities in role modeling, mentoring and coaching techniques/methods. Strive to achieve a common culture spanning didactic and clinical learning environments in which caring is exemplified and transmitted throughout teacher-learner and health care provider-patient interactions. Importantly, also incorporate methods of feedback, recognition and remediation, as well as reward exemplary performance.

Implement assessment strategies to monitor care facilitation in the learning environment and guide improvement efforts, as part of a comprehensive curriculum and program evaluation process

There are several instruments to choose from and/or adapt that are readily available in the literature for this purpose. Moreover, many learning environment instruments are brief, easy to administer, score and interpret (see for example, Cavanaugh & Simmons, 1997; Robins et al., 1997).

REFERENCES

American Board of Internal Medicine. (1992). *Guide to awareness and evaluation of humanistic qualities* (2nd ed.). Philadelphia, PA: Author.

American Board of Internal Medicine. (1999). *The ABIM recertification program: Introducing the new module on professional associate ratings (PARs) and patient satisfaction questionnaires (PSQs).* Philadelphia, PA: Author.

Anderson, P. C. (1999). Mentoring. *Academic Medicine, 74*, 4-5.

Arnold, E. L., Blank, L. L., Race, K. E. H., & Cipparrone, N. (1998). Can professionalism be measured? The development of a scale for use in the medical environment. *Academic Medicine, 73*, 1119-1121.

Baldwin, D. C., Daugherty, S. R., & Eckenfels, E. J. (1991). Student perceptions of mistreatment and harassment during medical school: A survey of ten United States schools. *Western Journal of Medicine, 155*, 140-145.

Bebeau, M. J., Rest, J. R., & Narvaez, D. (1999). Beyond the promise: A perspective on research in moral education. *Educational Researcher, 28*(4), 18-26.

Bevis, E. O., & Murray, J. P. (1990). The essence of the curriculum revolution: Emancipatory teaching. *Journal of Nursing Education, 29*(7), 326-331.

Branch, W. T. (2000). The ethics of caring and medical education. *Academic Medicine, 75,* 127-131.

Carmel, S., & Glick, S. M. (1996). Compassionate-empathic physicians: Personality traits and social-organizational factors that enhance or inhibit this behavior pattern. *Social Science & Medicine, 43,* 1253-1261.

Cavanaugh, S., & Simmons, P. (1997). Evaluation of a school climate instrument for assessing affective objectives in health professional education. *Evaluation & The Health Professions, 20*(4), 455-478.

Curry, R. H., & Makoul, G. (1998). The evolution of courses in professional skills and perspectives for medical students. *Academic Medicine, 73,* 10-13.

Feudtner, C., Christakis, D. A., & Christakis, N. A. (1994). Do clinical clerks suffer ethical erosion? Students' perceptions of their ethical environment and personal development. *Academic Medicine, 69,* 670-679.

Gaut, D. A. (1983). Development of a theoretically adequate description of caring. *Western Journal of Nursing Research, 5*(4), 313-324.

Gilligan, C. (1982). *In a different voice: Psychological theory and women's development.* Cambridge, MA: Harvard University Press.

Good, T. L., & Brophy, J. E. (1986). School effects. In M. C.Wittcock (Ed.), *Handbook of research on teaching* (3rd ed., pp. 570-602). New York: Macmillan.

Hughes, L. (1992). Faculty-student interactions and the student-perceived climate for caring. *Advances in Nursing Science, 14* (3), 60-71.

Hult, R. E. (1979). On pedagogical caring. *Educational Theory, 29*(3), 237-243.

Johnson, W. L., & Johnson, A. M. (1992). A study on the Kettering School Climate scale. *Education, 112,* 635-639.

Kaplan, G. (1964). *The conduct of inquiry.* Pennsylvania: Chandler Co.

Klessig, J., Robbins, A. S., Wieland, D., & Rubenstein, L. (1989). Evaluating humanistic attributes of internal medicine residents. *Journal of General Internal Medicine, 4,* 514-521.

Kohlberg, L. (1976). Moral stages and moralization: The cognitive-developmental approach. In T. Lickona (Ed.), *Moral development and behavior: Theory, research and social issues* (pp. 31-53). New York: Holt, Rinehart & Winston.

Kosowski, M. M. R. (1995). Clinical learning experiences and professional nurse caring: A critical phenomenological study of female baccalaureate nursing students. *Journal of Nursing Education, 34*(5), 235-242.

Kyle, T. V. (1995). The concept of caring: A review of the literature. *Journal of Advanced Nursing, 21,* 506-514.

Leininger, M. (1981). The phenomenon of caring: Importance, research questions and theoretical considerations. In M. Leininger (Ed.), *Caring: An essential human need* (pp. 3-16). Thorofare, NJ: Charles B. Slack.

Leininger, M. (1984). *Care: The essence of nursing and health.* Detroit, MI: Wayne State University Press.

Leininger, M. (1986). Care facilitation and resistance factors in the culture of nursing. *Topics in Clinical Nursing, 8*(2), 1-12.

Markakis, K. M., Beckman, H. B., Suchman, A. L., & Frankel, R.M. (2000). The path to professionalism: Cultivating humanistic values and attitudes in residency training. *Academic Medicine, 75,* 141-149.

Mayeroff, M. (1971). *On caring.* New York: Harper & Row.

Nkongho, N. O. (1990). The caring ability inventory. In O. Strickland and C. Waltz (Eds.), *Measurement of nursing outcomes* (pp. 3-16). New York: Springer.

Noddings, N. (1992). *The challenge to care in schools: An alternative approach to education.* New York: Teachers College Press.

Parker, G., Tupling, H., & Brown, L. B. (1979). A parental bonding instrument. *British Journal of Medical Psychology, 52,* 1-10.

Paterson, B., & Crawford, M. (1994). Caring in nursing education: An analysis. *Journal of Advanced Nursing, 19,* 164-173.

Peter, E., & Gallop, R. (1994). The ethic of care: A comparison of nursing and medical students. *Image: Journal of Nursing Scholarship, 26*(1), 47-51.

Reynolds, P. P. (1994). Reaffirming professionalism through the education community. *Annals of Internal Medicine, 120*(7), 609-614.

Robins, L. S., Gruppen, L. D., Alexander, G. L., Fantone, J. D., & Davis, W. K. (1997). A model of student satisfaction with the medical school learning environment. *Academic Medicine, 72*, 134-139.

SAEM Ethics Committee. (1996). Virtue in emergency medicine. *Academic Emergency Medicine, 3*, 961-966.

Schon, D. (1987). *Educating the reflective practitioner.* San Francisco: Jossey-Bass.

Simmons, P., & Cavanaugh, S. (1996). Relationships among childhood parental care, professional school climate and nursing student caring ability. *Journal of Professional Nursing, 12*(6), 373-381.

Simmons, P., & Cavanaugh, S. (2000). Relationships among student and graduate caring ability, and professional school climate. *Journal of Professional Nursing, 16*(2), 76-83.

Stobo, J. D., & Blank, L. L. (1994). Project professionalism: Staying ahead of the wave. *American Journal of Medicine, 97*(6), 1-3.

Testerman, J. K., Morton, K. R., Loo, L. K., Worthley, J. S., & Lamberton, H. H. (1996). The natural history of cynicism in physicians. *Academic Medicine, 71*, S43-S45.

Valentine, K. (1989). Contributions to the theory of care. *Evaluation and Program Planning, 12*, 17-23.

Van Hooft, S. (1996). Bioethics and caring. *Journal of Medical Ethics, 22*, 83-89.

Wolf, T. M., Randall, H. M., On Almen, K., & Tynes, L. L. (1991). Perceived mistreatment and attitude change by graduating medical students: A retrospective study. *Medical Education, 25*, 182-190.

32 Disseminating Educational Research and Implementing Change in Medical Educational Environments

SHEILA W. CHAUVIN
Tulane University School of Medicine

SUMMARY

Much of the medical education literature pertaining to change focuses on either descriptive accounts of new educational programs or the outcomes or effects of new programs. In contrast, much less attention has been given to the process of change and to the effective use of specific models and strategies for facilitating innovation implementation. Evidence from the literature suggests that simply disseminating the results of research does not translate into changes in physicians' practices (Dunn, Norton, Stewart, Tudiver, & Bass, 1994). Change strategies that work in one situation may not work in another, and maintaining new programs and practices beyond initial implementation is a persistent challenge (Lindberg, 1998). Individuals respond to and are involved in change from personal perspectives related to specific innovations (e.g., teaching techniques or faculty work processes) within specific contexts (e.g., teaching and learning environments or departments).

This chapter draws from diverse fields and across diverse educational settings and focuses on the professional literature pertaining to the process of change and the effective use of specific principles and change strategies for working with individuals within educational organizations; while chapter 33 focuses on implementing large scale changes. Key terms related to change process are defined and several predominant theories of individual behavior and systems within organizations are combined to provide a conceptual model of the change process within educational organizations. Using this model, one can understand the dynamic, interactive and systemic influences of personal, organizational, and environmental variables on implementing and incorporating specific innovations into everyday practice.

The effectiveness of specific change facilitation strategies is reviewed and examples from the professional literature are provided. The Concerns Based Adoption Model (CBAM) (Hall & Hord, 1987) is described and one of several change facilitating tools that are included in this model, the Stages of Concern (SoC), is used to demonstrate how individuals' implementation of innovation can be

997

International Handbook of Research in Medical Education, 997–1037.
G.R. Norman, C.P.M. Van der Vleuten, D.I. Newble (eds.)
© 2002 *Dordrecht: Kluwer Academic Publishers. Printed in Great Britain.*

facilitated to ensure long-lasting change. A key to successful individual change within educational organizations is the accurate assessment of individuals' concerns or focus of attention and the careful and appropriate matching of intervention strategies to identified concerns. Facilitating change successfully is also dependent on maintaining a balance between pressure for change and support for stability. The literature reviewed in this chapter documents clearly the important role of effective facilitative leadership strategies that include communicating a shared vision, providing necessary resources, investing in professional development, monitoring progress and providing feedback. The combined use of these strategies contributes to creating an environment that is conducive to change. The chapter closes with recommendations for future research; a summary of guidelines for practitioners involved in introducing, implementing, and sustaining change in medical education organizations; and short list of recommended readings.

INTRODUCTION

Change is so much a part of contemporary medical education that we sometimes overlook its complexity and influence on how we go about our day-to-day activities. Much of the medical education literature pertaining to change focuses on either descriptive accounts of new educational programs or the outcomes or effects of new programs, while much less attention has been given to identifying effective change processes that might be generalized across educational settings. Evidence from the literature suggests that simply disseminating the results of research (e.g., presentations, publications, lectures, traditional continuing medical education) does not translate into changes in physicians' practices (Dunn, Norton, Stewart, Tudiver, & Bass, 1994). Similarly, in attempting change in medical schools, what works in one situation may not work in another, and maintaining new programs and practices beyond initial implementation is a persistent challenge (Lindberg, 1998). Individuals respond to and are involved in change from personal perspectives related to specific innovations (e.g., curriculum design, teaching methods, instructional technology, assessment and evaluation, changes in faculty roles) within specific contexts (e.g., teaching and learning environments, departments, colleges/schools, universities, and communities). Therefore, this chapter focuses on the professional literature pertaining to the process of change and the effective use of specific principles and change strategies for working with individuals within educational organizations.

The basis for this chapter is drawn from diverse fields and across diverse settings. Much less research has been done regarding the process of change in medical education than in other educational settings (e.g., higher education, elementary and secondary education, organizational development). While change initiatives vary from small to large scale, each depends, in large part, on the extent to which individuals implement and sustain innovations (Dannefer, Johnston, & Krackov, 1998; Hall & Hord, 1987; Neufeld, Khanna, Bramble, & Simpson, 1995; Rubeck & Witze, 1998; Schwartz, Heath, & Egan, 1994); however, there is no single prescription or recipe for facilitating change successfully (Cohen et al., 1994; Fullan, 1993, 1999; Schwartz, Loten, & Miller, 1999; Wheatley, 1994; Wheatley & Kellner-Rogers, 1999). To realize successful implementation of innovations, one must consider the change process from multiple points of view: the people involved in implementing innovations, individuals who function as facilitative leaders or change agents, recipients of innovations, other key stakeholders, the characteristics of innovations, and the contexts of change.

This chapter begins with a discussion of important conceptual and theoretical underpinnings as a framework for thinking about and facilitating individuals' behaviors and responses to change within an organization (e.g., school of medicine) or an organizational unit (e.g., academic department). Specific change facilitation strategies are discussed and the chapter closes with a set of practical guidelines, recommendations for future research, and suggested resources and readings related to implementing change within educational organizations. Throughout the chapter, please pause periodically to reflect on and apply the concepts, principles, and interventions gleaned from the literature to your own situations. Finally, please use this chapter in combination with other chapters in the book to effectively disseminate medical education research findings and implement educational changes – a persistent challenge for medical educators and researchers around the globe.

CHANGE – THEORETICAL AND CONCEPTUAL UNDERPINNINGS

Individual and organizational change may be planned and purposeful, or it may be evolutionary, as in adaptive responses to societal demands. Regardless, change affects virtually every aspect of organizational structure and function (Christakis, 1995; Cuban, 1997; Hoy & Miskel, 1987; Owens, 1987). Similarly, change and calls for reform are not new to medical education, as essays, studies, and reform project descriptions are common in the professional literature (Association of American Medical Colleges, 1992; Christakis, 1995; Papa & Harasym, 1999).

Paul Mort, an early and avid student of educational change in the United States, reported in the late 1950s that there seemed to be a pattern in the diffusion of new ideas and technologies. Reflecting on initiatives and school-level responses to organizational change, Mort and Ross (1957) reported that schools typically lagged more than 25 years behind currently espoused "best" practice. In fact, Mort (1958) reported that approximately 15 years were necessary to achieve a 3% adoption of an innovation and that a lag of approximately 50 years was typical for an innovation to become generally incorporated into everyday school practice. More recently, Cuban (1997) states that only 5% of medical schools have realized fundamental change or radical reform of their curricula (i.e., a significant, permanent change from the traditional Flexner model of medical education – two years of basic science learning followed by two years of learning in the clinical setting).

Cuban (1997) and Bloom (1988, 1989) argue that medical schools, much like giant amoebas, absorb the effects of innovation and change initiatives in ways that preserve their traditional structures and functions. However, results and conclusions reported by Cuban (1997, 1999), Davis and White (1993), Lindberg (1998), Schwartz et al. (1994) and Schwartz et al. (1999) suggest that more change has occurred than one may realize at first glance. That is, by using a different lens, one focused on the process of change, rather than on just the effects or outcomes of change, our understanding of educational reform may be enhanced. Furthermore, these studies suggest that medical schools, as educational organizations, share similar characteristics with other types of educational settings (e.g., elementary and secondary education, higher education, and professional schools). Therefore, we should not limit our review of the literature on implementing change to that which has occurred only in medical education. After all, as Ludmerer (1985) quotes Abraham Flexner, "... *medical education is, after all, not medicine but education*" (p. 171). First, let's establish some common understandings of terms that are used frequently to discuss educational change processes.

Key terms related to change process

In this chapter, several important terms are used to discuss research pertaining to planned change and the use of research findings in facilitating the implementation of specific educational innovations. Working definitions of general terms are provided here to enhance the clarity and usefulness of this chapter. Reference citations have been included, where appropriate, to facilitate continuity and comparison among constructs and research findings. They are as follows:

1. Change and change process are used synonymously in this chapter and refer to planned, purposeful change efforts, as opposed to accidental change, natural diffusion or unintended changes. The terms also incorporate phrases found in the professional literature such as planned organizational change and organizational change. Specifically, change or change process refers to interactions among organizational members (e.g., faculty, staff, and students) within a particular context and the use of any method or specified strategies designed to change behaviors, attitudes, beliefs and/or orientations consciously and purposefully within a school. For the purpose of this chapter, change is examined specifically in terms of educational initiatives.

2. Incremental change and fundamental change are two categories of change process promoted by Cuban (1990, 1997, 1999). Incremental changes target refinements and enhancements (e.g., introducing a new module to a second year course or a new teaching method). Fundamental changes or reform target transformation, permanent alteration or complete overhaul of an educational program or process (e.g., restructuring an entire curriculum from a traditional to

a total problem-based learning approach). Altbach (1980) and Cuban (1990, 1997, 1999) use the term reform to describe fundamental change that occurs in the core structure and/or functions of educational organizations.

3. Innovation refers to any practice, process, or product that is, or was at one time, new to a potential user (Hall & Hord, 1984). Innovations are a subset of change that reflect a narrow focus on behavior and include clearly specified ways of behaving (e.g., altering work schedules or tasks). An innovation is typically represented as a specific and identifiable program or strategy (e.g., an organ systems-based course or curricula, problem-based learning, or hypermedia-assisted lectures).

4. Change facilitators refer to individuals within an organization who assume specific leader behaviors and combinations of behaviors. Change facilitators may evidence these behaviors using different styles that are influenced by belief systems, orientation toward organizational roles, knowledge and concerns regarding leadership role and tone with which behaviors are evidenced. Change facilitators may or may not hold positions of formal authority within the organizations, but organizational leaders often fill this role, at least in the beginning. In higher education and professional school settings, change facilitator roles might be filled by department chairs, program directors, academic deans, a director of a medical education research office, and/or faculty/instructional/organizational development specialists (Chauvin, 1992; Hall & Hord, 1987).

5. Receptivity to change is defined as the degree to which an individual is able or ready to accept or adopt an innovation. Conceptualized as a continuum, receptivity may range from strong, negative receptivity (i.e., absolute rejection) to strong, positive receptivity (i.e., absolute acceptance). to strong, negative receptivity (i.e., absolute rejection). An individual's level of receptivity or orientation toward change does not dictate how one may actually act in response to change initiatives. However, one who has strong, positive receptivity would be more likely to adopt and facilitate implementing a particular innovation. In contrast, an individual with strong, negative receptivity would openly resist and perhaps work overtly against implementing an innovation (Chauvin, 1992). Similarly, an individual with positive receptivity would be more likely to sustain implementation of an innovation without external pressure, than would an individual evidencing negative receptivity.

6. Intervention is an action or event, or set of actions or events, that influences use of an innovation. Interventions may be intended or unintended (Hall & Hord, 1984; Hord, Rutherford, Huling-Austin, & Hall, 1987).

7. Adoption, implementation, and incorporation are common stages of change through which individuals and groups progress. Adoption refers to the early stage when an innovation or change is introduced and contemplated, and receptivity plays a key role. Implementation refers to the stage during which the innovation or change is initiated and put into action. During the implementation

stage, considerable attention is given to managing the innovation and those involved in carrying it out within the existing organizational context. Incorporation refers to the stage of change when the innovation is no longer considered "new", but viewed as part of everyday life in the school (Bennis, Benne, & Chin, 1969; Rogers, 1995).

Having clarified the meanings of these key concepts, let's turn our attention to an important source of variability in implementing any type of educational change: individuals within educational organizations.

Individual behavior as a focus for change

Historically, a number of conceptions of human behavior from both psychological and sociological perspectives have been useful in attempts to explain and predict behavior within organizations. From a psychological perspective, Lewin (1947, 1951) and Bandura's (1977, 1986) view of human behavior, learning and change reflect reciprocal, dynamic interactions between person and environmental variables. Getzels and Guba's (1957) social systems theory of organizational behavior recognizes these dynamic interactions and represents them in terms of institutional and individual elements. Owens and Steinhoff's (1976) sociotechnical orientation reflects human behavior and change within an interactive and interdependent organizational systems model. Consistent with contemporary approaches used for understanding schools as complex, formal organizations (Hoy & Miskel, 1987; Owens, 1987), the dynamic interactions among these variables are apparent. Therefore, each of these perspectives is broadly discussed and then synthesized as a combined conceptual framework with which implementing change in medical educational environments can be understood.

Lewin's force-field theory

Influenced by Gestalt psychology, Lewin (1947, 1951) conceptualized individual behavior as resulting from a person's perception of the totality of facts within his/her psychological and physical environment at any specified moment in time. That is, the individual behavior (B) of a person can be explained as an interactive function of personal variables (P) and environmental variables (E): $B = f(P, E)$. For example, in a medical school, every faculty member has a particular and unique set of personal characteristics (e.g., age, gender, ethnic/cultural background, educational background, professional status, experience, values, beliefs, set of role orientations and so on). Likewise, the school has a unique set of contextual or environmental characteristics (e.g., student clientele, physical resources, school climate, organizational structure, communication patterns, leadership styles, governance policies and structures, performance expectations, and so on) that interact with a faculty member's personal characteristics.

Lewin explained individual behavior in terms of responses to the psychological environment in ways that attempt to balance opposing valences or forces (i.e., driving forces and restraining forces) that are necessary for one to maintain psychological equilibrium. That is, when driving and restraining forces are equal, behavior remains stable and no change occurs. When a change in personal or environmental variables strengthens or weakens driving or restraining forces, equilibrium is upset and individual behavior changes to equalize opposing forces and stabilize behavior again. Lewin theorized that an individual's behavior results from one's present perception of the environment at any given point in time, rather than any actual physical condition or event. For example, a faculty member might be inclined to implement an educational innovation in a school where incentives or rewards for innovation implementation are provided; whereas, without these incentives, s/he might not adopt and implement the innovation.

Bandura's social cognitive theory

Bandura (1977, 1986) conceptualized human learning and functioning as the continuing, reciprocal and dynamic interaction among three elements: the individual (personal characteristics), behavior, and the environment (situational characteristics). An individual's attributes are interacting continuously with his/her behavior. An individual and his/her behavior are also interacting constantly with the environment. Within this dynamic and reciprocal relationship, social cognitive theory also defines several underlying attributes that explain human behavior and change. First, individuals have the capability to recognize information and events based on their prior experiences (symbolic attributes). Second, individuals can formulate images or visions of desirable future events and use them to guide or motivate behavior (forethought attributes). Individuals can learn through observing others' behaviors and the consequences of those actions (vicarious attributes), use reflective evaluation to learn from past experiences (self-reflective attributes), and set standards for goals and behaviors (self-regulatory attributes). Therefore, using Bandura's conception, individuals are able to visualize their future, set goals, monitor and adjust their behavior and progress toward goals and desired future states, and reward themselves appropriately for achieving their goals. Throughout these processes, individuals' attributes, values and beliefs, their behaviors, and the environment are influencing, and are being influenced by, each other. For example, a faculty member with a record of success may perceive the benefits of implementing an innovation as greater than the associated potential risks. On the other hand, a new faculty member in the same school whose self-confidence in his/her role is still developing and who does not have much prior experience in the organization and with implementing educational innovations, may be more inclined to resist changes because risks are perceived to be greater than benefits.

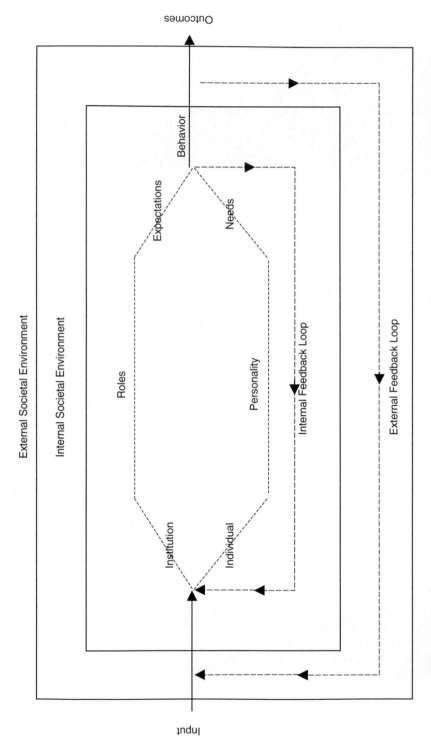

Figure 1. Structural elements (subsystems) of the organization: Getzels-Guba social systems model (1957)

Getzels and Guba's social systems theory

Getzels and Guba (1957) also explain organizational behavior as the result of the interaction between person and environmental variables: institutional/nomothetic and individual/idiographic. Getzels and Guba's model represents the influence of distinctive environmental features that are within and outside of an organization. As shown in Figure 1, behavior (B) within an organization is described as a function of the interaction of role (R) and personality (P): $B = f(R \times P)$. Feedback mechanisms, both internal and external to the organization, are distinctive features of this model that represent the ongoing and interactive, reciprocal relationships among the various elements.

Getzels and Guba (1957) argue that individuals do not enter the organization as "blank slates", but bring with them unique personalities, sets of personal beliefs, norms, values, experiences, and needs, which in part reflect the external environment of the organization. Person variables enter the model represented in Figure 1 as Input, and are reflected as the individual/idiographic dimension that contributes to an explanation of an individual's behavior within an organization. For example, faculty members come to a school organization with preconceived, personal beliefs regarding how they should act and interact with others. These individual beliefs contribute to individuals' perceptions of variables such as role orientations (e.g., faculty member as content expert, researcher, teacher, and/or mentor) and personal preferences (e.g., communication, work ethic, leadership and followership styles, and relationships with learners, administrators, colleagues and others).

Within the formal school organization, individuals interact with one another and their individual beliefs, norms and values influence, and are influenced by, the collective perspective. However, these interactions do not occur in isolation of the unique characteristics of the organization. Therefore, organizational characteristics are also represented in Figure 1 as Input, reflecting the institutional/nomothetic dimension that contributes to explaining individuals' behaviors within organizations. These organizational characteristics (e.g., organizational goals, prescribed structures and roles, and resulting expectations) are also influenced by the external environment (e.g., geographical, political, and professional communities).

Owens and Steinhoff's sociotechnical systems theory

Owens and Steinhoff (1976) describe school organizational structure and function as the dynamic interplay among four organizational subsystems (task, human, structure, and technology). The personal or individual/ideographic variables are represented by the human subsystem, while the other three subsystems (task, technology, and structure) represent the environmental or institutional/nomothetic variables. Schools are described as formal organizations in which simultaneous and interactive relationships occur among the four subsystems that are supplemented by input and output mechanisms and feedback loops. Such a model extends the individual-institutional relationship to reflect a realistic conception of the complex environment of educational organizations.

The human subsystem interacts with other human elements and the other three subsystems, and reflects individual skills (e.g., teaching and leadership abilities), values, beliefs and perceptions, and role orientations (e.g., educator, researcher, clinician, colleague, coach, mentor). This is the only one of the four subsystems that is affective and nonrational. The tasks subsystem is concerned with the various tasks necessary to achieve organizational goals. In one sense, faculty members' roles in colleges/schools are defined within this subsystem in terms of research, teaching, and service/practice (e.g., committee work and patient care). Essential elements of organizational structure such as authority, departments and offices, decision-making, planning, rules and communication patterns are reflected in the structure subsystem, which interacts with human and task elements. The technology subsystem reflects the "tools of the trade" and includes elements of organizational functioning such as knowledge and technical expertise, equipment and materials, order, and routine. Overall, faculty members' receptivity to proposed changes and their abilities to implement and sustain innovations may be significantly influenced by elements within this subsystem. If necessary resources are not routinely available, faculty members, as implementors of change (or students, as recipients of change), may be resistant to altering normative practice simply because they lack the tools, sufficient time, or access to the appropriate technical support and/or information (e.g., evidence, research findings) (Friedman, 1996). For example, Bowdish, Chauvin, and Vigh (1998) examined the initial implementation of hypermedia-assisted teaching in a gross anatomy course. Among their conclusions was that the degree to which faculty members implement hypermedia-assisted teaching depends a variety of factors, including the following: (1) the availability of appropriate hardware, software, and technical support services; (2) the organizational structure, goals, and role expectations; (3) individuals' abilities, beliefs, and needs (students and faculty); and (4) how these variables interact with each other as a dynamic system.

Reviews of past change efforts in medical education (e.g., Bussigel, Barzansky, & Greenholm, 1988; Davis, 1998; Davis, Thomson, Oxman, & Haynes, 1992; Davis & White, 1993; Rankin & Fox, 1997; Fox, Mazmanian, & Putnam, 1989; Schwartz et al., 1994) suggest that elements within the human subsystem are dominant factors that influence and interact with the other three subsystems (task, technology, and structure) during periods of educational change. Given the complex, interactive relationships among these subsystems in the change process and the resiliency of medical school structures to withstand continued efforts to change and maintain their systemic aspects (Bloom, 1988; Cuban, 1997; Schwartz et al., 1994), each theory described here seems insufficient when considered separately from the others. Therefore, how can these theories be combined as a conceptual framework to guide change facilitators' decision-making and use of interventions effectively for implementing educational change?

A conceptual model for understanding individuals' behavior and change within organizations

Figure 2 represents a way of thinking about how individuals perceive innovations and engage in change efforts within a school organization (Chauvin, 1992). This conceptual framework combines elements of the psychological, sociological, and sociotechnical perspectives on behavior and recognizes the multiple individual, social, and organizational factors that interact simultaneously in various ways to influence how change is adopted, implemented, and incorporated into everyday professional practice. Personal variables are shown as input variables and reflect the influence of individuals' prior knowledge, abilities, beliefs and values. Environmental variables are reflected in the subsystems, as well as the external environment in which the organization and its members exist. The broken double arrows are used in the model to represent the multiplicative ways in which each subsystem interacts with and influences itself, the other subsystems, and the external environment. These interactions contribute to change and stability in various aspects of personal and environmental variables, as patterns of structure and function evolve, change over time, and remain stable (i.e., resist change). For example, as an individual begins to identify with a particular school and becomes familiar with other individuals in the school, his/her beliefs and perceptions may influence, and be influenced by, the collective set of beliefs, values, and norms (i.e., organizational culture) within the school. Similarly, the environmental subsystems (i.e., task, structure, and technology) influence, and are influenced by, the organizational culture and the external environment. Such interactive relationships contribute to the development of informal, organizational norms or culture that guide how organizational members (e.g., faculty, staff, students) view "who we are" and "how we do things around here" (Corbett, Firestone, & Rossman, 1987). In turn, such norms and perspectives can influence individuals' receptivity to change and the extent to which individuals, and the organization as a whole, adopt and implement innovation (Bussigel et al., 1988; Cavanaugh, 1993; Cohen et al., 1994; Corbett et al., 1987; Schein, 1992; Schwartz et al., 1994).

Please note that this model does not represent a specific theory of change, but rather a conceptual framework for understanding, facilitating, and examining the change process in medical education environments. Michael Fullan (1999), an internationally recognized leader in change, argues that there will never be a definitive theory of change, since it is impossible to create a conceptual explanation that applies to all situations. However, he has argued for a general framework on which change facilitators can build practical wisdom, experience, and skills in how to understand and work with the unique combinations and interplay of

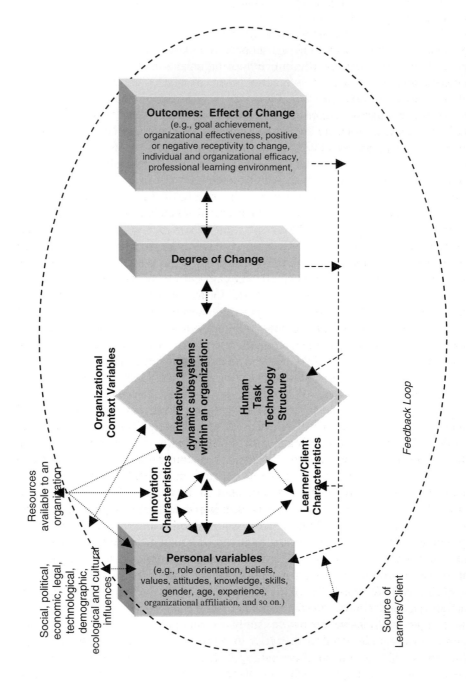

Figure 2. A combined conceptual model for understanding individuals' behavior and change within organizations

characteristics related to implementing change in organizations and incorporating change successfully into everyday practice.

As individuals and the organization, as a whole, are involved in educational change initiatives, these experiences influence receptivity to and involvement in future efforts to implement innovations. For example, in a school where educational innovation and creativity are the norm, faculty members are likely to stay abreast of educational advances and use research findings to identify better ways of doing things. However, faculty members may be less willing to embrace teaching innovations in situations where economic concerns are present, increased emphasis is given to research productivity over teaching effectiveness for career advancement, and/or priority or recognition has not been given to innovations over tradition in the past. Similarly, faculty and students will lack the motivation to implement innovations in situations where either group is satisfied with the status quo and students are successful in securing desirable residency training assignments. Similarly, educational innovations that encourage students' responsibility for learning (e.g., problem based learning) may not be easily adopted within a school where faculty members believe they are the deliverers of knowledge and students perceive their roles as passive receivers of information and services.

In summary, the conceptual framework shown in Figure 2 combines the theoretical perspectives previously described in a way that reinforces tenets of systems thinking and organizational learning that comprise contemporary views of organizational effectiveness (Cohen & Sproull, 1996; Senge, 1990; Wheatley, 1994; Wheatley & Kellner-Rogers, 1999). That is, from a systems perspective, a change in one part of the system results in a change in another part of the system, and at the same time may cause change (or stability) in at least one other part of the system. Organizational learning reflects a perspective where change is viewed as a way of life and the goal becomes an increased capacity for change, including flexibility and adaptability. Knowledge of the dynamic and interactive nature of these subsystems, and the influence of individuals' perceptions of an innovation and the context in which change occurs, can be used to design and implement interventions that facilitate and sustain individuals' involvement in managing change effectively. Similarly, the model can help those involved in implementing change (e.g., change facilitators and implementors) balance change and stability effectively. As systems, these complex, interactive, and cyclical patterns of behaviors within organizations develop and change over time; thus, through effective change facilitation, organizational learning and effectiveness can result. Noteworthy is that the Rand Study (McLaughlin & Marsh, 1978), one of the earliest and most recognized studies on change, reached similar conclusions. The Rand Study was conducted in the 1970s as a comprehensive follow-up study of federally funded programs and innovations that were initiated in the 1960s to determine the extent to which change and innovations had continued after funding ended. An important finding was that successful educational improvement initiatives were not specific projects, but part of an ongoing, comprehensive, problem solving and continuous improvement process. More recently, the results of a ten-year study of effective and ineffective schools by Teddlie and Stringfield (1993) and a five-year follow-up study of a statewide school improvement project (Lofton, Ellett, Hill, & Chauvin, 1998) also supported systems thinking and organizational learning perspectives regarding implementing change within organizations. While these longitudinal studies were conducted outside of medical education, the findings and conclusions are applicable. Such studies also demonstrate the important relationship between change and stability that is necessary to facilitate and maintain long-lasting success.

CHANGE AND STABILITY IN EDUCATIONAL ORGANIZATIONS

Larry Cuban's comprehensive study of educational change involving a history department and a school of medicine (Cuban, 1997, 1999), revealed that while educational organizations vary in terms of their goals, purposes, clientele and structure, they share many common structures and perspectives. For example, strong roots of tradition and history, long-standing norms, and beliefs about roles and professional practice (e.g., teaching, research, and service) provide organizational stability and are highly similar across the disciplines. Faculty experiences and beliefs about their roles, in many ways, are grounded first in past experiences as learners and protégés, then as teachers and mentors. Therefore, proposed changes in the ways faculty teach and students learn challenge individuals' beliefs about the effectiveness and credibility of past experiences and practices – experiences first as learners, then as professors. The same analogy can be drawn for changes in clinical practices, research methodology, or organizational operations within a medical school or academic department.

Faculty members in medical schools struggle to maintain stability in their roles, responsibilities, and ways of working and interacting with each other in the midst of rapidly changing healthcare practices, societal demands for meeting community needs, and rapidly expanding knowledge bases (Neufeld et al., 1995). For example, through an extensive set of interviews with medical educators from around the globe, Neufeld and his colleagues (1995) found that faculty members in medical schools who were involved in change initiatives attempted to keep up with advances in the field by reverting to familiar and routine ways of behaving. That is, they retreated to their discipline-specific settings, traditional forms of teaching (e.g., lectures), and research roles to maintain a level of predictability and stability in terms of "who we are" (i.e., how people define their roles and relationships within the organization) and "how we do things around here" (i.e., perceived norms, values, and beliefs within the organization, as a whole) (Corbett et al., 1987).

In a comparative case study of six United States medical schools that implemented broad-based medical education change, the unique organizational culture of each school played an important role in the extent to which change was implemented (Cohen et al., 1994). For example, while these schools shared a common goal of reducing the number of lecture hours in their respective M.D.

degree programs, they realized divergent outcomes. The diversity of change outcomes was influenced, at least in part, by the specific features of their respective local organizational cultures and the ways individuals made sense of and implemented change. Neufeld and his colleagues (1995) argued that an important challenge to medical educators is to find ways in which faculty can work together effectively, be responsive to changing societal needs, and make sense of change, given the contexts in which they work. Such efforts often mean moving toward establishing new roles and new ways of doing things. Changes in roles and functioning require involving faculty members and others in becoming knowledgeable about innovations and stages in the change process, their roles in implementing such changes, and achieving a good fit between their personal beliefs and the organizational mission and vision (Dannefer et al., 1998; Kaufman, 1998; Schwartz et al., 1994). Whether one is involved in implementing an individual change (e.g., implementing a new teaching method) or a large-scale organizational change (e.g., completely transforming a degree program), individuals are influenced by their environments and, in turn, influence, and are influenced by, others within the organization. These influences are important in assessing needs and determining appropriate change facilitation strategies and interventions as individuals progress developmentally: first, adopting innovation, then implementing it and finally making it part of everyday practice. Individuals' needs for stability and predictability in an organization, coupled with their receptivity to and capacity for implementing change, contribute to the importance of understanding change as a developmental, albeit not necessarily linear, process.

CHANGE AS A DEVELOPMENTAL PROCESS

Researchers have typically described the change process as a series of predictable stages or steps that are not necessarily linear or lock step progressions. For example, Rogers (1995) describes a two-stage process of change. The first stage is focused on initiating change (i.e., setting agenda, matching the problem with a solution), while the second stage is focused on implementing the change (i.e., redefining/restructuring innovation, clarifying expectations about change, and making change routine).

Levine (1980) explains change as a four-stage process that includes the following: (1) recognize a need for change, (2) plan the change, (3) initiate and implement the change plan, and (4) institutionalize the change. Levine's model was used recently as a basis for facilitating innovation in the eight United States medical schools that were part of the Robert Wood Johnson Foundation's Preparing Physicians for the Future: Program in Medical Education (Dannefer et al., 1998). In brief, their experiences revealed that broad-based involvement at all levels within the organization and clear, consistent means of communication are critical to achieving faculty members' adoption and implementation of educational change.

Havelock (1975), based on his extensive work with teachers, developed a situation-based approach to implementing change that focuses specifically on an individual's involvement in implementing change, as opposed to facilitating the change with groups. The change facilitator uses problem solving strategies and ongoing collaboration with an innovation user. Havelock identified six stages through which a change facilitator can effectively promote innovation implementation. These stages comprised the following: (1) build a relationship (change facilitator and user), (2) diagnose the problem, (3) acquire relevant resources, (4) choose a solution, (5) gain acceptance or resistance (use appropriate change facilitator diffusion strategies and define corresponding user adoption strategies), and (6) stabilize the innovation and generate self-renewing processes. While six stages are defined in this model, Havelock asserts that not every stage is necessarily a component of every innovation implementation, nor do individuals progress through the stages in a distinct, hierarchical order, since different stages may occur simultaneously. Although Havelock provides greater detail in his model than do others (e.g., Rogers, 1995; Levine, 1980), specific strategies are not identified.

Another perspective that has been useful in facilitating change is Rogers' (1995) taxonomy of individual responses to change. The five categories in this taxonomy comprise the following: (1) Innovators, (2) Early Adopters, (3) Early Majority, (4) Late Majority, and (5) Laggards. According to Rogers (1995), Innovators are eager to try new ideas and are comfortable with the ambiguities and occasional setbacks that are often a part of change. Innovators are not discouraged when interventions are unsuccessful. Early Adopters include those individuals who become involved with an innovation early on in the process of change. They are typically more integrated into the organization than are the Innovators, hold a high degree of credibility among their peers, and possess considerable opinion leadership. Individuals within an organization that represent these two categories are usually the first to suggest or introduce new ways of doing things and become involved in initiating change (Rogers' Stage I change strategies). However, involving Innovators and Early Adopters is insufficient to accomplish change implementation activities and achieve successful, long-lasting implementation of educational innovations.

The third category of individual responses, Early Majority, includes individuals who are cautious about change, but are willing to adopt and implement innovations, based on clues about the success or failure of an innovation that they get from observing and interacting with the Early Adopters. They are rarely in leadership positions, so are usually not among individuals charged with leading change. However, their participation in Rogers' Stage II change activities carries substantial weight among organizational members and is critical to overall success. Early Majority adopters can be important players in facilitating the group or organizational change activities.

Individuals who reflect Late Majority responses are skeptical and critical about change. These individuals rarely adopt and implement change until they feel pressure from others who have already adopted or implemented an innovation. Successful change can be threatened if the concerns and uncertainty expressed by Late Majority participants are not resolved. Finally, the Laggards are those individuals within the organization who are very traditional and invested in the past and the status quo. While they usually have no opinion leadership, they are the last persons to adopt or implement change, despite being knowledgeable about the innovation for some period of time. Often, by the time Laggards become involved with an innovation, Innovators are already moving on to another innovation and cycle of change. While Laggards should not be ignored, efforts to "bring them on board" must be expended carefully, as these individuals will be the last ones to adopt and implement innovation, if ever. Depending on the proposed change, some Laggards may drop out by retiring or moving on to other responsibilities or settings. Successful change facilitators use this taxonomy to facilitate the ongoing process of change.

MODELS OF PLANNED CHANGE STRATEGIES

A careful assessment of the various contextual characteristics that are reflected in Figure 2 and the use of one or more models of change strategies can enhance the manner in which strategies are used. These models can be used to achieve a good fit between the individual and organizational change needs and the interventions used to facilitate successful progress in adopting, implementing, and institutionalizing a specific innovation. This section summarizes three models of change strategies that have persisted in the literature, i.e. the following: (1) empirical-rational, (2) power-coercive and (3) normative-reeducative (Bennis et al., 1969; Owens, 1987).

Empirical-rational

Empirical-rational strategies are represented in the professional literature using several different labels, including research-development-diffusion (RDD), knowledge-dissemination-use (KDU), or research-development-dissemination-adoption (RDDA). This category of strategies assumes that someone is conducting research and creating new knowledge that is then disseminated and used to create new products or methods for enhancing current practices. The approach assumes that, because new knowledge is identified through qualified research, others will be rational, accept it as valuable and beneficial, and adopt it as part of their routine practices. Typical strategies include dissemination of information (e.g., research reports, print materials, conferences, and informational seminars).

Power-coercive

Power-coercive strategies are just as implied by this label. That is, change is prompted using power, internal or external to the organization, and sanctions, typically political, financial or moral. Shifts in organizational structure and authority, governance structures, legislative, licensure or accreditation standards, public pressure for change, or changes in funding and resource allocations are all strategies that effect change in behaviors and/or beliefs. These strategies rely heavily on formal authority, strict guidelines, and frequent monitoring. Rationality and human relations are secondary to the ability to achieve changes directly through the exercise of power and authority, often associated with central administrative (e.g., Dean's directives) or external agency mandates (e.g., program accreditation standards, funding stipulations, legislation).

Normative-reeducative

Normative-reeducative strategies (sometimes referred to as organizational development or renewal) is based on a systems theory perspective and a premise that the key to achieving successful planned change is through developing individuals' problem-solving capabilities, often through organizational development and renewal activities. This category also recognizes the strong influence of organizational culture and environmental idiosyncrasies, and emphasizes the importance of nurturing a continuous cycle of improvement. Change strategies in this category focus on individuals within organizations, target participants' learning through hands-on applications, real-life situations, and are used to achieve long-lasting change by developing the following three essential characteristics of an effective organization:
1. adaptability and responsiveness to change (e.g., open communication channels, high value on collaboration and problem-solving);
2. clear-cut, explicit, and clearly understood procedures for participants to engage in collaboration and problem-solving (e.g., committees, work groups, facilitator-user collaborative relationships); and
3. open system structure – individuals know when and how to seek appropriate ideas and resources for solving problems and facilitating change.

While there is no doubt that empirical-rational and power-coercive strategies are effective in some instances, they are based on the impetus for change originating from outside of the individual or the organization. Maintaining long-lasting change using either or both of these categories of strategies is difficult and usually not very successful. On the other hand, a normative-reeducative approach recognizes the resiliency of individuals and organizations to buffer attempts at change and retain their existing status or structure and function. This approach uses the organization's interaction-influence system of human, task, technology, and structure subsystems (Figure 1) to alter individual and organizational norms or "ways of thinking and doing", so that changes become incorporated into the everyday life of the organization. In reality, successful change initiatives typically reflect normative-reeducative strategies, even if empirical-rational and/or power-coercive strategies are also present. Regardless of the approach, the primary focus of change strategies is the focus on individuals in an organization.

FACILITATING INDIVIDUAL CHANGE

Keeping in mind the conceptual framework shown in Figure 2 and the predominant role of the human subsystem in an organization, let's revisit Lewin's psychological model of behavior (B = f[P, E]) specifically in terms of his force-field theory of change (Lewin, 1951) before examining any specific normative-reeducative approaches to facilitating change. Lewin explained behavior change as the result of stress or anxiety in the form of driving forces (i.e., factors that encourage change) and restraining forces (i.e., factors that resist change). Further, he described change as occurring in three stages: (1) Unfreezing – planning and creating a climate for innovation and change; (2) Moving – implementing change; and (3) Refreezing – reinforcing innovation. An imbalance between driving and restraining forces facilitates the unfreezing stage and continues to facilitate change in behaviors or beliefs during the moving stage. When driving and restraining forces become equalized or balanced again, individuals are in the refreezing stage and behavior stabilizes at this new level. For example, an individual perceives a proposed change as beneficial because current practices are satisfactory and the proposed change is perceived as a realistic improvement (i.e., moving toward a more effective or optimal situation). Similarly, an individual might perceive a proposed change as beneficial because current practices are problematic and the proposed change reflects a realistic and necessary remedy (i.e., moving away from an ineffective or sub-optimal situation).

Lewin explained that very high or very low levels of stress or anxiety might actually strengthen restraining forces and prevent implementation of change. For example, if an individual is very comfortable with the status quo, s/he will likely experience very low levels of stress; thus, feeling little or no urgency or need to change. Thus, a change facilitator would use strategies that heighten the individual's stress regarding implementing an innovation (i.e., strengthen driving forces or individual urgency or need to change). For example, a change facilitator might share information about and empirical evidence for why the new approach is better than current practices, to create urgency for change within the individual. On the other hand, an individual with a very high level of stress regarding implementing an innovation is not capable of coping with change. That is, the individual may be overwhelmed by the pressure for change (e.g., too much, too fast), the complexity of an innovation, the lack of skills or training, or a perception of unrealistic expectations for performance. In this situation the change facilitator would focus on strategies that reduce the individual's high level of stress or anxiety that is preventing adoption or implementation of an innovation (i.e., reduce restraining forces), so that driving forces may be strengthened to unfreeze behavior and promote change.

While Lewin's change theory seems straightforward, change facilitators must take care to maintain a reasonable balance between change and stability to ensure that individuals progress through the moving stage (i.e., implementing change) toward incorporating new behaviors or beliefs into everyday practice (refreezing stage). Also, a variety of factors can influence an individual's willingness to implement change, not all of which are within the professional setting. Perceptions of personal, social, political, and economic factors, to name a few, play an important role in an individual's adoption of change and willingness to implement and incorporate innovations into everyday practice. For example, Fox et al. (1989), in their comprehensive study of how and why physicians change their professional practices (referred to in the continuing medical education literature as the Change Study), revealed that the source of these driving and restraining forces can vary considerably. They identified ten personal, professional, and social forces for change that influenced physicians' goals for learning and their willingness to adopt, implement, and incorporate specific innovations into everyday practice. These forces included personal and financial well being, curiosity, stage of career, desire to enhance professional competency or achieve professional aspirations, pressure from patients and colleagues, and influences of the social and cultural contexts in which physicians work. Knowledge of these sources of influence and how they interact with the characteristics of a specific innovation can help change facilitators manage potential barriers to innovation and facilitate individuals' involvement in implementing change. In addition, Rogers (1995) described five characteristics of an innovation that influence the extent to which individuals are willing to adopt the change:

1. Complexity – How difficult is it to understand the innovation?
2. Compatibility – How similar is the innovation to the user's previous experience or beliefs?
3. Relative advantage – To what extent is the innovation viewed as better than current practice?
4. Observability – How easy is it for others to see the potential user implementing the innovation?
5. Trialability – Can the potential user implement the innovation on a trial basis?

Kaslow (1974), and Giacquinta (1975a, 1975b), Rogers (1995), and Rankin and Fox (1997) indicated that change facilitators might use the following four questions to determine the extent to which an individual might be willing to adopt an innovation (in terms of perceived benefits and risks):

1. What is the relative advantage of the innovation to the potential users/clients (benefit factor)?
2. How well will the innovation fit with individual beliefs and organizational norms (risk factor)?

3. What level of commitment is required up front (risk factor)? That is, can the innovation be implemented temporarily and eliminated later, if unacceptable?
4. To what extent will others know about and see the user attempt implementation (risk factor)?

Clearly, if risks are perceived to be greater than benefits, an individual will be less likely to adopt an innovation than vice versa. Change facilitators can use the five characteristics of an innovation and the four benefit-risk questions listed above to make informed decisions regarding the most effective dissemination and change facilitation strategies for an individual innovation user or a group of users.

Using principles of innovation and concerns theory (i.e., the Concerns Based Adoption Model that will be described later in this chapter), Rankin and Fox (1997) validated the influence of the above five characteristics of an innovation on Canadian radiologists' willingness to adopt innovation. Chute and Hancock (1982) demonstrated the effectiveness of situated learning (Lave & Wenger, 1990) and follow up coaching and feedback techniques for addressing these characteristics and facilitating adoption and implementation of teleconferencing as an instructional medium. Reports of curriculum change initiatives in medical schools (e.g., Dannefer et al., 1998; Davis & White, 1993; Wilkes et al., 1994) have identified several variables that contribute to successful change. For example, these reports support using several general strategies for facilitating individuals' willingness to implement change (driving forces) and minimize resistance (restraining forces): (1) providing information about educational advances (e.g., research reports), (2) demonstrating a clear vision and strong leadership for change, and (3) ensuring broad-based stakeholder involvement. Drawing on the results of the Change Study (Fox et al., 1989), Fox and Bennett (1998) conclude that physicians progress through four stages of self-assessment when faced with change. They describe these stages as follows:

1. Estimate where one should be in terms of knowledge, skills, and attitudes necessary to implement an innovation successfully;
2. Estimate one's current knowledge, skills, and attitudes in terms of their image of an innovation;
3. Estimate the discrepancy that exists between 1 and 2; and
4. Experience a level of anxiety or dissonance between where one should be and actually is, providing a potential motivator for learning and for adopting an innovation/change. However, too little or too much anxiety can prevent learning and adoption of change.

Fullan (1993, 1999) argues that there is no substitute for focusing on individuals for accomplishing change successfully, including situations involving large-scale, systemic change. Understanding how individuals perceive and orient themselves to specific organizational roles when implementing innovations, and how they make sense of innovations within this perceptual context, is critical to effecting long-lasting changes in professional practice (e.g., teaching and learning) (Corbett et al., 1987). As individuals progress through various stages of change, they alter their ways of thinking and doing. Change at the individual level involves anxiety and uncertainty, developing new skills, practice, feedback, and cognitive transformations with respect to why this new way works better.

Drawing on the results of extensive field studies involving teachers, Hall and Hord (1987) also concluded that individual perceptions, feelings, and concerns evolve and are resolved at each stage of incorporating innovation into practice. They developed the Concerns Based Adoption Model (CBAM) as a comprehensive approach to facilitating change in schools by focusing on individuals' responses to implementing educational change. At the Southwest Educational Development Laboratory at the University of Texas at Austin, Shirley Hord continues research and development activities that are based, in part, on the CBAM. For example, Hord and her colleagues have included the CBAM as an integral part of their Leadership for Change (LFC) project that has been funded by the United States Office of Educational Research and Improvement. In fact, the concept of change facilitation as one aspect of leadership style is a distinct area of study in the professional education literature that includes medical education (e.g., Chauvin, 1992, 1993; Evans & Chauvin, 1993; Evans & Teddlie, 1993; Hall & Hord, 1987; Neufeld et al., 1995; Tosteson, 1990). While this work focuses primarily on elementary and secondary school improvement, the CBAM and its components (e.g., the Stages of Concern [SoC]) have been used effectively in various educational settings (e.g., science education, elementary and secondary schools, higher education, nursing, dental, and medical schools and business education) and in various countries (e.g., United States, Australia, Canada, the Netherlands, South Africa, Afghanistan, Ghana, Sweden, and Belgium) (Chang, 1986; Chute & Hancock, 1982; Cicchelli & Baecher, 1989; Evans & Chauvin, 1993; Hall & Hord, 1987; Lewis & Watson, 1997; Snyder, 1983). Personal experiences using the CBAM and the LFC with faculty members and others in a variety of settings, including medical education, and ongoing collaboration with change facilitators reinforce the CBAM and LFC as an effective and comprehensive approach. Therefore, let's take a closer look at the CBAM and one of its components, the Stages of Concern (SoC).

The Concerns Based Adoption Model (CBAM)

Frances Fuller developed a concept of concerns theory in the late 1960s from her research with teachers. She observed specific patterns of needs and interests that differed, based on the career stage of the individuals. Beginning teachers were observed to evidence concerns about themselves first, followed by concerns about tasks or management. Later, as they gained experience, they expressed concerns about impact (i.e., concerns about outcomes such as student learning). Building on the work of Frances Fuller and her concept of concerns theory (1969), Gene Hall, Shirley Hord and other researchers at the University of Texas at Austin Research and Development Center for Teacher Education conducted extensive field work and expanded Fuller's original concerns model to include seven developmental stages, or Stages of Concern (SoC), in relation to implementation of innovations (Hall, Wallace, & Dossett, 1973; Hall, George, & Rutherford, 1979; Hall & Hord, 1984, 1987). The SoC is part of a larger model of change process, the Concerns Based Adoption Model (CBAM) that Hall and his colleagues developed.

The Stages of Concern: The Stages of Concern consists of seven developmental stages that function ideally as a continuous cycle of change. These seven stages are based on Fuller's original concerns theory (1969) that included the following three categories: self, task, and impact. As shown in Figure 3, the seven stages, from lowest to highest, include the following: awareness, informational, personal, management, consequence, collaboration, and refocusing. Individuals who are faced with an innovation progress through these stages and express corresponding concerns. Their movement through the stages is not as a lock step, one-way progression, but rather as a developmental pattern in which the relative intensity of concerns is the key to successful change facilitation. That is, knowing an individual's particular Stages of Concern in relation to a particular innovation and context facilitates the selection and use of appropriate intervention strategies to resolve current concerns and encourages an individual's movement toward incorporating the innovation into everyday practice. For example, at the beginning of a change process, an individual is a nonuser and concerns are likely related to self. For typical nonusers, self-concerns are relatively high in the earlier stages, first at Stage 0 (Awareness), developing to Stage 1 (Informational), and then to Stage 2 (Personal). As individuals begin to actually implement and use an innovation, task concerns about management and efficiency (Stage 3) evolve, as self-concerns are resolved. Individuals focused at Stage 3 (Management Concerns) may still have unresolved concerns at other stages, but the primary focus is managing the logistics of implementation. As shown in Figure 3, as individuals become skilled in using the innovation, management and lower level concerns diminish (i.e., self concerns) and impact concerns increase (i.e., Stage 4 Consequence, Stage 5 Collaboration, and Stage 6 Refocusing).

Throughout the change process, concerns at the various stages do not completely disappear, but the relative intensity changes as individuals progress with implementing an innovation. Individuals can revert to previously resolved concerns, should new organizational or individual characteristics emerge. Finally, individuals progress through the Stages of Concern at different rates, such as Innovators and Early Adopters (Rogers, 1995) resolving self concerns more rapidly than Early or Late Majority (Rogers, 1995) users. Change facilitators and innovation users can overcome barriers and implement change successfully within their organizations by combining knowledge of theoretical frameworks of change (e.g., Figure 2) with Hall and Hord's work on the CBAM, specifically the Stages of Concern.

Three methods for assessing individuals' stage(s) of concern are used in the CBAM. One-legged conferences are short, informal interactions (e.g., over coffee, during work breaks, hallway conversations, or walking down the hall, stepping with one leg at a time (thus, the name, one-legged conferences!). Open-ended statements are used to obtain written responses that can be analyzed later to determine an individual's stage(s) of concern. A 35-item Stages of Concern questionnaire (Hall, George, & Rutherford, 1979) is also available and provides a systematic method of assessing an individual's profile of the Stages of Concern with regard to a specific innovation. Two forms are currently available, one for users/implementers of an innovation and one for change facilitators. Skilled facilitators who are trained in using the various components of CBAM can use the Stages of Concern assessment data to determine the primary foci of concerns and offer intervention strategies that are appropriate for individuals' respective Stages of Concern.

The CBAM includes other components (e.g., the Levels of Use and Innovation Configuration Matrix) that can be used to observe, assess, and facilitate educational change systematically with individuals or groups of individuals in an organization. These are described in detail in Hord et al. (1987). The Levels of Use are used to assess and facilitate the extent to which individuals are using an innovation as intended. Change facilitators develop Innovation Configuration Matrixes with key stakeholders and users/implementers of innovation to specify, assess, and enhance the extent to which actual implementation reflects intended implementation.

Extensive field studies using quantitative and qualitative methods targeting implementation of educational innovations led to the refined Intervention Taxonomy and conceptual framework presented in Hall and Hord (1984). This taxonomy and framework was designed to be applicable to any change effort and to make sense to practitioners. Several levels of intervention have been identified in the taxonomy and include the following: policy, game plan, game plan component, strategy, tactic, and incident. These level distinctions accommodate intervention features such as scope, duration, and number of users affected. Therefore, at one end of the continuum the policy level represents global, general, and abstract interventions; whereas the incident level at the opposite end represents minute, concrete and specific intervention strategies. Many examples and detailed explanations that are grounded in extensive field studies are included Hall and Hord (1984) for each of the intervention levels. While the field-based examples are from elementary and secondary school settings, they can be used quite easily to identify parallel examples that would be highly appropriate for other contexts (e.g., medical education). Figure 3 also includes some examples of specific intervention strategies for each Stage of Concern. The examples shown in Figure 3 demonstrate how intervention strategies must fit the Stage of Concern expressed by an individual user. For example, a faculty member who has adopted and implemented a new teaching approach has likely resolved most self concerns and is focused on task or management concerns. At this Stage of Concern the user may express concerns about planning effectively, managing time and/or resources. Thus, suggesting an intervention that provides assistance with time management or planning tips would likely help to resolve management and efficiency concerns and facilitate movement toward being concerned about the effectiveness of implementation (i.e., concerns about impact or student learning). On the other hand, a nonuser who is aware of the innovation, but not interested in hearing about it (Stage 0 – Awareness), will not be encouraged toward adopting the innovation by engaging him/her in strategies to enhance planning and/or managing time for implementing the innovation (Stage 3 – Management). Such a tactic would likely increase negative receptivity (resistance) – not positive receptivity (adoption). Thus, an accurate interpretation of Stages of Concern assessment data is critical to selecting or designing an appropriate intervention strategy that helps an individual resolve concerns at one stage and move toward the next stage(s) of concern associated with implementing an innovation. In addition, assessing concerns at the individual user level affords change facilitators the flexibility to address implementation needs through both individual and group level interventions (see Figure 3 for examples).

Finally, the CBAM literature suggests that it is important for change facilitators to attend to the higher level stages (Stage 4-6) as much as they do to the lower ones (Stages 0-3). Attending to the full range of the Stages of Concern will maximize opportunities for nurturing the continuous processes of organizational learning (Hord, 1997; Senge, 1990; Wheatley, 1994; Wheatley & Kellner-Rogers, 1999). Similarly, broad-based involvement in continuous improvement processes facilitates the development of a climate that is conducive to change, adaptability, and flexibility – all desirable traits of effective organizations in today's world of rapid changes and ever-expanding knowledge. Effective leadership and change facilitation are critical to realizing a continuous cycle of improvement and an organizational climate of change.

USING EVALUATION TO FACILITATE CHANGE

In many respects the CBAM focuses on the behaviors, feelings, and concerns of an individual as an important stakeholder in evaluating, problem solving, and implementing educational change. While the CBAM is a useful approach to facilitating individuals' successful implementation of long-lasting change, it can be used in combination with other approaches and strategies to fit unique combinations of individual-innovation-context characteristics. For example, evaluation activities and the dissemination of the evaluation results can be used to promote and facilitate change. Examples include program or curriculum evaluation, the evaluation of traditional or innovative teaching/learning methods, the meta-analysis of the research literature to identify best educational practices in a particular area. Other chapters in this book address various aspects of evaluation and still others summarize the research pertaining to various aspects of medical education. This section summarizes important findings and insights gained from the professional

STAGES OF CONCERN	TYPICAL EXPRESSION OF CONCERN	EXAMPLES OF INTERVENTIONS
6 REFOCUSING	- I have a new approach that would work even better. - Now that the innovation is working well, where do I go from here?	- Encourage creative adaptations, expansions, and enhancements (e.g., How can we make this better?) - Share a vision of future directions - Use evaluation data to identify new targets/directions or higher levels of performance/achievement
5 COLLABORATION	- I would like to compare what I am doing with what others are doing in this area. - I am available to help new users of the innovation.	- Share ideas with others - Invite others to visit and observe - Create opportunities for experienced users to share tips with others - Provide opportunities to present new ideas or projects to others (e.g., workshops, demonstrations, professional meetings)
4 CONSEQUENCE	- In what ways is this innovation impacting my students? - How can we determine if this new method is better than what we did in the past?	- Invite the user to share success stories with you - Identify ways in which evidence of effectiveness can be measured - Collect pre and post test data to examine impact - Distribute a questionnaire to users (faculty) and clients (learners) to identify perceptions, evidence of success and areas in need of improvement - Facilitate sharing among users of "what works"
3 MANAGEMENT	- I am spending all of my time planning and getting materials ready. - I am having trouble managing the parts of this new approach and concentrating on my students at the same time.	- Provide demonstrations of logistical planning and implementation - Share management techniques and tips related to the innovation - Help organize planning and work groups - Provide assistance with setting timelines for implementation - Provide individual assistance with planning - Provide one-on-one assistance with initial implementation (e.g., experienced user team teaches with a new user)

IMPACT

TASK

STAGES OF CONCERN	TYPICAL EXPRESSION OF CONCERN	EXAMPLES OF INTERVENTIONS
2 **PERSONAL**	- How is my use of this innovation going to affect me?	- Recognize perceived risks and anxiety, and try to direct attention toward positive actions - Offer moral support and build confidence - Clarify information and correct misperceptions - Pair non-users with an experienced and successful user - Visit a site where the innovation is being used successfully - Point out "little successes" and provide support and assistance with new tasks
1 **INFORMATIONAL**	- I don't know much about this new approach, but would like to learn more. - Can you tell me more about it?	- Pair users of an innovation with non-users - Show a videotape about the "innovation" - Provide an orientation or awareness workshop - Provide printed materials to read or opportunities to observe demonstrations - Locate resources and provide number to contact
0 **AWARENESS**	- I'm not interested in hearing about the innovation. - I am not concerned about this innovation. - Something else will come along before I have to be concerned with it.	- Offer new ideas - Ask questions about what is "working" and what is not - Conduct needs assessment - Provide introductory materials and/or evidence that implementation of the innovation is imminent.

SELF

Figure 3. Stages of concern: Typical expressions of concern and examples of interventions appropriate to each stage. Source: Based on the Concerns Based Adoption Model (CBAM) Project (Hall & Hord, 1987)

literature regarding the effective use of dissemination and change facilitation strategies to translate new insights into improved medical education practices.

Knowledge-Dissemination-Use (KDU) strategies

Knowledge-dissemination-use strategies (also known as research-development-diffusion-adoption [RDDA]) reflect primarily an empirical-rational model of change. The use of knowledge-dissemination-use strategies has been common in medicine for many years, especially in traditional continuing medical education programs for practicing physicians. In recent years considerable efforts have focused on evaluating the efficacy of traditional and innovative continuing medical education methods (e.g., Davis et al., 1992; Davis, 1998; Fox et al., 1989). Results of continuing medical education evaluation studies are important, given the ongoing impetus to increase the use of community-based settings for teaching and learning in undergraduate and graduate medical education. Similarly, the results of continuing medical education evaluation studies can provide insights about implementing change effectively in medical education settings now and in the future.

Comprehensive evaluation studies (e.g., Fox et al., 1989) and systematic reviews of the professional literature pertaining to the effectiveness of continuing medical education methods (e.g., Cantillon & Jones, 1999; Davis et al., 1992; and Haynes, Davis, McKibbon, & Tugwell, 1984) reveal the following conclusions:
1. Strategies that are implemented within the everyday practice environment have the highest level of relevance for practicing physicians.
2. Strategies that include enabling or practice-reinforcing strategies are highly effective.
3. Strategies that link learning directly to practice, interactive educational meetings, outreach events, community-based strategies, and multiple-strategy interventions (e.g., outreach plus reminders, interactive meetings plus follow up reminders) are also highly effective in changing physicians' professional behaviors.
4. Audit, feedback, local consensus processes, and the influence of opinion leaders are less effective than strategies mentioned above.
5. Formal continuing medical education programs using traditional methods (e.g., lectures), disseminating unsolicited printed materials and practice guidelines, and formal continuing medical education activities that do not include enabling or practice-reinforcing strategies have little or no impact on changing physician practice behaviors.

Avorn and Soumerai (1983) and others (Evans, Haynes, & Birkett, 1986; Kosecoff, Kanouse, Rogers, McCloskey, Winslow & Brook, 1987; Lomas, Anderson, Dominick-Pierre, Vayda, Enkin, & Hannah, 1989) also document the ineffectiveness of passive dissemination strategies for changing physician practice behaviors. While these researchers argue that there are a sufficient number of studies on which to identify the most and least effective strategies for producing behavior and/or outcomes changes, few of these reflect rigorous evaluations of educational interventions. However, only a small percentage of studies were designed to promote long-term behavior change (Cantillon & Jones, 1999). For example, these researchers indicated that only a few of the 69 studies that met review criteria to be included in their study included any follow up activity beyond 3 months. They also questioned whether effective change strategies always produce immediate results. For example, Moran, Kirk, and Kopelow (1996) utilized group learning, and treatment and control subjects. At first the treatment subjects performed worse than the control subjects, but later improved significantly. My colleagues and I observed similar findings in a study of implementing hypermedia assisted lecture methods in a gross anatomy course for occupational therapy students (Bowdish et al., 1998). The analysis of quantitative and qualitative data in our study revealed that both teacher and learners experienced substantial changes in their roles and their perceptions of the learning environment and needed time to adjust to the new expectations and ways of behaving. This study and research by Moran et al., 1996 document this phenomenon referred to as the *implementation dip* in the Concerns Based Adoption Model and Leadership for Change project. Cantillon and Jones (1999) question whether these observations should be a concern for future investigations or simply an observation reflective of the challenges inherent in conducting educational research and evaluation. One might conclude that such concerns must be addressed study-by-study, so that researchers can balance and accommodate the unique characteristics of each investigation, and at the same time support high quality research methodology.

Educational evaluation strategies

Educational evaluation, often described as curriculum or program evaluation, is used frequently to identify the effectiveness of current methods, to recommend educational changes, and/or to assess the extent to which changes are made and are effective. Evaluation is a central component of educational change, but for which its design is often not considered until late in the implementation of an innovation, when participants are tired and frustrated and when resources are low or depleted. Grant funding for educational research is not easy to obtain and evaluation can consume a lot of time and resources (Carter, Battista, Hodge, Lewis, Basinski, & Davis, 1995; Gerrity & Mahaffy, 1998; Jolly & Grant, 1997). Consequently, the designers of new educational programs may prefer to spend their limited resources on developing and implementing the innovations, rather than on evaluating them. Evaluation is important for facilitating change, but it must be sound, multidimensional (i.e., multiple methods, multiple data sources, formative and summative purposes), and established at the onset of implementing change. Just as stakeholders must develop ownership for implementing innovations, they must also be committed to supporting and implementing high quality evaluation processes. Therefore, participants should be educated about evaluation processes and involved from the beginning in planning and implementing evaluation strategies. Educating individuals about the purposes and involving them in the processes associated with evaluation activities can help reduce anxiety about and resistance to participation. Finally, educating individuals about such processes can enhance their perceptions of the value of credible evaluation and facilitate candid responses from participants (Craig & Bandaranayake, 1993; Gerrity & Mahaffy, 1998).

When educational evaluation studies are implemented, attempts to disseminate the results via publications are also met with obstacles. For example, these types of reports are often not published in general readership journals. They are often rejected because they are either not sufficiently rigorous (e.g., not randomized controlled trials) or not deemed to be of general interest. Controlled trials of educational projects are particularly difficult (e.g., finding appropriate control groups, managing threats to internal and external validity). Similarly, results of evaluation studies are not easily generalized to other settings because of the unique features of each organizational and/or instructional setting. Reports that are disseminated are generally about positive outcomes and few examine failed change efforts. Despite these difficulties, evaluation is a critical component of change and the continuous improvement cycle, and concerted efforts to implement appropriate evaluation studies are necessary. Widespread dissemination of educational ideas is problematic without evaluation and others are less likely to attempt innovative approaches without some evidence of effectiveness. Similarly, valuable lessons from interventions resulting in less-than-successful outcomes may be lost; thus contributing to the potential for medical educators reinventing the wheel across the globe.

Educational evaluation models can take a variety of forms, such as student-, program-, institutional- or stakeholder-oriented. They may focus on indicators that are context-, outcomes- or process-based, or some combination. Measures can involve quantitative and/or qualitative methods, and some will likely require longitudinal data. Regardless of the format, evaluation plans must fit the change situation and answer the questions that are most important to stakeholders – locally and beyond. There are many aspects to planning and implementing credible evaluation plans and guidance is available in the professional literature (e.g. Sanders, 1994). Finally, evaluation results should be obtained and reported in a way that makes it easy for users and potential users to benefit from the information (Mennin, Friedman, & Woodward 1992; Rotem, 1992; Woodward, 1992).

Even when educational evaluations are well-designed, implemented rigorously, and reported appropriately, the use of results may not be very effective in facilitating long-lasting change. Why is this? First, as has been mentioned already, organizations, as a whole, are extremely resilient to change imposed from outside. Second, while evaluation studies may reflect valid designs and use rigorous methods, activities might be implemented by one group of individuals (e.g, an external evaluator or evaluation team) without involving those persons (e.g., program users or stakeholders) who may be asked or expected to use the results and implement recommended changes. Consequently, these users or stakeholders may question the evaluation purpose or focus, the method(s) of data collection, the findings, or the specific recommendations resulting from the evaluation processes.

That is, they may not perceive the evaluation as credible or necessary, believe there is a need for change, or have ownership for implementing recommended changes successfully. They may view evaluation and change being done to them, rather than with them. Third, because change efforts are influenced by specific features of an innovation, the individuals involved, and the particular contexts in which they are implemented, evaluation results that are relevant to one setting may or may not apply to another. Even if the results are relevant, stakeholders may still reflect a "... but that would never work here" perspective.

Kerbeshian (1986) reported a stakeholder approach to educational program evaluation that was used successfully in evaluating and enhancing basic science courses at the University of North Dakota School of Medicine. Based on a follow up evaluation conducted three years following the initial program review, results indicated that the recommendations for changes made in the original review had been implemented. Kerbeshian outlined strategies that contributed to the successful use of a stakeholder approach to program/curriculum evaluation that included the following:

1. Identify the decision makers;
2. Define clearly the nature, character and purpose of the evaluation;
3. Establish congruence between the evaluator's goals and objectives and those of the audience;
4. Legitimize the various stakes in the program;
5. Provide information to appropriate individuals in a format that is acceptable and useful;
6. Ensure that clients/users have a sense of input and control; and
7. Offer recommendations for change that are broad enough to allow clients/users the flexibility to determine how they can bring about the recommended change (an important element of ownership for change and implementation success).

While educational evaluation studies can be used effectively to determine the need for change and to facilitate the implementation of change (e.g., Kerbeshian, 1986), they can also be used to assess the effectiveness of innovation or planned changes. Several recent contributions to the professional literature on using research and evaluation to facilitate continuous improvement and long-lasting change summarize common barriers that interfere with users/implementors accepting and using research and evaluation results effectively (Kotter, 1996; Harvey, 1990; Kanter, Stein, & Jick, 1993; Shatzer, 1998). Among these authors' observations are the following:

1. Stakeholders are not identified and involved at the beginning of evaluative processes and their commitment is not secured and maintained throughout the change process. Consequently, change is perceived as something done to individuals, not with them.
2. Information systems and communication channels are used ineffectively (e.g., individuals are unaware of advances in the field and innovative efforts by others).
3. Individuals cannot implement evaluation recommendations because they lack specific skills or knowledge.

4. Insufficient resources are available to support and sustain actions and initiatives related to the innovation (e.g., necessary personnel, expertise, training, materials, technology, or finances) or they are discouraged or blocked.
5. Formal organizational structure and function make it difficult to implement the innovation (e.g., lack of clear vision and leadership; insufficient commitment to change; competing performance expectations; no or insufficient release time).
6. The timelines for implementing change(s) are unrealistic or the formats of the recommended changes are too complex or rigid to afford sufficient flexibility or adaptation to fit in with existing practices. Therefore, individuals' perceive the level of chaos and unpredictability associated with implementing an innovation to be greater than their ability to maintain sufficient stability and predict day-to-day roles and expectations.

COMBINED APPROACHES AND MULTIPLE CHANGE STRATEGIES

Kerbeshian's report and the common barriers to using evaluation effectively that are cited above reinforce the importance of balancing change and stability, open communication, and the use of combined approaches (e.g., empirical-rational and normative-reeducative) and multiple change strategies (e.g., stakeholder, program evaluation, and concerns-based). Others have reported similar observations and conclusions. For example, Wilkerson (1994) and Wilkes, Slavin, and Usatine (1994) highlight successful experiences at the University of California at Los Angeles School of Medicine's implementation of their Doctoring curriculum. Newman (1994) shares lessons learned at the University of Toronto School of Medicine. Tosteson (1990) describes insights about facilitating change resulting from Harvard Medical School's implementation of their New Pathways curriculum. Davis and White (1993) report insights associated with implementing large-scale curriculum changes at the University of Michigan Medical School. Lindberg (1998) provides a collective account of change experiences in the eight Robert Wood Johnson Foundation project schools. DesMarchais, Bureau, Dumais, and Pigeon (1992) document experiences in implementing problem-based learning. In each instance, change is described as a developmental process and multiple, simultaneous strategies are selected or designed based on context-dependent needs of innovation users in the organization.

Clearly, these accounts of educational change demonstrate across multiple contexts the importance of both top-down and bottom-up support, broad-based stakeholder involvement and combined approaches to facilitating change throughout all stages of the change process. In each instance, these authors reiterate the importance of stakeholder involvement in facilitating educational changes successfully and planning for both initial implementation and long-term maintenance. Guiding principles resulting from these reports are summarized as follows:

1. Initiate the change process with strong leadership, a clearly articulated vision, realistic perspectives of educational and organizational features, broad-based

faculty input and involvement, and sufficient resources to support innovation planning, implementation, and ongoing support.

2. Generate a comprehensive and clear description of the innovation that includes broad-based stakeholder involvement (e.g., committee meetings, faculty retreats, working groups); an adopted philosophy and plan for the innovation; adequate attention to organizational issues (e.g., time, organizational boundaries); and formal endorsement from key individuals and groups (e.g., formal leaders, curriculum committee).
3. Plan for and provide support for initial implementation of the innovation that includes the use of local champions/change facilitators; visual support from central leadership, technical, logistical, and resource support; assessment and monitoring; training and consultation; and broad-based stakeholder involvement.
4. Plan for and provide support for facilitating long-lasting change that maintains visible leadership support, adequate resource, technical, and logistical support, and stakeholder involvement that facilitates continued forward movement and enthusiasm.

Bussigel et al. (1988) and Mennin and Kaufman (1989) offer similar recommendations for facilitating change, and Schwartz, et al. (1994) describe in detail what can happen when things go awry. These and other reports illustrate the important role that context plays in selecting and combining strategies to effectively facilitate successful change. For example, Benor and Mahler (1989) describe a multiphase, developmental training program for medical teachers at Ben Gurion University (Israel) in which they reinforce the general principles of successful individual change listed previously. However, they also documented the importance of accounting for individual and institutional needs and resources, and individual needs for the pace or rate at which individuals progress toward incorporating long-lasting changes. In this study, specific change strategies that were effective included the following: (1) a strong and visible institutional commitment to supporting faculty members' roles as teachers; (2) active learning, simulations, and real-life application in program components; and (3) faculty collaboration, assessment, and ongoing coaching and feedback to accommodate the range of faculty needs. Rankin and Fox (1997) used the CBAM Stages of Concern to study how Canadian radiologists adopted innovations using survey methodology. Of the 1005 radiologists surveyed, 372 responded (37%), of whom 278 indicated that they had adopted an innovation within the preceding year. Compatibility of the innovation with current practice and perception of a clinical advantage over existing practice were reported as the most important innovation characteristics that facilitated adoption.

These reports and others (e.g., Havelock, 1975; Hord et al, 1987; Neufeld et al., 1995; Rogers, 1995) reiterate the principles of effective change facilitation and add the following points relevant to achieving a good fit between an innovation and person and environmental variables for a given context:

1. Change is influenced by characteristics of the innovation more than the characteristics of the context in which the user considers adopting the innovation (particularly in terms of benefits and costs to the individual user). However,

individuals are more likely to adopt and implement changes in practice that they perceive to fit well with existing norms and values of the local group.

2. Local champions can be significant change agents, particularly to encourage and support others' adoption and implementation of an innovation within a particular setting.

3. Innovations should be presented in ways that allow reasonable local and individual adaptation (i.e., too many restrictions on implementation will hinder individuals' willingness to adopt and stick with implementation efforts).

4. Interventions must be individualized to fit the stage of change at which an individual is operating (e.g., Stages of Concern, see Figure 3 for specific suggestions) to be effective at facilitating the process of change.

5. Monitoring and assessment throughout implementation is critical, so that individual adaptations do not deviate too far from the intended innovation and appropriate interventions can be offered to meet individual needs.

6. Change facilitators must provide continuous assistance and support to maintain an ongoing, effective balance of change and stability, and to facilitate individuals' progress toward incorporating long-lasting change. Keep in mind, too much support can cause individuals to stall, withdraw, or rely on others to move implementation forward. Similarly, too much pressure to move forward with implementation (e.g., too much change, too fast) can raise personal concerns and cause distress and frustration. Heightened and prolonged personal concerns can result in individuals either withdrawing from participation or backsliding to old patterns of behaviors and/or beliefs.

Studies reviewed in this chapter suggest that, once the innovation starts to become routine within the organization, users will be concerned with whether this new way of doing things is better and worth continuing. Change facilitators who have included evaluation processes from the onset will be able to use the results of initial implementation to support the higher Stages of Concern identified by Hall and Hord (1987). Over time, the consistent use of evaluation strategies and context-appropriate interventions similar to those shown in Figure 3 will contribute to creating a context that is conducive to change within the organization.

RECOMMENDATIONS FOR FUTURE RESEARCH

Given the recurring calls for change and the complexity of organizational and educational processes in contemporary medical education, understanding how to use the results of research and facilitate the process of change effectively within these environments is as important as assessing the outcomes and effectiveness of educational innovations. Compared to studies of change process in general education, there are fewer investigations targeting this phenomenon in medical education settings. Of the reports that are available, many reflect single-site, descriptive reports of change efforts in which the researchers were also the leaders, implementors, or participants of the target change initiative (introducing a potential for bias). Few studies of implementing change in medical education reflect theory-based studies or draw on the much larger literature base of educational change studies conducted in other settings (e.g., elementary and secondary education, higher education). Threats to internal validity and external validity are persistent concerns and there is a need to strive for comprehensive studies that utilize multivariate analyses, rigorous qualitative research, or combined quantitative-qualitative methodology. Despite these limitations, many consistent themes emerged from the literature reviewed in this chapter that can serve as an initial set of guiding principles and suggested strategies for implementing change successfully. So, where do we go from here? Below are recommendations for future research pertaining to implementing change in medical education.

Comprehensive, theory-based investigations that accommodate the complex nature of the change process are needed. Studies should reflect appropriate research design and measurement rigor, including the complementary use of quantitative and qualitative methods and adequate attention to examining potential threats to internal validity and external validity. There is a need to refine existing measures (e.g., CBAM measures) that have promise for studying the change process in medical education. There is an equally important need to develop new quantitative and qualitative instrumentation where valid and reliable measures are not available. Instrument development and refinement is an area of study related to change process that will require substantial expertise, resources, and time. Collaborative studies involving different units of analysis and multiple sites are needed to expand our conceptual frameworks for understanding the change process as it applies generally across school settings and as it is evidenced in terms of within-school idiosyncrasies. Such studies in medical schools will certainly require strong leadership; inter-institutional collaboration; and commitments of time, resources, expertise and patience, but the payoff seems worthwhile.

Medical education researchers should consider investigating the process and outcomes of change as a series of longitudinal studies. Normative, cultural change is slow and success is not always immediately apparent, but emergent some time after innovations are implemented. Educators often have only a few years within which to target change efforts, because of either organizational directives or external funding parameters. Timelines are frequently too short to realistically study the full cycle of adoption, implementation, and incorporation of innovation into everyday practice. Future reports of such efforts should argue for the need to examine educational innovations beyond the stages of initial implementation. Well-grounded arguments might facilitate extramural funding increases sufficient to support long-term investigations and follow up studies.

Medical educators are encouraged to use the professional education literature base beyond those studies in medical education settings to guide educational change initiatives and the study of change process and outcomes. Results and conclusions from studies of change in other educational environments can be used to enhance change facilitation effectiveness and to prompt the development of research questions pertaining to the various aspects of implementing change in medical education. Several research questions come to mind immediately, for which systematic studies across time and settings might reveal highly valuable insights.

For example, what individual beliefs and values influence adoption, implementation, and incorporation of innovative approaches to medical education? To what extent do other individual variables (e.g., career stage, tenure status, self-efficacy, dogmatism, receptivity to change, role orientation) influence adoption, implementation, and/or incorporation of innovation into everyday practice? What is the relationship between specific leadership behaviors and the extent to which innovations are adopted, implemented, and incorporated into everyday practice? What is the relationship between specific organizational variables and the extent to which innovations are adopted, implemented, and incorporated into everyday practice? What are the relationships between student receptivity and faculty receptivity to educational innovation, and the extent to which innovation is implemented? What is the relationship between individuals' prior experiences with change and the extent to which they adopt, implement, and incorporate innovation into their everyday practice?

Last, but not least, medical educators should seize opportunities to educate colleagues and decision makers in a variety of internal and external arenas (e.g., institutional funding agencies, regulatory agencies, professional organizations and societies) about the importance of educational research, generally, and research pertaining to change and innovation, specifically. At present the infrastructure within institutions and the extramural funding available for medical education research is limited. Because the change process is often slow and highly resource dependent, project periods and funding allocations are often insufficient to adequately design and implement educational innovations and the desired research and evaluation plans. Therefore, medical educators must seize opportunities to educate internal and external communities and decision-makers about the expertise, technical support, and financial resources that are necessary to design and implement high quality educational innovations and the corresponding research studies that are necessary.

These recommendations do not diminish the value of studies currently reported in the literature, nor should such efforts come to a screeching halt. Although the above recommendations carry with them significant challenges, these are expectations that we should strive to achieve. Of course, the realities we face are constant reminders that we must do the best we can with the resources available, and recognize publicly the limitations to our efforts as they occur. To close this chapter some general points on facilitating change that have been gleaned from the literature reviewed are here.

GUIDELINES FOR PRACTITIONERS: LINKING EDUCATIONAL RESEARCH AND PRACTICE RELATED TO INNOVATION AND CHANGE

Throughout this chapter you have had opportunities to reflect on and apply to your own situation the results of studies targeting disseminating educational research and implementing change. Grounded in a systems framework for thinking about individual change within organizations (Figure 2), guiding principles, examples, and change facilitation strategies have been gleaned from the professional literature. The points emphasized in previous sections of this chapter provide a ready set of guidelines for practitioners. This section summarizes the various principles and guidelines in terms of the Sacred Six of Facilitative Leadership (for Change) that is reflected in the work of Hord and her colleagues in the Leadership for Change project. These six elements are as follows:

1. Develop and communicate a shared vision
2. Provide resources
3. Invest in training and professional development
4. Provide continuous assistance
5. Monitor and assess progress
6. Create a context for change (results from applying the other five principles).

The above elements of facilitative leadership provide a basis for selecting and designing change strategies that can be instrumental in strategic planning, decision-making, and day-to-day tactical interventions focused on individual implementors or groups of implementors. The Stages of Concern framework that is part of the CBAM provides a useful tool for supporting and facilitating individuals' implementation of change. Although not fully described in this chapter, the Intervention Taxonomy (Hall & Hord, 1984) and other CBAM tools (e.g., Levels of Use and Innovation Configuration Matrix, Hord et al., 1987) are highly useful and complementary tools for facilitating individual and organizational level changes in a variety of educational settings worldwide. These resources are available through the Southwest Educational Development Laboratory (SEDL). Although the SEDL work currently focuses on elementary and secondary education, user manuals for the CBAM tools, information about the Leadership for Change project, and monographs related to facilitative leadership are valuable resources available through their website (http://www.sedl.org). Please consult these references and others listed below to support your learning about and efforts in disseminating educational research and implementing change effectively.

REFERENCES

Altbach, P. G. (1980). *University reform: An international perspective.* AAHE-ERIC Higher Education Research Report No. 10. Washington, DC: ERIC Clearinghouse on Higher Education, The George Washington University.

Association of American Medical Colleges. (1992). *Educating medical students: Assessing change in medical education. The road to implementation.* ACME-TRI Report. Washington, DC: Author.

Avorn, J., & Soumerai, S. B. (1983). Improving drug-therapy decisions through educational outreach. *New England Journal of Medicine, 308,* 1457-1463.

Bandura, A. (1977). *Social learning theory.* Englewood-Cliffs, NJ: Prentice Hall.

Bandura, A. (1986). *Social foundation of thought and action: Social cognitive theory.* Englewood-Cliffs, NJ: Prentice Hall.

Bennis, W. G., Benne, K. D., & Chin, R. (1969). *The planning of change.* New York: Holt, Rinehart & Winston.

Benor, D. E., & Mahler, S. (1989). Training medical teachers: Rationale and outcomes. In H. G. Schmidt, M. Lipkin, Jr., M. W. deVries, & J. M. Greep (Eds.), *New directions for medical education: Problem-based learning and community-oriented medical education* (pp. 2408-2459). New York: Springer-Verlag.

Bloom, S. W. (1988). Structure and ideology in medical education: An analysis of resistance to change. *Journal of Health and Social Behavior, 29*, 294-306.

Bloom, S. W. (1989). The medical school as a social organization: The sources of resistance to change. *Medical Education, 23*, 228-241.

Bowdish, B. E., Chauvin, S., & Vigh, S. (April 1998). Comparing student learning outcomes in hypermedia and analog assisted lectures (HAL & AAL). Paper presented at the annual meeting of the American Educational Research Association, San Diego, California.

Bussigel, M. N., Barzansky, B. M., & Grenholm, G. G. (1988). *Processes in medical education*. New York: Praeger.

Cantillon, P., & Jones, R. (1999). Does continuing medical education in general practice make a difference? *British Medical Journal, 318*, 1276-1279.

Carter, A. O., Battista, R. N., Hodge, M. J., Lewis, S., Basinski, A., & Davis, D. A. (1995). Reports on activities and attitudes of organisations active in the clinical practice guidelines field. *Canadian Medical Association Journal, 153*, 901-907.

Cavanaugh, S. H. (1993). Connecting education and practice. In L. Curry, J. Wergin, and Associates (Eds.), *Educating professionals: Responding to new expectations for competence and accountability* (pp 107-125). San Francisco: Jossey-Bass.

Chang, B. (1986). Adoption of innovations: Nursing and computer use. *Nursing Computing, 2*, 119-235.

Chauvin, S. W. (1992). An exploration of principal change facilitator style, teacher bureaucratic and professional orientations, and teacher receptivity to change. (Vols. I and II). Dissertation Abstracts International (University Microfilms Order No. 9316956).

Christakis, N. A. (1995). Implicit purposes of proposals to reform American medical education: A report written for the Acadia Institute and the Medical College of Pennsylvania Project on Undergraduate Medical Education. Philadephia, PA: Acadia Institute and Medical College of Pennsylvania.

Chute, A. G., & Hancock, B. W. (1982) Training and evaluation strategies for teleconferencing. Paper presented at the annual conference of the Association for Educational Communications and Technology, Dallas, Texas. (ERIC Document Reproduction Service No. ED 224471).

Cicchelli, T., & Baecher, R. (1989). Microcomputers in the classroom: Focusing on teacher concerns. *Computing Education, 13*, 37-46.

Cohen, J., Dannefer, E. F., Seidel, H. M., Weisman, C. S., Wexler, P., Brown, T. M., Brieger, G. H., Margolis, S., Ross, L. R., & Kunitz, S. J. (1994). Medical education change: A detailed study of six medical schools. *Medical Education, 28*, 350-360.

Cohen, M. D., & Sproull, L. S. (1996). *Organizational learning*. Thousand Oaks, CA: Sage.

Corbett, H. D., Firestone, W. A., & Rossman, G. B. (1987). Resistance to planned change and the sacred in school cultures. *Educational Administrative Quarterly, 23*(4), 36-59.

Craig, P., & Bandaranayake, R. (1993). Experiences with a method for obtaining feedback on a medical curriculum undergoing change. *Medical Education, 27*, 15-21.

Cuban, L. (1990). Reforming again, again, again, and again. *Educational Researcher, 19*(1), 3-13.

Cuban, L. (1997). Change without reform: The case of Stanford University School of Medicine, 1908-1990. *American Educational Research Journal, 34*(1), 83-122.

Cuban, L. (1999). *How scholars trumped teachers: Change without reform in university curriculum, teaching, and research, 1890-1990*. New York: Teachers College Press.

Dannefer, E. F., Johnston, M. A., & Krackov, S. K. (1998). Communication and the process of change. In S. P. Mennin & S. K Kalisman (Eds.), Issues and strategies for reform in medical education: Lessons from eight medical schools. *Academic Medicine, 73*(9), S16-S23.

Davis, D. A. (1998). Does CME work? An analysis of the effect of educational activities on physician performance or health care outcomes. *International Journal of Psychiatry and Medicine, 28*(1), 21-39.

Davis, D. A., Thomson, M. A., Oxman, A. D., & Haynes, R. B. (1992). Evidence for the effectiveness of CME: A review of 50 randomized controlled trials. *Journal of the American Medical Association, 268*(9), 1111-1117.

Davis, W. K., & White, B. (1993). Centralized decision making in management of the curriculum at the University of Michigan Medical School. *Academic Medicine, 68*(5), 333-335.

DesMarchais, J. E., Bureau, M. A., Dumais, B., & Pigeon, G. (1992). From traditional to problem-based learning: A case report of complete curriculum reform. *Medical Education, 26*, 190-199.

Dunn, E. V., Norton, P. G., Stewart, M., Tudiver, F., & Bass, M. J. (1994). *Disseminating research/changing practice,* Vol. 6 in *Research methods for primary care series*. Thousand Oaks, CA: Sage.

Evans, C., Haynes, R., & Birkett, N. (1986). Does a mailed continuing education program improve physician performance? *Journal of the American Medical Association, 225*, 501-504.

Evans, R. L., & Chauvin, S. W. (1993). Faculty developers as change facilitators: The concerns-based adoption model. In D. L. Wright & J. P. Lunde (Eds.), *To improve the academy* (pp. 165-178). Stillwater, OK: New Forums Press.

Evans, R. L., and Teddlie, C. (1993). Facilitating change: Is there one best style? Paper presented at the annual conference of the American Educational Research Association, Atlanta, GA.

Fox, R. D. (1990). Lessons from the Change Study: A case for collaborative research in continuing medical education. *Teaching and Learning in Medicine, 2*(3), 126-129.

Fox, R. D., & Bennett, N. L. (1998). Continuing medical education: Learning and change: Implications for continuing medical education. *British Medical Journal, 316*, 466-468.

Fox, R. D., Mazmanian, P. E., & Putnam, R. W. (Eds.) (1989). *Change and learning in the lives of physicians.* New York: Praeger.

Friedman, R. B. (1996). Top ten reasons the World Wide Web may fail to change medical education. *Academic Medicine, 71*(9), 79-81.

Fullan, M. (1993). *Change forces: Probing the depths of educational reform.* London: Falmer Press.

Fullan, M. (1999). *Change forces: The sequel.* London: Falmer Press.

Fuller, F. F. (1969). Concerns of teachers: A developmental conceptualization. *American Educational Research Journal, 6*(2), 207-226.

Gerrity, M. S., & Mahaffy, J. (1998). Evaluating change in medical school curricula: How did we know where we were going? In S. P. Mennin & S. K Kalisman (Eds.), Issues and strategies for reform in medical education: Lessons from eight medical schools. *Academic Medicine, 73*(9), S55-S59.

Getzels, J. W., & Guba, E. G. (1957). Social behavior and the administrative process. *School Review, 65*, 423-441.

Giacquinta, J. B. (1975a). Status, risk, and receptivity to innovation in complex organizations: A study of the responses of four groups of educators to the proposed introduction of sex education in elementary school. *Sociology of Education, 48*, 38-58.

Giacquinta, J. B. (1975b). Status risk-taking: A central issue in the initiation and implementation of public school innovations. *Journal of Research and Development in Education, 9*(1), 102-114.

Hall, G. E., & Hord, S. M. (1984). Analyzing what change facilitators do: The intervention taxonomy. *Knowledge: Creation, Diffusion, Utilization, 5*(3), 275-307.

Hall, G. E., & Hord, S. M. (1987). *Change in schools: Facilitating the process.* New York: State University of New York Press.

Hall, G. E., George, A., & Rutherford, W. L. (1979). *Measuring Stages of Concern about the innovation: A manual for use of the SoC questionnaire* (Report No. 3032). Austin: University of Texas at Austin, Research and Development Center for Teacher Education. (ERIC Document Reproduction Service No. ED 147 342).

Hall, G. E., Wallace, R. C., & Dossett, W. A. (1973). *A developmental conceptualization of the adoption process within educational institutions* (Report No. 3006). Austin: University of Texas at Austin, Research and Development Center for Teacher Education. (ERIC Document Reproduction Service No. ED 095 126).

Harvey, T. R. (1990). *Checklist for change: A pragmatic approach to creating and controlling change.* Boston, MA: Allyn & Bacon.

Havelock, R. G. (1975). *The change agent's guide to innovation in education.* Englewood Cliffs, NJ: Educational Technology Publications.

Haynes, R. B., Davis, D. A., McKibbon, A., & Tugwell, P. (1984). A critical appraisal of the efficacy of continuing medical education. *Journal of the American Medical Association, 251*(1), 61-64.

Hord, S. M. (1997). *Professional learning communities: Communities of continuous inquiry and improvement.* Austin, Texas: Southwest Educational Development Laboratory.

Hord, S. M., Rutherford, W. L., Huling-Austin, L., & Hall, G. (1987). *Taking charge of change.* Alexandria, VA: Association for Supervision and Curriculum Development.

Hoy, W. K., & Miskel, C. G. (1987). *Educational administration: Theory, research and practice* (3rd ed.), New York: Random House.

Jolly, B., & Grant, J. (1997). *The good assessment guide.* London: Joint Centre for Education in Medicine.

Kanter, R. M., Stein, B. A., & Jick, T. D. (1993). *The challenge of organizational change.* New York: Free Press.

Kaslow, C. (1974). Resistance to innovations in complex organizations: A test of two models of resistance in a higher education setting. Dissertation Abstracts International, 3130A-3131A (University Microfilms No. 74-24, 999).

Kaufman, A. (1998). Leadership and governance. In S. P. Mennin & S. K Kalisman (Eds.), Issues and strategies for reform in medical education: Lessons from eight medical schools. *Academic Medicine, 73*(9), S11-S15.

Kerbeshian, L. A. (1986). *A curriculum evaluation using the stakeholder approach as a change strategy.* ERIC Document ED 295 997.

Kosecoff, J., Kanouse, D., Rogers, W., McCloskey, L., Winslow, C., & Brook, R. (1987). Effects of the National Institutes of Health Consensus Development Program on physician practice. *Journal of the American Medical Association, 258*, 2708-2713.

Kotter, J. P. (1996). *Leading change.* Cambridge, MA: Harvard Business School Press.

Lave, J., & Wenger, E. (1990). *Situated learning: Legitimate peripheral participation.* Cambridge, UK: Cambridge University Press.

Lewis, D., & Watson, J. E. (1997). Nursing faculty concerns regarding the adoption of computer technology. *Computers in Nursing, 13*(2), 71-76.

Levine, A. (1980). *Why innovation fails.* Albany, NY: State University of New York Press.

Lewin, K. (1947). Frontiers in group dynamics. *Human Relations, 1*, 5-41.

Lewin, K. (1951). *Field theory in social science.* New York: Harper & Brothers.

Lindberg, M. A. (1998). The process of change: Stories of the journey. In S. P. Mennin & S. K Kalisman (Eds.), Issues and strategies for reform in medical education: Lessons from eight medical schools. *Academic Medicine, 73*(9), S4-S10.

Lofton, G. G., Ellett, C., Hill, F., & Chauvin, S. (1998). Five years after implementation: The role of the district in maintaining an ongoing school improvement process. *School Effectiveness and School Improvement, 9*(1), 58-69.

Lomas, J. (1994). Teaching old (and not so old) docs new tricks: Effective ways to implement research findings. In E. V. Dunn, P. G. Norton, M. Stewart, F. Tudiver, & M. J. Bass (Eds.), *Disseminating research/changing practice,* Vol. 6 in *Research methods for primary care series* (pp. 1- 18). Thousand Oaks, CA: Sage.

Lomas, J., Anderson, G. M., Dominick-Pierre, K., Vayda, E., Enkin, M. W., & Hannah, W. J. (1989). Do practice guidelines guide practice? The effect of a consensus statement on the practice of physicians. *New England Journal of Medicine, 321*(19), 1306-1311.

Ludmerer, K. (1985). *Learning to heal.* New York: Basic Books.

McKinlay, J. B. (1981). From "promising report" to "standard procedure": Seven stages in the career of a medical innovation. *Milbank Memorial Fund Quarterly/Health and Society, 59*(3).

McLaughlin, M. W., & Marsh, D. D. (1978, September). Staff development and school change. *Teachers College Record*, 69-94.

Mennin, S. P., & Kalishman, S. (1998). Issues and strategies for reform in medical education: Lessons from eight medical schools [Supplement]. *Academic Medicine, 73*(9), S46-54.

Mennin, S. P., & Kaufman, A. (1989). The change process and medical education. *Medical Teacher, 11*(1), 9-16.

Mennin, S. P., Friedman, M., & Woodward, C. A. (1992). Evaluating innovative medical education programmes: Common questions and problems. *Annals of Community-Oriented Education, 5*, 123-133.

Moran, J. A., Kirk, P., & Kopelow, M. (1996). Measuring the effectiveness of a pilot continuing medical education program. *Canadian Family Physician, 42*, 272-276.

Mort, P. R. (1958). Educational adaptability. In D. H. Ross (Ed.), *Administration for adaptability.* New York: Metropolitan School Study Council.

Mort, P. R., & Ross, D. H. (1957). *Principles of school administration.* New York: McGraw-Hill.

Neufeld, V., Khanna, S., Bramble, L., & Simpson, J. (1995). *Leadership for change in the education of health professionals.* Maastricht, The Netherlands: Network Publications.

Newman, A. (1994). Additional dividends of curriculum change. *Academic Medicine, 69*(2), 127.

Owens, R. G. (1987). *Organizational behavior in education* (3rd ed.). Englewood Cliffs, NJ: Prentice-Hall.

Owens, R. G., & Steinhoff, C. R. (1976). *Administering change in schools.* Englewood Cliffs, NJ: Prentice-Hall.

Papa, F. J., & Harasym, P. H. (1999). Medical curriculum reform in North America. 1765 to present: A cognitive science perspective. *Academic Medicine, 74*(2), 154-164.

Rankin, R. N., & Fox, R. D. (1997). How Canadian radiologists adopt innovations: A survey. *Canadian Association of Radiology Journal, 48*(5-6), 313-322.

Rogers, E. M. (1995). *Diffusion of innovations* (4th ed.). New York: Free Press.

Rotem, A. (1992). Evaluation to improve educational programmes. *Annals of Community-Oriented Education, 5*, 135-141.

Rubeck, R. F., & Witzke, D. B. (1998). Faculty development: A field of dreams. In S. P. Mennin & S. K Kalisman (Eds.), Issues and strategies for reform in medical education: Lessons from eight medical schools. *Academic Medicine, 73*(9), S32-S37.

Sanders, J. R. (1994). *The program evaluation standards: How to assess evaluations of educational programs* (2nd ed.). Thousand Oaks, CA: Sage.

Schatzer, J. H. (1998). Instructional methods. In S. P. Mennin & S. K. Kalisman (Eds.), Issues and strategies for reform in medical education: Lessons from eight medical schools. *Academic Medicine, 73*(9), S38-S45.

Schein, E. H. (1992). *Organizational culture and leadership* (2nd ed.) San Francisco, CA: Jossey Bass.

Schwartz, P. L., Health, C. J., & Egan, A. G. (1994). *The art of the possible: Ideas for a traditional medical school engaged in curricular revision.* Dunedin, New Zealand: University of Otago Press.

Schwartz, P. L., Loten, E. G., & Miller, A P. (1999). Curriculum reform at the University of Otago Medical School. *Academic Medicine, 74*(6), 675-679.

Senge, P. M. (1990). *The fifth discipline: The art and practice of the learning organization.* New York: Doubleday.

Snyder, J. R. (1983). Managerial intervention to facilitate organizational change. *American Journal of Medical Technology, 49*(7), 513-518.

Teddlie, C., & Stringfield, S. (1993). *Schools make a difference: Lessons learned from a ten-year study of school effects.* New York: Teachers College Press.

Tosteson, D. (1990). New pathways in general medical education. *New England Journal of Medicine, 322,* 234-238.

Wheatley, M. J. (1994). *Leadership and the new science: Learning about organization from an orderly universe.* San Francisco, CA: Berrett-Koehler Publishers.

Wheatley, M. J., & Kellner-Rogers, M. (1999). *A simpler way.* San Francisco, CA: Berrett-Koehler.

Wilkerson, L. (1994). Ideas for medical education. *Academic Medicine, 69*(3), 190.

Wilkes, M. S., Slavin, S. J., & Usatine, R. (1994). Doctoring: A longitudinal generalist curriculum. *Academic Medicine, 69*(3), 191-193.

Woodward, C. A. (1992). Some reflections on evaluation of outcomes of innovative medical education programmes during the practice period. *Annals of Community-Oriented Education, 5,* 181-191.

33   Achieving Large-Scale Change In Medical Education

LYNN CURRY

CurryCorp

SUMMARY

"The problem is the reconciliation of unbridled radicalism and inert conservatism into reasonable reform". (Dewey, 1898)

INTRODUCTION

Human beings are a questing lot. The idea of finding "a better way" has motivated mankind across cultures, time, space and adversity. All areas of human knowledge have benefited from this drive to know more, to predict more accurately, to act more effectively and to produce more efficiently. This increase in human capacity has not been achieved in a smooth ascending curve. There are irregular intercept jumps corresponding to new understandings, more useful paradigms or wider generalization from previous knowledge. We are living during one such "intercept jump" characterized by significant new capacities in biology (i.e. genomics) and in informatics (i.e. the Internet). This chapter makes the case that these accomplishments and others portend radical change in the form, function and content of medical education.

We are also a social species. We organize into collectivities and we create institutions to carry out functions on behalf of society at large. Institutions are regularly formed and reformed to follow changes in social needs and human capability. The pressures for institutional adjustment may wax and wane, and may require implementation of small or large-scale modifications, but the requirements for adjustments are ubiquitous and inexorable. The question is not whether social institutions will change, but how frequently and by how much.

Medical schools are one such socially sensitive institution. The societal function fulfilled by medical schools has existed from the beginning of medicine: to provide a reliable supply of suitably trained physicians to replace those individuals currently in practice serving the health needs of society. To date, the responsibility to satisfy the social demand for new physicians has been entrusted solely to the profession of

1039

International Handbook of Research in Medical Education, 1039–1084.
G.R. Norman, C.P.M. Van der Vleuten, D.I. Newble (eds.)
© *2002 Dordrecht: Kluwer Academic Publishers. Printed in Great Britain.*

medicine. This is one of the responsibilities in the social contract that medicine, like other professions, have with the society they serve. In exchange for the right to decide who will be allowed to enter the profession, as well as the means and conditions of that entry, the profession undertakes to train those chosen individuals to standards defined by the profession and to guarantee that anyone legitimately awarded professional status is competent to serve society in that capacity. Society at large enforces this contract with significant sanctions against anyone purporting to practice a profession without status attested to by that profession. For example, "practicing medicine without a license" is a prosecutable offence in most of the developed world.

Medical schools slowly come to reflect significant gains in human knowledge and capacity by making constant small adjustments in pertinent areas. The initial scientific breakthroughs in bacteriology were eventually reflected in professional medicine and medical schools. That quantum gain in human knowledge had many effects, one of which was to provide the practice of medicine with a scientific base, increasing both the predictability and efficacy of medical interventions. Writing in 1915 Cabot described this shift:

> The "big men" of twenty years ago, had without exception, gone through the school of general practice and had risen from the ranks to eminence by sheer force of character, being largely without assistance of the laboratory, and having fewer instruments of precision than we possess. They had trained their faculties of observation in the hard school of experience and had come to rely far more than we do today upon their individual judgment, unsupported by clearly demonstrable fact. They were more astute judges of men, with a larger comprehension of the strength and weakness of human nature and a wider sympathy. They were characterized by a certain boldness less seen today, bred of the necessity of staking their reputations upon much less certain evidence. They seem to me to have been broader-minded, and rather more in touch with affairs other than those of medicine. Their devotion to the ideals of medicine I believe to have been more profound. *(p. 65).*

Thus the emphasis on the quality of the human interaction in the provision of care became increasingly overshadowed by the importance of correctly understanding, interpreting and employing the relevant science. As a consequence, the medical school changed significantly from an apprenticeship model to one that could more easily guarantee sufficient exposure to the requisite sciences. The Flexnerian (1910) revolution in medical education codified this trend by requiring that all medical education take place in research universities and be composed of two years of "basic medical sciences", taught by scientists currently engaged in research in these "basic" sciences, before any clinical application or exposure to clinicians would be allowed.

The structure for medical education promulgated by Flexner satisfied social needs for increasing standardization of medical graduates and brought together a sufficiently strong constellation of interests to be both initially cohesive and self-sustaining within the medical profession. The Flexnerian structure for medical education has been replicated across the world and has remained essentially unchanged from that time. Such is the resiliency of that entrenched organizational model that new educational technologies (i.e. "problem-based" medical curricula) can be accommodated within the standard medical school structures without change to the operative divisions by academic discipline or between basic and clinical sciences.

This comfortable equilibrium in medical schools is, however, likely to destabilize over the next decade. The limits of the organizational resiliency within medical schools to maintain the current structure will be challenged by a massive reformation that is occurring in our capabilities and in our expectations. These social changes, outlined in the next section, are sufficiently fundamental to impinge directly on medical schools as individual and collective organizations. In response to these pressures, new organizational structures with corresponding new functions will transform medical education. Again, the question is not whether, but how soon and by how much. Perhaps more important is a second level question: what can we do to participate in shaping this transformation?

IMMINENT LARGE-SCALE CHANGE IN MEDICAL EDUCATION

Many of the following signs and symptoms of impending large-scale change have been noted for some time in the literature (for example, Inglehart, 1997; MacLeod, 1997). These and other authors have repeatedly documented the following forces for significant change in the nature, structure and content of medical education:
1. Internal and external dissatisfaction with the system
2. Increased challenge in practice scope
3. Shifts in primary stakeholders: physicians
4. Shifts in secondary stakeholders: patient/clients
5. Success of new models for higher and professional education
6. Development of alternate models for medical education
7. Informatics technology supporting increased access to information.

Internal and external dissatisfaction with medical schools

Both the mission and the mandate of medical education are being actively questioned from inside the profession and by society. There are increasingly vocal complaints from practitioners about the result, the process and the content of initial professional education and training. Medical students are becoming more organized and are lobbying locally and nationally for guarantees that their education will be "relevant" on graduation, that they will be employable in their preferred locations and specialties. Medical schools are being challenged by students to justify all aspects of the training: the content, the process, the structure, the timing and the cost.

There is much debate within the medical disciplines, sometimes in contradictory directions, about the most appropriate structure for the knowledge and skill base and the format for delivery of that knowledge and skill to the public. One form of this pressure for structural change is the perennial debate about generalization versus specialization in discipline-based knowledge and skills. For example, in North America the discipline of pathology divided in the 1980s into anatomical, forensic and laboratory pathology. Each required a specialized course of studies, separate examinations and separate certifications. Now the separate fields are re-generalizing, perhaps in part due to the fact that the employment market is very narrow for sub-specialized pathologists, but adequate for general pathologists. Similar pressures are seen in surgery and internal medicine. Worldwide, the biggest defined need for physicians is for general practitioners (WHO, 1966).

The public, acting through their agents in elected and public office, is showing significant signs of dissatisfaction with current medical school structures. In the United States most states have restricted university education budgets for the last decade and recently many states have enacted balanced budget legislation. The effect of these measures has been to effectively remove almost all direct government subsidies for higher education including medicine. All higher education, including medicine, reacted by passing more costs along to students. As that strategy began to produce negative results (such as a dwindling applicant pool), the search began for opportunities to create new revenue streams such as catering to industrial research partners, training foreign students on contract and aggressively entering the health care provision market. Medical schools sought to control referral chains by buying the practices of independent physicians, particularly general practitioners. Corporate mergers were undertaken to control geographic segments of the managed care market. These revenue enhancing strategies have been less than successful, at least partially because state and federal governments have attempted to control costs in health care.

The costs of health care are of grave concern throughout the world. Economic analyses (e.g. Evans & Stoddard, 1990) indicate an inverse relationship in the developed world between social spending on provision of health care and indicators of health status at a population level (i.e. premature mortality, infant mortality, low birth weight babies). This effect has been documented by the Organization for Economic Cooperation and Development (OECD, 1999) across 23 countries. Only in countries that currently spend very little on health care (such as Mexico where less than $500US is spent on health care per person per year) would an increase in health care spending result in increased population health. Countries with currently higher rates of spending on health care provision, such as Canada at $2200US and the USA with $4000US per person each year, would receive almost no increase in population health status from increases in spending on health care.

Given those results, government office holders acting for the public across many countries have tried various means to control the costs of health care provision. In Canada the monopsony power of governments, derived from their role as the only source and payer of hospital and medical care, allows relatively direct control over both the costs (i.e. drug costs, physician costs) and the utilization of costly interventions (i.e. MRIs). As costs grow within restricted budgets, Canadian governments restrict the rate of growth in both costs and access to interventions. These dual restrictions have immediate negative effects on Canadian medical schools from uncompetitive salaries for faculty to vastly increased acuity in teaching hospitals. In the US this cost containment is seen in the significant reductions in direct government support for health care programs (i.e. Medicare and Medicaid) and a sharp increase in government tolerance for the aggressive cost-cutting measures taken by privately funded programs. These measures have severely restricted revenues to medical schools from health care provision.

Attempts to increase medical school revenues through other sources have been similarly problematic. The successful training of foreign students requires more faculty and administrative support than usual and thus nets fewer dollars than expected. Revenues from industrial research partners or government grants and contracts tend to be increasingly directed towards very specific research issues, personnel and processes. In addition to this curtailing and forced shaping of interest-based research, the increased importance of private enterprise research funding has had further negative effects. Blumenthal et al. (1997) reported that 20% of surveyed faculty members delayed publication of at least one study for at least six months to serve proprietary needs. Results that are negative or unfavorable are less likely to be published when research is sponsored by private industry (Stelfox et al., 1998; Friedberg et al., 1999; Bodenheimer, 2000). Both effects are the result of researcher conflict of interest, violate the basic tenets of science and imperil the public trust. Added to the already myriad methods of industry influence in academic medical centers, the general effect is a threat to the integrity of these institutions, the professionals within them, and the medical profession as a whole (Angell, 2000).

The public, and their agents in government, have poorly understood medical schools and academic medical centers, at least partly due to the confused rhetoric put out by these medical centers and the mismatch between the objectives stated by academic medical centers and the observable actions taken. Richard Lamm, former Governor of Colorado writes:

> Academic health centres have their place in the health care system, but they are also fiscal black holes into which society can pour endless resources and often get little in return. – For 12 years as governor of Colorado, I listened to self-serving statements from our medical centre, which did little or nothing about our major health challenges: increasing primary care; expanding coverage to the uninsured; dealing with smoking, alcohol abuse, dietary excesses, and deficits; non-medical drugs; and violence. Their biomedical model had little room for the chronic degenerative diseases that are the predominant health issues of the elderly. *(Science, 1993, p. 1497)*

In summary, medical schools provide high cost education in circumstances where those high costs are no longer being met. Either costs will have to be reduced or revenue increased to sustain the current structure. All obvious mechanisms to do the latter have been implemented without solving the shortfall. The biggest portion of any education budget is faculty costs. Therefore, reducing faculty costs would be the most effective way to reduce overall costs in medical education. However, any significant change in faculty numbers will require a major change in the structure and function of the medical school. For example, in many North American medical schools the clinical earnings of faculty significantly subsidize the costs of medical education (practice earnings are often pooled and redeployed to satisfy departmental needs including education). This is rationalized in part because the apprenticeship nature of medical training allows faculty significant delegation latitude to students at varying levels of training. Clinical faculty members, for example, are not often seen in the on-call rota. Reducing faculty numbers would, at least, force recalibration of work and reappraisal of the true displacement cost of medical education on a departmental basis. It remains to be seen whether clinicians will continue to be willing to participate in cross-subsidizing departmental practice plans when their personal incomes are squeezed by the paying agencies. Pardes (1997, 2000) argues convincingly that American clinical faculty may not be eager to use clinical revenue to cross subsidize medical education given the likely context of bankruptcies, massive deficits, layoffs and merger dissolutions that will follow the negative balance sheets seen in 60% to 70% of US hospitals (Lewin Group, 2000).

Challenges to traditional scope of practice

The scope of practice in medicine has expanded exponentially to match the growth in medical capability. New medical sub-disciplines are being invented annually and compete for medical personnel through the creation and funding of residencies and related research programs. Even during the period (1980 to 1995) of substantial increase in the number of medical graduates produced (49% in Canada [*Globe & Mail*, 1999] and 62% in the US [Finocchio et al., 1995]), there was active competition among specialties for new personnel. Medical schools in North America were downsized during the latter half of the decade, so the competition has only increased.

One of the side effects of this competition among medical disciplines for personnel has been that some areas of medicine do not attract replacement physicians in sufficient numbers to meet social obligations for service provision. Areas such as pregnancy, delivery and well baby care, foot care for diabetics, geriatric monitoring, primary care in specialized populations (for example, the homeless, the indigent, the home-bound) are perennially short of medical manpower. Health care agencies have recognized the cost of not providing early and preventative care to each of these populations and in the absence of physicians have legitimized alternate providers: midwives, advanced practice nurses, podiatrists and community care workers. This trend is perceived with alarm from within medicine, particularly as evidence accumulates indicating that results obtained by these alternative providers are equal to or better than those obtained by physicians (for example, Koch, Pazaki, & Campbell, 1992; Mitchell et al., 1993; and Hylka & Beschle, 1995).

What is the appropriate response from medical schools to this erosion in control of practice scope? A number of possible responses would be legitimate measures to meet the social contract: the schools could insure that replacement medical personnel are available in these underserved areas; they could incorporate the training of the alternative providers within the medical school; or they could restructure the training of physicians to cede this practice scope to the other providers and teach appropriate interactions with them. Any of these responses represents a significant change in the medical school structure, values, curricula and operations.

Shifts in the primary stakeholders: physicians

For the past two decades increasing numbers of women have entered medical training. At present fully half of the physicians under the age of 35 in Canada are female. This gender rebalancing is perceived to have positive effects: the majority (79%) of physicians believe that patients will benefit from the increase in counseling associated with female physicians' practice. Ninety-two percent of female and 72% of male physicians shared that opinion (*Medical Post*, 1998). This expectation appears to be supported in differential patient outcomes. Younger women general practitioners were more effective in lowering the rate of teenage pregnancies in their practices than were male physicians of any age (Hippisley-Cox et al., 2000). This effect was attributed to provision of more effective counseling.

In addition to changing the content of their practices, women are changing the structure of practice as well. Historically women physicians have worked fewer hours per week than their male colleagues (Powers, Parmella, & Wisenfelder, 1976; Kehrer, 1976; Heins et al., 1977; Gray, 1980; Bobula, 1980; Day, 1982). This pattern continues: in 1999 women physicians in Canada worked an average of nine hours less each week than did their male counterparts (*Globe & Mail*, 1999). Male physicians in Canada now work an average of 2426 hours annually (*Globe & Mail*, 1999), one third more than average male earners. Female physicians work 1970 hours, 43% more than the average for female workers in Canada. Women physicians were also three times more likely than male physicians to work part time (*Globe & Mail*, 1999), a pattern documented by other observers over the past thirty years. This configuration of part-time work and fewer hours has long been attributed to the conflicts women physicians must manage among their competing primary roles of physician, wife and mother (Johnson & Johnson, 1976; Levinson, Tolle, & Lewis, 1989 and Cooper, Rout, & Faragher, 1989). The effects of these role conflicts continue as well: Woodward, Cohen, & Ferrier (1990) report that becoming a parent had no effect on the practice patterns of male physicians but was associated with a significant reduction of working hours for women physicians. Studying gender roles and family pressure among British physicians Dumelow et al. (2000) found that 15% of female physicians as opposed to only 3% of male physicians chose to live single or divorced and childless as a consequence of their careers. Thirty percent of female physicians and 12% of male physicians significantly restricted their work involvement to allow more time for family roles. The majority of physicians (55% of female physicians and 85% of male physicians) try to manage both full-time careers and family roles.

So, in general the higher percentage of women in medical practice indicates steadily fewer hours of available medical expertise. These effects are not predictably linear however. Partly due to a more generalized desire for better-balanced lifestyles, average total work hours have been dropping for both male and female physicians over the past decades. In fact male physicians have reduced their work hours by a significantly higher percentage than have female physicians (14% versus 2% fewer hours in 1999 [*Globe & Mail*] than in 1969 [Powers, Parmella, & Wisenfelder, 1976]). Regardless of the cause, less physician availability has implications for medical manpower planning and will contribute to the substitution rate of other health care professionals in any and all releasable aspects of the medical scope of practice. Demand for more physician services may lead to an increase in medical school entering class size, but the degree of matching financial support will be questionable. Equally likely are other solutions such as increased use of foreign medical graduates and tightly focused training programs to produce physician-like skills in narrow targeted areas.

Also associated with managing their role conflicts, women physicians have tended to practice in hospital settings or in institutional situations with fixed salaries and fixed hours (Wilson, 1979). The higher percentage of women in medical practice, all seeking stability, predictability and controllability in their work life in order to better manage their other roles, has provided willing staff for a range of formerly novel financial arrangements. Salaried physicians, for example, are essential to the community clinic models in North America.

Female physicians have been less inclined to join medical professional organizations (Relman, 1980). This lack of involvement is at least part of the reason that organized medicine now represents less than 50% of practicing physicians in Canada or in the USA. This reality narrows the points of view available within organized medicine and thus hampers policy formation. Being less representative makes medical organizations less relevant. It also makes organized medicine less powerful in renegotiating the social contract. Individual paying agencies are therefore much more successful in negotiating variances with local physicians irrespective of positions taken by national or regional medical professional associations. Some of the variances currently in place as pilot programs will be adopted more widely as cost saving measures: capitated funding for identified practices; consolidation of sole practitioners into larger groups supported by alternative health care providers.

Lastly, there appears to be a gender difference in how physicians learn (Curry, 1991) when they are given the freedom to choose methods as occurs in continuing medical education. Male and female physicians also have different patterns of cognitive style (Curry, 1991) indicating that rigidly structured learning situations, such as most medical schools, systematically disadvantage one gender or the other most of the time.

In sum, the fact that female physicians will shortly form half of the available medical personnel is a profound pressure for change in medical education, medical professional organization, and the structure for delivery of medical care and remuneration for that care.

Shifts in secondary stakeholders: the public

A broader base of society is educated, even well educated. A much wider segment of the population has direct and sustained access to what was "guild" information a generation ago (MacLellan, 1998). Increased information availability has provided interested patient/clients the access to study symptoms, conditions, treatments and the exotica of risk-benefit studies in significant detail. Patient/clients are routinely able to seek alternative opinions, medical and otherwise, from across the globe. The Cochrane Collaboration (http://hiru.mcmaster.ca/cochrane) has been explicitly established as an international organization to encourage *"clinicians and consumers to work together, mainly through the internet, to design, conduct, report, disseminate and criticize systematic reviews in all areas of health care"* (Jadad, 1999, p. 761).

One result of this equalization of access to medical knowledge has been the democratization of medical action and intervention. Citizens now have the access to educate themselves as narrowly or as broadly as they might wish to, and are acting on that knowledge. Insisting on equal status for their own knowledge in their interactions with physicians and with the health care system, citizens are making their own diagnoses and initiating their own treatments. This phenomenon has been noted for some time in over the counter (OTC) remedies, the use of herbs and the use of alternative therapies, all of which has been enhanced by the race among pharmacies to have a sales presence on the Internet (Zoeller, 1999). Now, however, even prescription drugs are obtainable over the Internet with questionable, if any, medical input (Bloom, 1999; Larkin, 1999; *PJ* 1999 and 2000). Pharmaceutical firms have responded to this self-diagnosis and self-intervention trend with direct to consumer advertising (Pirisi, 1999; Levy, 1999). *Business & Health* (1998) reports on the success of this direct advertising tactic: eight of ten physicians write a prescription for the requested drug. Furthermore, they state that consumers with drug plans are less likely to accept generic substitutes.

The "baby-boomers" and all subsequent generations have developed relationships to authority differently than did the generations that went before them. People now have less automatic respect for authority figures of all kinds; they are more likely to question and even openly challenge authority. This widely observed change has representation in patient/client attitude and approach to interaction with their physicians. Patient/clients now expect, unless they specifically request otherwise, to be primary decision makers in all matters of health care for themselves and their families. This attitude places all health care professionals in consulting roles and requires them to be patient-centered in a much broader way. Patient autonomy now requires responsibility to be taken by providers of care for what the whole health care system has, or has not, delivered and the specific outcomes obtained by each patient/client, including their degree of satisfaction with the health care system and the outcomes they obtained. Most medical curricula do not currently prepare physicians for that role.

This shift away from deference to health care authority might be expected to produce more patient/client self-responsibility for health status. But, because patient/clients are not generally health economists, this self-responsibility is often ill informed and counter-productive. For example, when faced with a low-level health situation (any perceived health crises will go directly to hospital emergency rooms) and a bureaucratized delivery system in a social context that emphasizes choice and convenience, a growing proportion of patient/clients utilize the "quick medicine" options such as walk-in clinics. This pattern results in less continuity of care and foregoes the opportunity to build truly supportive relationships with a health care team of providers. It also costs more, both directly to the patient/client at the time of use and indirectly to the patient/client through increased premiums or increased taxes to maintain the rest of the health care system. Because there is no central medical record system that follows the client, all tests are repeated, further escalating costs and increasing risk.

We live in an era of assessment and accountability that affects all segments of society. This is a positive development if it leads to increased information flow to inform decision making at all levels, including that of patient/clients. If, however, the emphasis on assessment and accountability produces only simplistic data compilation and unreasonable comparisons, then neither the patient/clients, the health care providers, education systems nor society at large has gained anything worth the massive increase in costs involved to collect and analyze ineffective data.

These and other social changes are forcing renegotiation of the social contract held by the profession of medicine with society and with its members. The renegotiation is occurring at the level of individual patient/client interactions with professionals, student interactions with educators and staff and student or user interaction with administrators. The renegotiation is also occurring at collective levels in the legislative, policy and regulatory processes by which society periodically codifies its values. All of this presents a direct and significant challenge to the structure and function of medical schools and medical education.

Success of new models for higher and professional education

Consumer pressure and new technical capabilities are producing other models of higher and professional education that will have significant impact on medical education. In 1997 Traub described the exponential growth of "distance learning" programs offered by a range of organizations, some of which are licensed as higher education institutions. Described as "para-universities" they operate without tenured professors, without campuses and without libraries. They do, however, have students, teachers, classrooms, examinations and degree granting programs. The students are primarily working adults. Teachers are predominantly from practice, not academic or research settings. Courses are compressed in time, are often offered in the evenings or on weekends in convenient sites or over the Internet. Examinations for content knowledge are provided via computer in secure sites allowing authentication. Practical examinations are conducted in dispersed practical settings under the supervision of a practice mentor or examiner. The degrees granted are often not in traditional academic graduate career tracks, but are used to directly advance employment.

Corporations (e.g. Motorola in Tempe, AZ and General Motors in Detroit) establish extensive programs like these to efficiently educate and motivate their own workforce. Others are set up as frankly profit-making institutions (e.g. the University of Phoenix in the US) as non-profit independent institutions (e.g. Athabaska University in Canada, and the Open University in the UK) or as profit-making sections of traditional universities. Within each of these ownership models the focus remains on improving practice in some field of applied work. During the 1990s, a decade that saw the closure of traditional colleges and enrollment erosion in many others, the demand for this alternate model continues to grow exponentially. For-profit degree programs continue to proliferate, although to date they have been self-confined to the areas of commerce and technology (e.g. the new Unexus University's Executive Masters of Business Administration owned and operated by Learnsoft Corp, announced in the February 18th 2000 *Financial Post*). The growth cannot be attributed to lower costs as the cost per credit in these programs ranges from $500 to $1000US for a total of $15,000 to $35,000 for a degree. This range is higher than the majority of traditional degree programs in similar content. The advantages that attract increasing numbers of students are the shortened training time, the practical focus, the state-of-the-art equipment and the increased interaction provided by the personalized course structures and the technology that supports those structures.

Informatics capabilities have allowed development of another alternate model with implications for medical education: World Wide Web-based access to information with and without interaction. US high tech billionaire Michael Saylor has recently launched one such model. Saylor will establish a free Internet university to offer *"an 'Ivy League' education online to anyone in the world at no cost"* (*Ottawa Citizen*, March 16th 2000). The model is built upon a cyberlibrary of videotaped lectures to be provided pro bono by thousands of leading educators and great thinkers. The Web would also supply FAQs (frequently asked questions) and examinations. While agreeing that the technical capacity exists to support this venture, *Science (*2000) questions the willingness of the invited speakers to participate on a pro bono basis as was initially suggested. Even if some sort of licensing or access fee is required to remunerate lecturers, this model offers learners anywhere the opportunity to learn from the best in the world in any field at any time.

Other more focused Web-based information repositories (see the NetWatch section of any *Science* issue) provide graduated levels of information and links to related repositories and topics. Many of these sources offer a range of additional features including on-line chat rooms and monitored listservs that allow users to query experts and other users. How long can it be until some collection of these information sources and services are organized into sequences similar to the content coverage in medical schools? How long after that will it take for one or more entrepreneurial universities or medical schools to recognize a market opportunity and offer a partnership arrangement exchanging its degree-granting capacity for some share of revenues?

Development of alternate models for medical education

The development of alternate models for medical education has historically taken an evolutionary course. Early reform efforts are reviewed in the following section.

More recently the Association of American Medical Colleges (AAMC) sponsored two rounds of self-reflection within the North American medical school community designed to develop new models for medical education. If not entirely new, the models were at least supposed to address some of the noted weaknesses and challenges in the current structure for medical education. The first of these attempts, the ACME-TRI (*Educating Medical Students: Assessing Change in Medical Education—The Road to Implementation*, 1993) was largely judged ineffectual in producing the recommended change in medical schools, although there was widespread support for both the analysis and the resulting recommendations for change. The second effort, the Medical School Objectives Project (MSOP), begun in 1996, took a more descriptive approach by inviting a group of 23 medical schools to develop change processes within their own schools consistent with goals set out by the project. The central goal was to establish medical school curricula based on identified learning objectives and responsive to contemporary issues in medicine (AAMC, 1998a, 1998b, 1999). Each school was asked to document its progress and share information through the change process. It was hoped that these 23 individual case studies would yield insights into "best practices" in curriculum change. Review of the posters presented at the 1998 AAMC session by the 23 participating schools indicates that the change projects undertaken included only modest aspirations for change and no radical departures from accustomed structures and practice. Most projects are efforts to rationalize current curricula by making the curricula more transparent and more accountable across all local stakeholder groups.

Regan-Smith (1998) advocates a more fundamental approach to needed change in medical education with her strong assertion that educational reform efforts in medical schools have failed, and will continue to fail, due to the deleterious effects of the unacknowledged hypocrisy in the structure of present medical schools. For a range of reasons that do not generally include the quality of medical education, medical schools compete to hire researchers and clinicians as faculty members. These reasons usually revolve around staffing research programs or clinical services. The contribution these faculty members will make to general medical education is assumed, but this is not central to their recruitment and selection. The reward structure continues this clear message for faculty about the relative insignificance of education. Promotions in academic rank, salary, office space, staff support and all other tokens of appreciation are awarded for above average clinical income, peer-recognized research funding and publications. Clinicians and researchers are thus understandably conflicted about the time required to teach. Regan-Smith contends: *"time spent providing effective education equals time away from research necessary to maintain their careers"* (p. 505) concluding that: *"[r]esearch's stranglehold on medical education reform needs to be broken by separating researchers from medical student teaching and from curriculum decisions"* (p. 507). DeAngelis (2000) extends this argument to the conflict that clinical instructors have between taking time to teach versus seeing patients more efficiently themselves which would lead directly to increased income. The alternative supported by Regan-Smith is medical education provided by individuals entirely, or at least primarily, focused on education, not research or clinical service. Adopting the Regan-Smith proposition would mean a redefinition in the "three-legged stool" metaphor (research, education and clinical service) that has been reified within medical education since Flexner (see for example, Carey, Wheby, & Reynolds, 1993). The three role expectations would remain valid missions for academic health centers as a whole, and perhaps for faculty members over the course of their careers, but not simultaneously. Research, for example, could receive undivided attention in early career stages when the majority of scientists make their contributions. As this early stage winds down (ideas, staff or funding becomes harder to come by), career attention could move to other forms of scholarship.

There is considerable rhetorical support for a rebalancing of faculty roles in higher education. The Carnegie Foundation for the Advancement of Teaching (Boyer, 1990) recommended a broader conception of legitimate faculty erudition. The Boyer Commission outlined four types of scholarship to be equally valued, assessed and rewarded in higher education:
1. The scholarship of discovery;
2. The scholarship of integration;
3. The scholarship of teaching and learning; and
4. The scholarship of practice.

The first and last of these (research and clinical practice) are well known and highly esteemed within the current structure of medical education. Efforts have been made within some academic medical school settings (Jones & Gold, 1998) to create a separate promotion track or specific promotion criteria for clinician-educators. Others (Levinson & Rubenstein, 1999) point out the problems with these clinician-educator promotion tracks: often these are non-tenure tracks and some of the requirements modeled on research faculty are not realistic for clinicians (i.e. national or international reputations, publications in peer-reviewed journals).

The middle two types of scholarship do occur in medical schools, but are not valued as highly, and as a consequence are not well supported relative to the attention and funding apportioned to discovery (research) and practice. The scholarship of integration, which produces a novel synthesis of existing information, is hampered by the traditional disciplinary boundaries in medical schools. Even more rare is any sort of rigorous scholarly synthesis between medical school disciplines and disciplines from the arts and humanities.

The third type of scholarship Boyer identified was the scholarship of teaching and learning, belied by the widely shared misconception that anyone can teach. Rice and Richlin (1993) describe three necessary features as foundations for the scholarship of teaching and learning: synoptic capacity, pedagogical content knowledge and learning theory. Only the second of these dimensions might be assumed in recruiting leading researchers and clinicians as medical school faculty. The Boyer Commission on Educating Undergraduates in the Research Universities (1998) continued the emphasis on re-establishing teaching as a valued role for faculty on par with research in tenure and promotion decisions. However, serious attention to the scholarship of teaching and learning is rare in medical schools where most offices of medical education, if they exist at all, are pressed into primarily service functions such as managing the logistics for curricula and assessment functions.

The present and the promise in informatics

The breakthrough increase in human capability represented by the Internet and the World Wide Web (WWW) is an "intercept jump" for higher and continuing education. The original concept of a university as a community of scholars was founded on the technical limitations in accessing learned texts. The texts were hand copied, very expensive to produce and therefore very rare. Usually texts were owned and protected by powerful agents in noble families (e.g. the Medicis in Rome; the succession of dynastic families in China), governments (e.g. King Alfred's in Winchester) or the churches (e.g. the cathedral school at Paris). Scholars traveled to seek the patronage of those powerful protectors and access to the texts in exchange for translating, copying or illustrating them, and, incidentally, making their contents useful to their patrons. The students came to study with the scholars and thus the communities of scholarship grew up in a few places centered on the existence of learned works. The Oriental traditions were similar, eventually establishing a mandarin class that served the local power base and controlled access to highly prized, manually produced, written information sources. Only those few individuals chosen to enter these communities of scholars could expect to have access to the texts. Accessing texts from another community of scholars required traveling to their physical location and meeting conditions imposed to join their community.

In contrast, the Web supports access by anyone to the learned works: ancient, modern and everything in between. There is no test of bone fides prior to granting access to this information; all information is available to anyone, at any time, anywhere in the world. Part of the educational appeal of Web supported information is the accessibility during "teachable moments" when the learner is aware of the need or desires to learn something. Content is available by individuals or small groups as might occur in on-the-job problem solving.

Faculties in traditional higher education have opposed incorporation of these electronic access methods. At the University of Washington in Seattle, over 900 professors signed a protest letter to the governor, and the faculty at York University in Canada went on strike over the use of on-line courses or components (*Science,* 1998). Difficulties with incorporating these electronic methods are almost gleefully well documented by faculty (Cravener, 1999). Faculty have attempted to create guidelines (*Science,* 2000) for these new education models which are noteworthy only in the likely futile attempt to preserve the hegemony of the faculty member as the arbiter of content and the university as the controller of access.

There is a proposal in development by a partnership of the Open University in the UK with at least eight existing traditional medical schools to create a distance learning medical school (Southgate & Grant, 2000). Plans at this time are for the first two years of medical training to be offered via distance methods to students distributed across the country. The students will be organized and supported by local health service facilities (district health councils, general practices and other community facilities), which will also be the source of clinical faculty. Students will move among the localities during the course of their training to experience practice in different settings. Curricular content will be derived from a matrix of the health needs of the UK population (General Medical Council, 1997) and a range of common and important clinical problems. Strong central management is planned, responsible for the educational function (quality control, assessment, staff development and support), the clinical components and the research function. Assessment is envisioned to both show progress toward, and achievement of, competence standards. Maastricht-like computer-based progress tests are suggested. Local staff will do in-training assessment of clinical skill. Observed long cases and structured clinical examinations will occur before the end of the training period to assure that all learners have reached standards necessary for beginning clinical practice. Guided expansion of an assessable personal portfolio will assure development of professional attitudes and professional skills beyond the clinical.

This UK experiment is a timely response to opportunities for large-scale change in medical education. The demand for informatics supported medical education is well articulated (Bacon, 1999), the models exist (Berge & Collins, 1995; McCormach & Jones, 1998), they are well developed, well supported by learner demand in other areas of higher education and sufficiently efficacious to be promulgated by corporate structures dependent on constantly improving workplace knowledge and skills. There is nothing particular about the content of medical knowledge that makes it immune to transmission by these methods (Hersh, 1999; Barnes, 1998). Pruitt, Underwood, and Surver (2000) in collaboration with the National Science Foundation have produced a higher education level biology course that combines text, CD-Rom and Web-based technologies to enable both personalized courses of study with immediate access to the most current information. Continuing medical education has begun experimenting with these technologies (Dillon, 1996). Chan, LeClair, and Kaczorowski (1999) have managed interactive problem based learning formats through the Internet for continuing medical education. As with other innovations in medicine, the use of Web capabilities in medical practice will force their adoption in medical education. Goldstein (2000) suggests that 90% of emergency room visits could become unnecessary with online triage using Internet telephony and interactively linked Web cameras.

WHY EDUCATORS SHOULD LEARN TO MANAGE LARGE-SCALE CHANGE

It is widely reported, and generally believed, that all change in human institutions is incremental. In a seminal essay Lindblom (1959) offered the following explanation for this phenomenon: the reality of policy makers (and by extension academic administrators) is characterized by limited information about present conditions and results, restricted information on available alternatives and their consequences, perceived limitations on possible courses of action and limited support for change. In this context the decision maker "*muddles through*" successive constrained comparisons between alternatives which are already "*familiar from past controversies*" (p 79). Decisions are made using past experience to predict consequences; therefore similar decisions continue to be made. Little change is ever ventured and, if forced, is approached in small enough steps to allow past practice to be reflected in expected results.

Even within evolutionary change it is useful to distinguish two varieties of change: operational and strategic (Bryson, 1988, 1995). Changes are more operational if they must occur immediately, have impact only within a section of the organization, involve relatively small fiscal risks (10% of organizational budget or less), require few and obvious strategies for resolution, can be managed by lower level administrators, are not politically charged and have few negative consequences if not addressed.

In contrast, a strategic or large-scale change will significantly impact the organization and all related organizations over a multiple year timeframe. Large-scale change is highly politicized, carries significant financial risk (more than 25% of organizational budget), has no immediately clear resolution strategies and, if not addressed adequately, will result in major, long-term, negative organizational results or organizational dissolution.

No change from status quo is easy. Implementing incremental change in medical schools to accomplish the enhancements outlined elsewhere in this volume will require significant effort within the current structures of medical schools and academic health centers. What if that basic structure has to change? What if the current global struggle to contain burgeoning health care costs results in a severance in the relationship between medical schools and university-based tertiary care academic medical centers? What if the development of the Internet and digitization make medical school classes, even laboratories, comparatively too slow, too expensive, too unresponsive and ultimately redundant? These challenges are large-scale; the type of change addressed in this chapter.

Managing the future of medical education by "muddling through" is no longer acceptable. As medical educators we should model the behavior we teach as preferable in students and practitioners. We describe the "reflective practitioner" as the ideal result of medical schooling; one that reflects on less than satisfactory outcomes, searches for additional information, consciously adjusts approach and monitors results until satisfactory outcomes are obtained. Such an approach could be effectively applied to large-scale change in medical competence definition, inculcation and assessment throughout medical careers. Radically new social expectations for physicians have been documented for at least a decade (Neufeld, 1993; Hastings Centre, 1996; General Medical Council, 1996; AAMC, 1998c and Anderson, 1999). The significant change in social needs, market opportunities and working conditions for medical graduates should be reflected in their education and training.

If medical education refuses to manage, or is unsuccessful in managing, the large-scale change required by the forces outlined here, then the profession of medicine will lose control of the education structure. The medical profession has already lost control of the medical information base: as of January 2000 there were between 10,000 and 15,000 health related Internet sites (Jupiter Communications, 2000). Reputable institutions and organizations that attest to the accuracy of the provided information by associating access with their own reputations host a growing proportion of these sites. Much like the discipline-based committees in medical schools, information specialists (formerly librarians) are issuing guidelines to assist the public in evaluating health information obtained on the Internet and elsewhere (Murray, 1998). Social conditions and informatics capabilities will continue to evolve affecting medical education as has already occurred in other areas of higher education. Even the practicum period can be out-sourced to a series of appropriate sites and appropriate supervisors. The only legitimate role remaining for the medical profession to meet its social obligations would be in organizing, justifying and operating an examination system to assure competence to practice. The profession would no longer control who presented themselves for examination, or how their education was achieved. However, by controlling the examination content and process, the practice standard to be demonstrated prior to certification could remain the purview solely of the profession. At least that part of the social contract could be preserved. But this attenuation of medical education need not occur. Medical education leaders could effect significant change across the system that would adequately respond to the forces requiring adjustment in medical education. Leadership and astute change management could reconcile inert conservative and the unbridled radical elements into reasonable reform that both could support, and that could support medicine's social contract. To be successful, however, medical education leaders must become much more successful as change agents than they have been in the past.

WHAT CAN WE LEARN FROM PAST REFORM FAILURES?

The Flexner model was a fundamental shift for medical education. But even there, only selected aspects of the model were successfully implemented. Flexner's recommendations about integrating basic and clinical sciences, active learning in favor of lectures, and emphasis on problem-solving and critical thinking over memorization were not implemented. These shortcomings were noted at the time (Enarson & Burg, 1992) but not corrected until those elements reappeared in the slow adoption of problem-based learning by organized curricula.

The next effort at significant structural change was the Case Western Reserve curriculum of the 1950s. This was an attempt to integrate basic and clinical sciences and introduce the behavioral sciences in the service of medicine. A few medical schools adopted these concepts, but not many and not centrally (Funkenstein, 1971). The reductionist, rational, science focus remained central to the self-definition of medicine and medical schools.

Medical schools were affected only slightly by the social upheavals of the 1960's. Again the "social ecology" or "humanist" approaches to medicine were suggested for inclusion in medical school curricula (Pellegrino, 1978). Again, a few medical schools experimented with implementation (Beer-Sheva, Maastricht, McMaster, Michigan State, New Mexico) but no large-scale change occurred in medical education.

These debates and isolated change experiences were eventually reflected in a much-referenced series of reports on the need for paradigmatic change in medical education. These included:

- Future Directions for Medical Education (1982)
- The New Biology and Medical Education: merging the biological, information and cognitive sciences (Friedman & Purcell, 1983)
- Physicians for the 21st Century (1984)
- Adapting Clinical Medical Education to the Needs of Today and Tomorrow (1988).

The reports outlined a number of environmental changes impinging on medical education; all of which have grown stronger and more influential with time: exponential growth in the science base of medical knowledge; increasing importance of computer assisted information management in health care, increasingly informed public and increasing demands for patient/client-oriented care.

During this same period academic leaders exhorted the community to evolve (Jonas, 1984; Roddie, 1986; Bussigel et al., 1986; Weldon, 1986; Light, 1988; Cantor et al., 1991) but provided little guidance on direction or method. Reform was attempted without result in various ways around the world. For example, Mårtenson described innovations attempted at the Karolinska Institute as "*modest, but what has been achieved positively is a climate increasingly in favor of change*" (1989, p.17). Cuban (1997) documented 80 years of attempted change from 1908 to 1990 without significant reform at the Stanford University School of Medicine.

At the close of that decade Bloom (1988, 1989) published a review of the various attempted curricular reforms in medical education to that date. He concluded that the educational reforms were doomed to fail for two structural reasons:

1. the positive results from reform of medical school curriculum in the first years is quickly erased and made pointless by the "brutalizing" effect (quoting Mizrahi, 1986) of hospital-based clinical education, thus nullifying any net change achieved; and
2. because research, not education, was the central mission of medical schools.

The structure and demands of the research enterprise in medical schools at the time Bloom was writing, and even more so today, demands full-time attention and commitment to remain sufficiently competitive to attract outside funding at the scale necessary to support the large laboratories, large research staffs and expensive machinery required for cutting-edge science. Bloom quotes personal correspondence from Stevens (1988), *"medical education has become a minor activity of the American medical school. One could take the view that medical schools need medical students, not so much to teach them but to give the entire apparatus of the school a justification for being"*. Ten years later in 1998 Regan-Smith came to the same conclusions (Regan-Smith, 1998).

Our history as ineffectual managers of change is not reassuring about our abilities to shape the needed change given the mounting pressures on medical education. Is there an alternative to "muddling through" other than the ever-popular position with head in the sand, avoiding all responsibility, and focusing on reactive strategies to minimize personal inconvenience? There is, if we take a proactive position toward change in medical education and actively employ our training as clinicians and as researchers to the study and application of the accumulated knowledge about change management. As in clinical practice and research, we need to be familiar with both the relevant theory and results in practice. The next section categorizes and reviews current change theories illustrated by examples from medical education.

MANAGEMENT OF CHANGE MODELS

A great deal has been written about change management. The literature varies in tone, scope and scientific rigor because well known contributors come from such varied backgrounds: academia (e.g. Rosabeth Kanter, 1988), for-profit policy consultants (e.g. Osborne & Gaebler, 1993); human resource consultants (i.e. Smye, 1993) and front-line managers (e.g. Andrews et al., 1994). Viewed as a mass the literature on change management is a contradictory morass of exhortive prose with only occasional attempts at evaluation or validation of claims made. Epistemological evidence in this field comes from reported case studies, some merely anecdotes. Still, there is value in understanding the range, assumptions and potential of the different approaches to managing change.

Mintzberg, Ahlstrand, & Lampel (1998) produced an integrated compilation and critique of planned change models (labels have been altered here to improve recognition at the cost of de-emphasizing parallels between them). The first three are described as prescriptive, focused on how change should occur rather than how it actually happens. The last six have been derived from descriptions of how change actually occurs.

The SWOT analysis

Selznick (1957), Chandler (1962) and Andrews (1982) developed the SWOT analysis (strengths, weaknesses, opportunities, threats) to guide change processes. The theory guides data collection and displays the results in a 2×2 grid (strengths and weaknesses crossed with opportunities and threats). Changes likely to be effective are indicated by the intersections of measured strengths and perceived opportunities. This approach assumes that each analysis will be exclusive to its setting and time; each change process is considered as unique. Little or nothing will therefore be applicable from a SWOT analysis performed in one medical center to any other medical center. The principal criticisms of this approach are the assumptions of certainty about the data, the analysis and the stability of the operating environment.

The curricular reform at the University of Michigan medical school (Davis & White, 1993) and the larger changes at Emory University medical center (Saxton et al., 2000) both involved a formal SWOT analysis in the early stages.

The planning approach

This model builds on SWOT analyses by developing detailed implementation plans as a response to SWOT conclusions (Ansoff, 1965; Steiner, 1979; Lorange, 1980). These plans are carefully detailed in increasing levels of specification: goals, objectives, budgets, action items, timelines and feedback loops to monitor progress. In full implementation this model requires full-time planners quite separate from those responsible for the work of the organization. This is also one of the principal weaknesses: the division between planning and operations. A second significant limitation is the rigidity that sets in with detailed change specifications. The carefully constructed road map may quickly become irrelevant to actual evolution in needs and opportunities.

Many academic health centers in North America were structured along this model with full-time planners during the past years when funding was more plentiful (Andrews, 1994).

The analysis of position

Following detailed analysis of military and marketplace descriptions, this approach posits a fixed number of generic change strategies to be selected from to suit any organizational situation. Selection of appropriate strategies is viewed as a deductive process based on an analysis of the "competitive position" of the organization. This group of theories presumes that organizational environments are generic, or at least sufficiently similar to allow strategies perceived to be successful in one situation to be applied in other situations judged to be analogous. Michael Porter (1980) became a well-known proponent of this approach to change management when the governments of Poland and Russia engaged him to advise on their large-scale change to market economies. The orientation of this model is towards economic and territorial goals and does not account well for other social or political objectives such as education, group cohesion or population health.

Medical schools and academic health centers that perceive their context as a zero-sum competitive marketplace are using this type of change theory. The suggestions outlined by Griner and Danoff (2000) for reform in academic health centers derive from positional analysis.

Entrepreneurial management

This model focuses change strategy on the leader and his or her "vision". Vision is defined as a personal construct within the leader based on his/her intuition, judgment, wisdom, experience and insight. Leaders develop or change their vision through the three-stage process (unfreeze, change, refreeze) described by Lewin (1951). Drucker (1970), Collins and Moore (1970) and Bennis and Namus (1985) have all written descriptions of this change management type. Specific change plans are not articulated in this model, leaving the details vague to be adapted by the leader on the fly in the course of moving the organization in the direction of the vision.

Charismatic leaders are more successful with this change management approach because this model requires the leader to inspire others to implement his or her vision. This model is most successful in organizations with simple power structures, such as a single owner (e.g. Richard Branson's Virgin companies), a startup organization (e.g. McMaster medical school) or effectively leaderless due to considerable turmoil (e.g. Apple Computer immediately prior to the second reign of Steve Jobs). The strength of this model is also its greatest weakness: the dependence on the visionary leader. Others within the organization may resent such dependence and such concentration of power. Furthermore, visionaries are often particular to specific situations, i.e. specific industries, specific time periods, specific personal contexts. When the situational variables change, the vision, the entrepreneurial change style, and the leader him/herself may be inappropriate.

Giardino et al. (1994) describe a change process in clinical skills assessment and evaluation from this perspective and advocate this approach for other reforms in medical education. Aspects of the curricular change at Sherbrooke medical school (Des Marchais, 1992), particularly the initiation, were clearly entrepreneurial change strategies.

Applications of cognitive science

Well described by Makridakis (1990) and by Huff (1990), this group of change management theories explains how change makers reason through the choices they make. Knowing how choices are made, assert these theorists, better informs future choices and avoids pitfalls in thinking. Cognitive theory is employed in analyzing how people reason (e.g. biases in the use of analogies and metaphors that can distort decision-making), the effect of biasing action (e.g. articulating a plan tends to bind the speaker to that plan) and biases due to cognitive style. Although there are many measures of cognitive style available (Curry, 1999), one of the most widely used is the Myers-Briggs instrument (Myers, 1962).

Other writers in this type of change analysis examine change agent information processing as individuals or in groups within an organization undergoing change. Following Simon's (1957) and March and Simon's (1958) theories of cognitive psychology applied to information processing within organizations, these analyses are justified by a belief that specific, knowable mental structures (also referred to as frames, schema, concepts, scripts, mental models or causal maps) organize and process information. Knowledge and use of these mental structures provide predictability to decision-makers forced to operate in the real world with less than perfect information. This cognitive science model is faulted primarily because so far it is only descriptive, providing little prescriptive assistance to change agents.

Harris' (1993) descriptions of the deliberative curriculum inquiry process applied to support reform in medical education curricula illustrate the cognitive science approach to change management. Gruppen (1997) advocates for reform in ambulatory care education following cognitive science concepts.

Applying learning theory

This model enjoyed much attention in the popular press (Senge, 1990) as well as in the academic press (Argyris, 1991) during the 1990s. The central ideas, however, can be traced to Lindblom (1959) who described policymaking in government as a set of incremental and fragmented decision/reaction/learning steps. The Tuckman (1965) stages of group development (forming, storming, norming, performing) are stages in group learning. Quinn (1980) described a reason for incremental change, and then codified this logic into prescriptions for rational incrementalism based on stages of learning (Quinn, 1982). Nonaka and Takeuchi (1995) emphasized the importance of converting tacit knowledge into explicit knowledge within individuals, work groups and the organization as a whole to enable the acquisition, creation, accumulation and exploitation of knowledge. Argyris and Schön (1974, 1978) distinguished single-loop organizational learning (learned improvement in an action, response or intervention) and double-loop learning (change in both the underlying construct or variable and the associated response or action). Dick and Dalman (1990) outlined an "information chain" to describe the relationship among organizational learning and action stages, and recently extended the theory to include actions in planned change (Dick, 1996).

The learning approach to change is criticized because it may seem expensive and inefficient: it looks like trial and error, which is not usually perceived as quality management. Because it is impossible to predict which learning strategy might be effective in producing change, many are started at the same time, observed, evaluated, learned about and modified. All this takes participants' time and organizational resources. Much of the organizational learning process will be confusing to participants, destabilizing to the organization and frustrating to those in leadership positions because the learning has to occur before the change can begin. However, the learning approach is well suited to professional organizations operating in complex environments with diffuse power bases and ill-formed problems. In these circumstances change management often defaults to a process of collective learning by trial and error because there is no central authority to impose an analysis, a vision or an alternate change strategy.

Boverie and Blackwell (1993) describe use of the Tuchman model to assist faculty through an organizational change. Both the ACME-TRI (1993) and the MSOP (AAMC, 1999) projects of the American Association of Medical Schools were learning theory based change efforts.

Political power techniques

Change formation in this model is shaped by power and politics both inside an organization and between an organization and its external environment (Macmillan, 1978). Change is managed inside the organization through political processes such as persuasion, bargaining and, occasionally, direct confrontation among parochial interests and shifting coalitions. Change is managed across organizations by controlling, co-opting or cooperating with other organizations (Baldridge, 1975). This is accomplished through strategic maneuvering and political collectivizing strategies such as forming networks and alliances.

Political approaches to change are notable in periods of significant power restructuring and in situations, such as universities and professional organizations, composed of complex, highly decentralized experts with essentially equal power and strong vested interests. The principal critique of the power approach is that it tends to ignore the content of arguments and the integrating effects of learning and leadership.

The model developed by Gale and Grant (1997) for the Leverhulme Trust and published as an AMEE Medical Education Guide is an illustration of the power approach to change management. The external, formative evaluations as part of the change process at Sherbrooke medical school (Des Marchais & Bordage, 1998) were a deployment of political power technique in change management. They used carefully selected and briefed prestigious outsiders as evaluators to focus faculty preparations and participation. The status of the evaluators also gave extra weight to their recommendations. The story of Harvard Medical School's effort to modify its curriculum (Tosteson, Adelstein, & Carver, 1994) is an example of applied political power in the service of change. The complete lack of, or unsuccessfully applied, political power techniques clearly contributed to the failed curricular reform at Otago, New Zealand (Schwartz, Heath, & Egan, 1994).

The cultural analysis

This group of theories focuses on the attributes of organizational culture that preserve organizational stability and success. Culture is defined as those features shared by members. Critical cultural features are usually values, beliefs, traditions, habits, stories and symbols, which might include buildings, titles and products. These same cultural features can actively resist change and render an organization impermeable to even evolutionary adaptation. Cultures are generally stable, closely tied to individual identities and therefore extremely hard to change. These cultural analyses are more often used to explain why organizational cultures vary in terms of imperviousness to particular changes or change in general. A large number of these cultural change analyses were documented by Norwegian scholars (e.g. Rhenman, 1973 and Normann, 1977) but the method was eventually popularized in the 1980s by the comparative analyses of Japanese and American corporate cultures (Deming, 1986).

Mennin and Kaufman (1989) present a cultural analysis of barriers to change in medical education. Schwartz, Heath, and Egan (1994) identified mostly cultural factors in their analysis of the failed curricular reform at Otago, New Zealand.

The environmental imperative

There are some approaches to change that view the organization as essentially passive, with only reactive options in response to events that occur in the organizational context. Context features such as stability, complexity, market diversity and hostility are analyzed to inform choice of appropriate responses and/ or appropriate leaders (Miller, 1979, 1988).

As an aid to building commitment to change Harris (1993) calls for a series of descriptive studies of the effects on the immediate economic, political, social and cultural environment of medical schools' curricula. Schwartz, Heath, and Egan (1994) attribute one source of their failed curricular reform to environmental instability.

Combined approaches

A logical conclusion to any review of change management theories is to recommend a combination approach. Both the organization and its context should be analyzed and that information used to suggest transformations necessary to achieve desired results. Organizations should be viewed as stable and in equilibrium with their environment for periods of time until something changes in the organization or the environment that requires the organization to reconfigure. This process of "renewal" requires guidance to be efficient and should utilize any of the techniques listed above, as they are appropriate to the situation (Dickhout, Denham, & Blackwell, 1995). The challenge then is to match technique to circumstance (Beatty & Ulrich, 1991). Functional overall change strategies must support initiation from anywhere in the organization: from the bottom, or middle (Beer, Eisenstat, & Spector, 1990) or from the top down (Kotter, 1995). Combined approaches offer more likelihood of sustained change than any one method.

There has been some use made of combined strategy change management in medical education. Mårtenson (1989) indicates awareness of, but did not deploy, a range of techniques in his description of a modest change in an established medical school, the Karolinska Institute in Sweden. He suggested the following as necessary elements of change strategy in medical schools: analysis of the external environment, analysis of the internal culture, detailed planning as well as application of the basics in power manipulation. Shahabudin and Safiah (1991) report use of political power techniques and applications of learning theory in the institutionalization process for a curriculum change at the Universiti Kebansaan in Malaysia. The Sherbrooke School of Medicine conversion to problem based learning was primarily an entrepreneurial driven exercise (Des Marchais et al., 1992; Des Marchais, 1996), but had recourse to a range of political power techniques at a few key points in implementation (Des Marchais & Bordage, 1998). The case study of curriculum change at Michigan Medical School (Davis & White, 1993) outlines use of SWOT analysis, planning, and the deployment of political power to implement changes. Reflecting on the evidence as compiled across eight American medical schools, Lindberg (1998) describes a preferred change process that begins with entrepreneurial management (primacy of vision), then utilizes the learning approach, and includes elements from the political power approach. Reviewing the same schools, Kaufman (1998) describes preferred leadership in terms of the entrepreneurial and political power approaches. Saxton et al. (2000) followed a classic SWOT analysis with an intensive planning effort and reported use of a range of political power techniques to alter member behavior in planned directions.

BARRIERS TO CHANGE

Before any organized approach to change can be implemented, stakeholders have to agree on the necessity for reform. Reform may be mandated externally by national professional bodies or internally by opportunity or disaster; still each faculty group must decide for themselves whether, what and how to reform their curriculum and their organization. Usually there is a strong element of self-preservation in this choice. Stakeholders will not support organizations, programs or curricula that cannot demonstrate cutting edge relevance. For professional programs these critical stakeholders include the present and future faculty, students, administrators, funders (of the school, of faculty research, of the students), those supplying or supervising student training placements, employers, certifying and accrediting bodies.

A myriad attitudinal hurdles must be overcome before any large-scale change process can be initiated. One of the most common is a belief among stakeholders that they are individually over committed and too busy to take on any other project, most particularly *not* anything as large and complex as curriculum or organizational reform. Older stakeholders will have been involved in previous reforms; some of which would have been badly managed, resulting in hurt feelings and frustration, sometimes without achieving any real change. Those participants will have no enthusiasm for "going through that again". Others may not be convinced of the need for reform. This complacency, or willful misperception, or arrogance is indefensible because the context for professional school graduates has changed so rapidly and so thoroughly in the past decade the likelihood is great that both curricula and organization need attention.

Even if convinced of the need for reform, many stakeholders prefer the "wait and see someone else do it" approach, which they will then attempt to copy in their own situation, intentionally ignoring the facts that distinguish each professional school from the others. What works in an urban-based school with a number of other professional schools in the area, will not likely work in a less populated region where the professional schools are more isolated. Faculty composition, their values, professional interests and skills, and the school's culture are also critical to implementing change. Each setting will have a unique combination of these factors making the wholesale importation of a curricular solution unlikely to be successful. This caution is similar to the philosophy in the SWOT analysis change management model.

Sometimes reform is suppressed by "concept phobia": an unwillingness to seriously examine or learn about unfamiliar ideas. This occurred in many traditional medical schools at the end of the 1980s when they were forced by the success of the problem-based learning (PBL) model promulgated by McMaster University to understand and evaluate a set of adult education concepts and practices with which they were unfamiliar. Some say this "concept phobia" is occurring again in many health professions in their reaction against the public's demonstrated interest in alternative/complementary health interventions and the concomitant demand that these interventions be included in training curricula for all mainstream health professionals (Dacher, 1995). Similarly, many faculties remain phobic about aggressive application of informatics in education and competence assessment (*Science*, 1998; Cravener, 1999; *Science*, 2000).

"Mental locks and idea killers" have also hampered the processes of reform. There are a lot of these, and any well spoken, well respected faculty member using one or any selection can effectively derail a reform process by expressing, for example, the belief that "there is only one right (or most right) answer which will be identifiable by rigorous proof, preferably multiple randomized controlled trials and meta-analysis, published in the top-rated journals", (at least in the ones that the speaker happens to read)! Appeals to "be practical", to "avoid ambiguity" and "it's not my area of expertise" all function to constrain reform and dampen the energy needed to accomplish and sustain the reform process.

A related barrier is the often inaccurate concept of creativity held by professional school faculty; they rarely see a role for creativity, or "experimentation" in professional training, practice or assessment. Most professions proudly point to their training in science, or well-established canons of practice. Professional value systems tend to reward predictability. Even research ideas too far from current understandings are not well accepted by peers, and therefore not likely funded. Creativity is considered to be a "gift" more suitable to the performing arts than the practice of a profession. These attitudes and values make it difficult for professional school faculty to see themselves as "creating" curricula and "re-creating" their organizations to better meet a rapidly changing professional work context, the details of which they can never know for sure.

Overcoming all these barriers is necessary to curricular or organizational reform. Reminding faculty of the risks of not reforming their curricula is often sufficient to get the process started. The first, and most significant, risk has already been discussed: having a curriculum or an organization viewed as irrelevant or out-of-date will result in a loss of support from stakeholders in and beyond the professional school or organization. There will be other negative occurrences if needed reform is ducked or deferred. Frustration with under-performance will grow as news of more change requirements comes from within and beyond the profession. Unresolved political and personal conflicts will emerge in more virulent forms. Decision-making will be based on strong personalities rather than analyzed information and professional reflection. Both staff and administration/management tend to become disengaged from their work under these circumstances, leading to mediocre performance from both. There is a deadening of creativity and social interaction in all areas. Once a group recognizes the horrors of not proceeding with required reform, an educative process can begin to introduce the rudiments of curricular theory, organizational design and the models, processes and techniques involved in managing large-scale change.

Managing change through Facilitated Deliberative Inquiry (FDI)

How can a change agent make an intelligent choice among all these theorists and fervent testimonials? How can strands from any of the theories and experiences be identified and utilized as required in new circumstances? An integrated method is required that provides decision-makers sufficient distance from the situation to allow awareness, reflection, generation and weighing of alternatives. An effective method must test alternatives in context, allow for renegotiating alternatives, and re-testing. If this cycle is repeated sufficiently the eventual decision-making and implementation becomes a great deal easier because the method itself blurs the demarcation among trials, decisions and implementation. At the end of the process so many alternatives have been discussed, tried out and modified in use that the formal adoption of the change is a simple ratification of change already in place.

However, to get that far the ideal process must have enough forward momentum to avoid being filibustered or mired in endless inconclusive trials and pilot projects.

A process that meets these specifications, Facilitated Deliberative Inquiry, has been developed and tested by the author (Curry, 2000, 1998, 1997, 1996, 1995) in a range of large-scale change projects. FDI presents a real alternative to the "muddling through" approach to change by requiring both articulation and confirmation of central values and objectives, and their relative weightings, across key stakeholders. The method also requires generation of a range of alternative solutions or directions, and then provides guidance on processes to match up alternatives with weighted values and objectives.

Although FDI was initially developed as a model to direct curricular reform, it became immediately clear that to sustain curricular change the educational organization also had to change. The same reasons that FDI is effective in guiding curricular change makes it effective in managing organizational change as well. Elements of the FDI process are similar to features in the various management of change models previously reviewed. These correspondences are noted in the following description of FDI operations.

Theoretical Roots

Facilitated Deliberative Inquiry (FDI) was developed from a pragmatic synthesis of three strands of scholarly curricular thought: Tyler, Schwab and Schön-Cervero. Tyler's empirical-analytic paradigm (1949) was useful because that approach allows systematic analysis and organization of curricular elements, elements of arguments or political positions. Most faculties are familiar with this model for curriculum analysis and most of the national professional bodies encouraging curricular reform are presenting required analysis within that paradigm. The curricular concepts developed by Schwab (1969a, 1969b) contributed to FDI because his concept of deliberative curriculum inquiry focuses on fixing curricular problems in a way that puts boundaries on the reform/revision task. Harris (1986, 1990) expanded on the Schwab concept and the implications she drew for professional education (1991) were more understandable to faculty than Schwab's original concept development, which took examples only from the K-12 years. A second aspect of Schwab's writing proved helpful: the rationale for including a wider range of stakeholders (i.e. employers, regulators) in the reform process. Otherwise, faculties perceive this wider inclusion of participants as a purely politically motivated demand, and therefore an illegitimate encroachment on their academic responsibilities and freedoms. The research and writings of Schön (1983, 1987) and Cervero (1988) were helpful in the development of the FDI model because they articulate aspects of professional competence (i.e. professional judgment) that are not amenable to analytic fragmentation.

FDI Defined

Facilitated Deliberative Inquiry (FDI) is a logical framework for focused participation in review and reform particularly well suited to situations with multiple legitimate stakeholders or stakeholder groups, and ill-defined problems without obvious solutions. It allows systematic consideration of all perspectives and is enhanced by the existence of multiple viewpoints. The structure has a built in drive for completion as it organizes iterations through identification and weighting of critical problem facets, solution strand development and solution testing. The method is self-limiting, and cannot be filibustered. FDI organizes problem identification, solution development, implementation planning, testing and modification.

The FDI process has three objectives:

1. That all stakeholders in the issues to be deliberated understand their role and contribution, and also the role and contribution of every other stakeholder.
2. That the eventual consensus result be consistent and aligned from design through delivery, assessment and outcome.
3. That the result accomplishes what the stakeholders intend that it should.

FDI Process

There are eight steps to the FDI process organized to engage all the critical curricular and organizational dimensions in the review and reform considerations. This coverage insures that the review includes sufficient segments of the curriculum and the organization to actually effect a change if considered necessary. Noted in italics are the change management theories incorporated at each step. The steps are:

1. Identify problems through analysis *(SWOT)*:
   - definition of quality indicators (curricular and organizational intention) through internal or external standards and/or outcomes *(Positioning)*,
   - alignment of this quality intention with current internal mastery definitions (educational content and sequencing, and/or organizational design) *(Learning)*,
   - alignments of mastery definitions with teaching/learning methods and/or with actions taken and work done within the organization *(Learning)*,
   - alignments of mastery definitions with assessment mechanisms, content and criteria for individuals and organizational units. *(Learning)*.
2. Specify and document inadequacies involved in each identified problem *(SWOT; Positioning)*.
3. Specify criteria and constraints on possible solutions *(Positioning, Environmental and Cultural analysis)*.
4. Generate a creative range of possible solutions *(Planning)*.
5. Choose a preferred solution by consensus *(Entrepreneurial, Political power)*.
6. Identify specific changes necessary to effect preferred solutions. Identify and negotiate ownership and responsibility for those changes *(Cognitive science, Political power)*.
7. Develop detailed change plans showing real and potential impacts inside and outside the organization *(Planning, Learning, Environmental and Cultural analysis)*
   - on other curricular areas

- on other organizational areas
- on each stakeholder group.

8. Group consideration, acceptance or modification of each proposed change (*Entrepreneurial, Political power, Learning, Cognitive science*).

These Steps are obviously iterative: any change at step 8 will require re-working, or at least re-confirming, all previous decisions.

"Roll-outs" to stakeholder constituencies can occur at any time, and are advisable at each major decision point (i.e. when the Deliberative Group has agreed on the quality indicators, the problem list, the solution list, and when trade-offs are made among solutions). Throughout the FDI process, and particularly at each of these decision making occasions, it is necessary that all the stakeholders be aware of what the Deliberative Group is doing, how they are approaching the issues, what they are considering, and what they are deciding. As this information comes out of the Deliberative Group to the stakeholders, reaction, advice and information go back in; an exchange that has to be initiated and managed to best effect. Everyone learns in the process. (See similar concepts in the Learning Theory models of change management.)

It is important to keep the Deliberative Group together through this process. Do not be seduced by the possibility of subdividing the review task by curricular dimensions, or segments (i.e. years or disciplines). If the curriculum is to be integrated throughout, then consideration of the curricular dimensions must cumulate through iterative consideration, not by merging separate processes at the end. The curricular review process, and the resulting curriculum reform, is best thought of as a compound, not a mixture.

The same admonition applies to organizational change: do not atomize the apparent problems; do not assign different individuals or groups to work on fragments separately. This is a false economy that cannot result in an integrated solution. Keep the whole group deliberating on the whole problem. Even if they work at it piece by piece, they are responsible for continuously fitting pieces back into the whole by constant testing through the "roll-out" process.

Create a "Capstone" Statement of Commitment

In a final, but critically important FDI step, the Deliberative Group, working back and forth through their stakeholders, must articulate and adopt a summary statement that encapsulates their commitment to the new direction. In organizational change this could be in drafting a new mission statement. In the case of a curriculum reform, the FDI process should conclude with development of a concise consensus statement that summarizes what the curriculum promises to learners, to teachers and to other stakeholders. The statement should indicate evidence that those same stakeholders share this commitment. There should also be an indication of how stakeholders will determine if commitments are being met all the way through the reform implementation and specify remedies if the commitments are found to not be met.

This "capstone" is a statement of philosophy, a mission, a statement of purpose for the change undertaken. The "capstone" articulation and consensus process also gives all stakeholders the opportunity to reflect on, codify for themselves, and publicly affirm their personal commitment to the same ends. Or not, if that is the case! If any stakeholder cannot support the end product summary, his/her opposition or apathy is better surfaced and dealt with before the change goes into operation. Some minor tweaking or presentation detail may resolve the problem, but if not, that individual had best be separated from the process to avoid active or passive sabotage. This result should also be recognized as a failure of the FDI procedure to this point if such opposition is only discovered at the summary stage of the change process. These commitment techniques are reflected in the Political Power group of management change models.

FDI Working Group

A carefully chosen group facilitated by an individual familiar with the relevant content and experienced in facilitating working groups conducts the work of deliberation about the curriculum, and any other desired change. This Deliberative Group is made up of either all stakeholders, if this is a manageable number, or individuals chosen to represent the thinking of various stakeholder groups.

The total number in the Deliberative Group is important because that number constrains the nature of discussion and deliberation. There is too much work to be done for a group of five or fewer, but a group of more than 15 members will find themselves fighting for sufficient "air-time" to have their views aired, understood and elaborated upon. People need to feel that they have "had their say", been heard, and respected by others, particularly when the issue under examination is personal: one's courses, one's curriculum, one's school, one's career. Skilled facilitation can balance the "air-time" among as many as 30 members, but this is intrusive to the group process and doesn't fully resolve the tracking problem, as new ideas will still be initiated before other ideas already on the table are fully developed. A Deliberative Group of 9 to 15 members is ideal.

Answering the following question identifies the key stakeholders or groups that must be included in the Deliberative Group: *who cares about (and who is affected by) this problem/issue and what this organization is or does?* The obvious stakeholders in a professional school curriculum reform project would include the following: faculty, students (current and recent past), employers, administrators (in the school), support staff (in the school), professionals in practice, regulatory/certifying bodies (for graduates and for the school), professional associations, and collaborating schools/faculties. In any particular situation there may be more or other stakeholders. All these voices and viewpoints are valuable to the deliberation because they each see the school from a different angle, interact with it from and for different reasons. Each will see different problems and have different solutions, the combination of which will likely be the strongest solution. This is a concept similar to a technique in the Political Power change management model.

Individuals from these various groups of stakeholders should not be chosen by those stakeholders, or at least not alone. The Deliberative Group must function well as a group from inception if the process is to be time and resource efficient. Therefore members should be chosen from the stakeholder types, not to represent that constituency in any political sense of the term, but to contribute to the deliberations the perspective of that stakeholder group. Individuals should be chosen because they are broadly educated, have broad interests, are seen as influential within their stakeholder group (have qualities of character and experience valued in that group), have relevant education and experience, demonstrate "connoisseurship" (Eisner, 1977, 1985) about professional education and professional practice and have proven skills in working with a group. Skilled exercise of this choice among potential group members is a technique application from the Political Power group of change management models.

The duties of Deliberative Group members are to participate fully in the deliberations set out in the FDI Process, to prepare by reading material assigned for each session and updates periodically distributed on changes agreed to, and by leading "informational roll-outs" to the various stakeholder groups if requested. Because they have the detailed information from the Group's deliberative work the members of the Deliberative Group are the obvious, but not the only possible, individuals to lead these roll-out sessions, or communications (newsletters, telephone trees). Consideration should be given, however, to *not* assigning members to do the "roll-out" to the stakeholder group from which they came. Working with a different stakeholder group will force both sides to listen more carefully and communicate more clearly because they will less likely share attitudes, experiences, verbal shorthand, or jargon. This careful communication will benefit all concerned, particularly the Deliberative Group. (This concept relates to the Cognitive Science group of change management models.)

Facilitating the Deliberation

Large-scale review and reform processes are too complex to function well without a facilitator. A Deliberative Group without a designated facilitator will be dominated by the more powerful members, the group will flounder, waste time with repetition, non-productive work, aimless discussion and, as a consequence, become frustrated very quickly with their lack of progress. Members will not be willing to participate in a process that cannot guarantee results for their investment of time and respect for their individual contributions.

If the Deliberative Group designates one of its own members as the facilitator, that individual becomes effectively removed from the deliberative process. The person chosen in this manner is usually someone with legitimate authority in the Group, like the Curriculum Coordinator or the Dean. In order to be perceived as "fair" by the others, the facilitator can have no opinion to sell, no point of view to defend. If one of the Deliberators becomes the facilitator, that point of view is lost to the Group and is "not part of the solution". Being an outsider in a new curriculum launch or organizational renewal is no place for a faculty member, the Curriculum Coordinator or the Dean.

The tasks of the facilitator are in three areas: to maintain balance among the participants in the Deliberative Group (a Political Power model technique); to monitor and adjust the tempo of the Group (Cognitive Science model application); and to coordinate the secretariat functions. The first task is required because there is a wide power differential within Deliberative Groups: some curricular reform Groups will include Deans; all such groups should include students. It is critical that the students be listened to as much, and their viewpoints considered with the same gravity as the Dean's. The Group and its members must also be protected from vituperation, blame and the continuation of old, or extraneous arguments. Many of the "barriers to change" reviewed in the previous section will occur within the Deliberative Group. The facilitator must assist the Group to overcome each of those constraints.

Monitoring the tempo of the Deliberative Group is the most challenging task for the facilitator. This involves being constantly aware of each Group member, their affect, their personal styles, their intentions, their pervasive biases and their current tactics or arguments. Based on this tide of information, the facilitator judges how to help the Group accomplish the defined work. Sometimes this is leaving the Group alone, sometimes it is introducing more or diminishing the level of complexity the Group is dealing with. A facilitator must know how to break up "log-jams" for the Group. For example, it may be helpful to summarize repetitive arguments to move the Group to another point. This could involve diagramming a situation; sometimes getting more information or confirming information; possibly breaking the Group up into individual or small group projects for a short period and then insuring the integration of the parts.

The secretariat functions must also occur fluidly to support the Deliberative Group work. The change situation must be displayed in many different ways throughout the process to encourage the Deliberative Group, and their stakeholder constituencies, to always perceive the situation as a whole. Everyone must apprehend how any particular solution, or idea, affects that whole. For example, any adopted solution to an over-crowded curriculum will necessarily alter the whole curriculum, so Groups can easily get lost in the welter of paper and amendments. A good secretariat process uses a spreadsheet based computer program that can handle text (such as Lotus Notes, or equivalents) to easily make interactive changes in the descriptive documents and instantly re-issue overviews to the Deliberators. Careful documentation results in a "book" that succinctly, but thoroughly, describes the emerging consensus solution. At the end of the FDI process the "book" can be used to orient future stakeholders, funding, licensing or accrediting bodies to the curriculum or organization as a whole and to any specific component. The same requirements apply to organizational change: change in any existing function or unit requires adjustment in all other functions and units. Tracking and displaying these potential implications are critical to the accuracy of their interpretation and evaluation and to subsequent learning within the organization.

Given the complexity of the task, identifying and engaging a professional facilitator is a worthwhile expenditure, particularly if the individual is experienced in managing Deliberative Groups. An experienced facilitator can maximize the efficiency and the productivity of the process. The job description is:

1. to conclude the review and reform process proficiently,
2. make the most efficient use of Deliberators' time,
3. protect their interests,
4. fully engage the stakeholders in the "roll-out" process (and therefore keep them supportive of the changes as they occur),
5. assure that the situations/problems/issues and consensus resolutions are thoroughly reviewed, revised and
6. described in exquisite detail at both macro (organizational context or whole curriculum) and micro (course, experience or behavior change) levels.

CONCLUSIONS

The world in which professionals practice, and especially the "helping professions", has changed radically within one generation. In response, we as educators of the professions have a range of responsibilities: to current and future generations of professionals and to society at large. First of all to the next generation of professionals we must fairly represent the context into which they must fit as practitioners. What do they actually need to know, to be able to do and what attitudes are appropriate (requisite knowledge, skills and attitudes). We must develop efficient and effective curricula to inculcate this needed knowledge, skills and attitudes, and assessment structures that assure these capabilities exist at the point of entrance to practice. Our analysis of needed knowledge, skills and attitudes, the curricula, the assessments and the organizational structure that delivers all this must address the forces presently distorting medical education. The current dissatisfaction with medical schools will be diminished when a new equilibrium is reached regarding the medical scope of practice issues, the changed physician workforce and the altered social forces. These solutions will doubtless involve informatics capabilities in a significant way and will likely incorporate at least some aspects of the newer models for higher and professional education.

To the current generation of practitioners we must fairly represent the context into which they must fit as practitioners and how that has changed from what they are used to and were trained for. We must develop curricula effectively designed for practitioners (individuated, accessible, dispersed across time and location) to inculcate this needed knowledge, skills and attitude, and the change adaptation process. We must create assessment structures that allow the individual practitioner, his or her professional bodies, and the licensing bodies to be assured that these changed competencies have been achieved.

To society we own a duty to study and articulate changes in the social contract the profession has with society and to take responsibility to initiate change in all educational structures that bear on that changed contract. This will include systems of curricula, assessment, credentialing and licensing as well as the organizational structure of medical schools, practical training and continuing education.

Taking any one of these responsibilities seriously requires significant change in the present organization, structure and content of medical education. So medical education leaders must be in the change management business. To be effective we must avoid "bandwagon thinking" and mindless hopeful adoption of changes initiated elsewhere. The objective of useful change management must not be to recommend, or facilitate any particular change. A more appropriate enduring solution is to build *"flexible organizations responsive to environments, organizations with reserves of expertise and resources to sustain long-range problem solving. ... [W]e must be in the business of creating organizations with built-in capacities for assessing needs and creating viable alternatives"* (Baldridge & Deal, 1975). This chapter has reviewed a number of approaches to large-scale change that have at least some history of application in the professions. Facilitated Deliberative Inquiry (FDI) is a combined approach that guides coordinated identification and use of selected change management theories and techniques. Having used the FDI approach as a consultant to change processes over the past decade I can attest to its utility.

Bottom line:

1. Regardless of what you are told, the reason for change avoidance is never about money. Amazing things can happen when people want to change something. Lack of money won't stop it; a little extra money makes it a lot easier; too much money acts as a distraction.
2. Get help. Don't try to change the world by yourself. Some of your help will come from inside the organization, but a lot more is available. Learn how to use consultants effectively, and find one you can trust to be there personally, and for the long haul if needed.
3. Change is a marathon, not a sprint. Take care of yourself. Know the source of your energy, your spirit. Take pains to constantly renew the supply. Protect and nourish those sources.
4. Regardless of how dark it seems on occasion: have courage, faith in your abilities, and persevere. The sun will rise again tomorrow.

In the Appendix a number of practical recommendations are given.

AREAS NEEDING FURTHER RESEARCH

Most of the evidence supporting change management theories, including the FDI method, is anecdotal. It would be useful if change managers would be more conscious of their choice and application of any selected change theory or technique. They should more carefully monitor and describe implementation to note deviations or necessary modifications and results obtained over time. This research design could involve an ongoing change process archivist/historian/anthropologist to compile a detailed description of events including the reflective mental processing of participants. This effort would be aided by increased use of process assessment through the course of the change intervention to monitor the evolution in components, understandings, goals, methods and behavior.

REFERENCES

AAMC (1998a). The Medical School Objectives Project. Report I: Learning Objectives for Medical Student Education: Guidelines for Medical Schools. Washington, DC: Association of American Medical Schools.

AAMC (1998b). The Medical School Objectives Project. Report II: Contemporary Issues in Medicine: Medical Informatics and Population Health. Washington, DC: Association of American Medical Schools.

AAMC (1998c) What Americans Say About the Nation's Medical Schools and Teaching Hospitals: Report on Public Opinion Research, Part II. Washington, DC: Association of American Medical Schools.

AAMC (1999). (Association of American Medical Schools) The Medical School Objectives Project. *Academic Medicine, 74*(1).

AAMC (2000). The Medical School Objectives Project. Report III: Contemporary Issues in Medical Education: Integrating Spirituality, End of Life Issues and Cultural Issues into the Practice of Medicine. Washington, DC: Association of American Medical Schools.

ACME-TRI Report. (1993). Educating Medical Students: Assessing Change in Medical Education – The Road to Implementation. *Academic Medicine, 68*(6) Supplement.

Adapting Clinical Medical Education to the Needs of Today and Tomorrow. (1988). New York: Josiah H. Macy Jr. Foundation.

Anderson, M. B. (1999) In progress: reports of new approaches in medical education. *Academic Medicine, 74,* 562-618.

Andrews, H., Cook, L. M., Davidson, J. M., Schurman, D. P., Taylor, E. W., & Wensel, R. H. (1994). *Organizational transformation in health care.* San Francisco: Jossey Bass.

Angell, M. (2000). Is academic medicine for sale? *New England Journal of Medicine, 342*(20).

Ansoff, H. I. (1965). *Corporate strategy.* New York: McGraw-Hill.

Argyris, C. (1991). Teaching smart people how to learn. *Harvard Business Review, 69*(3) May-June, 99-109.

Argyris, C., & Schön, D. A. (1974). *Theory in practice: increasing professional effectiveness.* San Francisco: Jossey-Bass.

Argyris, C., & Schön, D. A. (1978). *Organisational learning: A theory of action perspective.* Reading, MA: Addison Wesley.

Bacon, N. C. (1999). Modernizing medical education. *Hospital Medicine, 60,* 54-56.

Baldridge, J. V. (1975). Rules for a Machiavellian change agent: transforming the entrenched professional organization. In J. V. Baldridge & T. E. Deal (Eds.), *Managing change in educational organizations* (pp. 378-388). Berkeley, CA: McCutcheon.

Baldridge, J. V., & Deal, T. E. (1975). Overview of change processes in educational organizations. In J. V. Baldridge & T. E. Deal (Eds.), *Managing change in educational organizations* (pp. 1-23). Berkeley, CA: McCutcheon.

Barnes, B. E. (1998). Creating the practice-learning environment: Using information technology to support a new model of continuing medical education, *Academic Medicine, 73,* 278-281.

Beatty, R. W., & Ulrich, D. O. (1991). Re-energizing the mature organization. *Organizational Dynamics, Summer,* 16-30.

Beckhard, R., & Pritchard, W. (1992). *Changing the essence.* San Francisco: Jossey-Bass.

Beer, M., Eisenstat, R. A., & Spector, B. (1990). Why change programs don't produce change. *Harvard Business Review, Nov-Dec,* 158-166.

Bennis, W. G. (1989). *Why leaders can't lead.* San Francisco: Jossey-Bass.

Bennis, W. G., & Namus, B. (1985). *Leaders: Strategies for taking charge.* New York: Harper & Row.

Bennis, W. G., Benne, K. D., Chin, R., & Corey, K. E. (1976). *The planning of change.* New York: Holt Rinehart & Winston.

Berge, Z. L., & Collins, M. P. (Eds.). (1995) *Computer mediated communication and the online classroom.* Cresskill, NJ: Hampton Press.

Bloom, B. S. (1999). Internet availability of prescription pharmaceuticals to the public. *Annals of Internal Medicine, 131,* 830-833.

Bloom, S. W. (1988) Structure and ideology in medical education: an analysis of resistance to change. *Journal of Health and Social Behavior, Dec,* 294-306.

Bloom, S. W. (1989). The medical school as a social organization: the sources of resistance to change. *Medical Education, 23,* 228-241.

Blumenthal, D., Campbell, E. G., Anderson, M. S., Causino, N., & Louis, K. S. (1997). Withholding research results in academic life science: evidence from a national survey of faculty. *Journal of the American Medical Association, 277,* 1224-1228.

Bobula, J. D. (1980). Work patterns, practice characteristics, and incomes of male and female physicians. *Journal of Medical Education, 55,* 826-833.

Bodenheimer, T. (2000). Uneasy alliance: clinical investigators and the pharmaceutical industry. *New England Journal of Medicine, 342*(20), 1539-1544.

Boyer, E. L. (1990). *"Scholarship reconsidered" priorities of the professorate.* Princeton, NJ: Carnegie Foundation for the Advancement of Teaching.

Boyer Commission on Educating Undergraduates in the Research University. (1998). *Reinventing undergraduate education: a blueprint for America's research universities.* Stony Brook, NY: State University of New York.

Bryson, J. M. (1988). *Strategic planning for public and nonprofit organizations.* San Francisco: Jossey-Bass.

Bryson, J. M. (1995). *Strategic planning for public and nonprofit organizations.* San Francisco: Jossey-Bass.

Bulger, R. J. (1998). *The quest for mercy.* Charlottesville, VA: Jennings.

Bulger, R. J. (2000). The quest for the therapeutic organization. *Journal of the American Medical Association, 283*(18), 2431-2433.

Business & Health. (1998). DataWatch: Rx coverage and consumer ads: a costly combo. October, 68.

Bussigel, M., Barzansky, B., & Grenholm, G. (1986). Goal coupling and innovation in medical schools. *Journal of Applied Behavioral Sciences, 22,* 425-451.

Cabot, H. (1915). Medicine: a profession or a trade. *Boston Medical and Surgical Journal, Nov 4th,* 685-688.

Cantor, J. C., Cohen, A. B., Barker, D. C., Shuster, A. L., & Reynolds, R. C. (1991). Medical educators' views on medical education reform. *Journal of the American Medical Association, 265,* 1002-1006.

Carey, R. M., Wheby, M. S., & Reynolds, R. E. (1993). Evaluating faculty clinical excellence in the academic health science center. *Academic Medicine, 68,* 813-817.

Chan, D., LeClair, K., & Kaczorowski, J. (1999). Problem-based small-group learning via the Internet among community family physicians: A randomized controlled trial. *MD Computing, 16*(3), 54-58.

Chandler, A. D. (1962). *Strategy and structure: Chapters in the history of the industrial enterprise.* Cambridge: MIT Press.

Collins, O., & Moore, D. G. (1970). *The organization makers.* New York: Appleton-Century.

Cooper, C. L., Rout, U., & Faragher, B. (1989). Mental health, job satisfaction and job stress among general practitioners. *British Medical Journal, 298,* 366-370.

Cravener, P. A. (1999). Faculty experiences with providing online courses: thorns among roses. *Computers in Nursing, 17,* 42-47.

Cuban, L. (1997). Change without reform: the case of Stanford University School of Medicine, 1908-1990. *American Educational Research Journal, 34*(1), 83-122.

Curry, L. (1991). Patterns of learning style across selected medical specialties. *Educational Psychology, 11*(3&4), 247-277.

Curry, L. (1998). *Blueprint for the future: Educational enhancement project report and recommendations.* Washington, DC: The Liaison Committee for Podiatric Medical Education and Practice.

Curry, L. (1999). Cognitive and learning styles in medical education. *Academic Medicine, 74*(4), 409-413.

Davis, W. K., & White, B. A. (1993). Centralized decision making in management of the curriculum at the University of Michigan Medical School. *Academic Medicine, 68*(5), 333-335.

Day, P. (1982). Women doctors: choices and constraints in policies for medical manpower. Project Paper #28. London: King's Fund Centre.

DeAngelis, C. D. (2000). The plight of academic health centers. *Journal of the American Medical Association, 283*(18), 2438-2439.

Deming, W. E. (1986). *Out of the crisis.* Cambridge: MIT Center for Advanced Engineering Study.

Des Marchais, J. E. et collaborateurs. (1996). *Apprendre à Devenir Médecin: Bilan d'un Changement Pédagogique centre sur l'étudiant.* Sherbrooke, Québec: Université de Sherbrooke.

Des Marchais, J. E., & Bordage, G. (1998). Sustaining curricular change at Sherbrooke through external, formative program evaluations. *Academic Medicine, 73*(5), 494-503.

Des Marchais, J. E., Bureau, M. A., Dumais, B., & Pigeon, G. (1992). From traditional to problem-based learning: a case report of complete curriculum reform. *Medical Education, 26,* 190-199.

Dewey, *Journal Monist* (1898), 8, 335.

Dick, B. (1996). *Managing change.* [On line] Available at http://www.scu.edu.au/schools/sawd/arr/change.html.

Dick, B., & Dalman, T. (1990). *Values in action: applying the ideas of Argyris and Schön.* Brisbane: Interchange.

Dickhout, R., Denham, M., & Blackwell, N. (1995). Designing change programs that won't cost you your job. *McKinsey Quarterly, 4,* 101-116.

Dillon, C. L. (1996). Distance education research and continuing professional education: reframing questions for the emerging information infrastructure. *Journal for Continuous Education in the Health Professions, 16,* 5-13.

Drucker, P. E. (1970). Entrepreneurship in business enterprise. *Journal of Business Policy, I*(1), 3-12.

Dumelow, C., Littlejohns, P., & Griffiths, S. (2000). The inter-relationship between a medical career and family life for hospital consultants: an interview survey. *British Medical Journal, 320,* 1437-1440.

Enarson, C., & Burg, F. D. (1992). An overview of reform initiatives in medical education: 1906 through 1992. *Journal of the American Medical Association, 268,* 1141-1143.

Evans, R. G., & Stoddart, G. L. (1990). Producing health, consuming health care. *Social Science in Medicine, 31*(12), 1347-1363.

Financial Post. (2000). Advertisement: Get your Executive MBA Online. Friday, February 18th: D8, columns 2 &3.

Finocchio, L. J., Dower, C. M., McMahon, T., Gragnola, C. M., & the Taskforce on Health Care Workforce Regulation. (1995). *Reforming health care workforce regulation: Policy considerations for the 21st century.* San Francisco: Pew Health Professions Commission.

Flexner, A. (1910). Medical Education in the United States and Canada: a report to the Carnegie Foundation for the Advancement of Teaching. Bulletin no. 4. Princeton, NJ: Carnegie Foundation for the Advancement of Teaching.

Friedberg, M., Saffran, B., Stinson, T. J., Nelson, W., & Bennett, C. L. (1999). Evaluation of conflict of interest in economic analyses of new drugs used in oncology. *Journal of the American Medical Association, 282,* 1453-1457.

Friedman, C. P., & Purcell, E. F. (Eds.). (1983). *The new biology and medical education: merging the biological, information and cognitive sciences.* New York: Josiah H. Macy Jr. Foundation.

Funkenstein, D. H. (1978). *Medical students, medical schools, and society during five eras.* Cambridge, MA: Ballinger.

Future Directions for Medical Education: a report of the Council on Medical Education. (1982). Chicago: American Medical Association.

Gale, R., & Grant, J. (1997). AMEE Medical Education Guide No. 10: managing change in a medical context: guidelines for action. *Medical Teacher, 19*(4), 239-249.

General Medical Council. (1996). *Tomorrow's doctors: recommendations on undergraduate medical education.* London: GMC

General Medical Council. (1997). *The new doctor.* London: GMC

Giardino, A. P., Giardino, E. R., MacLaren, C. F., & Burg, F. D. (1994). Managing change: a case study of implementing change in a clinical evaluation system. *Teaching and Learning in Medicine, 6*(3), 149-153.

Globe and Mail. (1999). Statscan study shows doctors raking it in. Thursday, December 2nd.

Goldstein, D. (2000). *e-Health care: Harness the Power of Internet e-Commerce and e-Care* as quoted in "Online relief for health care overload", *Financial Post,* Monday May 1st: E1.

Grant, J., & Marsden, P. (1992). *Training senior house officers by service-based learning.* London: Joint Centre for Education in Medicine.

Gray, C. (1980). How will the new wave of women graduates change the medical profession? *Canadian Medical Association Journal, 123,* 798-801.

Griner, P. F., & Danoff, D. (2000). Sustaining change in medical education. *Journal of the American Medical Association, 283*(18), 2429-2431.

Gruppen, L. D. (1997). Implications of cognitive research for ambulatory care education. *Academic Medicine, 72*(2), 117-120.

Harris, I. B. (1993). Perspectives for curriculum renewal in medical education. *Academic Medicine, 68*(6), 484-486.

Hastings Centre Report. (1996) The Goals of Medicine: Setting new standards. Special Supplement, Nov-Dec.

Heins, M., Smock, S., Martindale, L., Jacobs, J., & Stein, M. (1977). Comparison of the productivity of women and men physicians. *Journal of the American Medical Association, 237*(23), 2514-2517.

Hersh, W. (1999). A world of knowledge at your fingertips: The promise, reality and future directions of on-line information retrieval. *Academic Medicine, 72,* 240-243.

Hippisley-Cox, J., Allan, J., Pringle, M., Ebdon, D., McPhearson, M., Churchill, D., & Bradley, S. (2000). Association between teenage pregnancy rates and the age and sex of general practitioners: cross sectional survey in Trent 1994-7. *British Medical Journal, 320,* 842-845.

Huff, A. S. (Ed.). (1990). *Mapping strategic thought.* Somerset, NJ: Wiley.

Hylka, S. C., & Beschle, J. C. (1995). Nurse practitioners, cost savings and improved patient care in the Department of Surgery. *Nurse Economist, 13*(6), 349-354.

Inglehart, J. (1997). Forum on the future of academic medicine: Session 1 – Setting the stage. *Academic Medicine, 72*(7), 595-599.

Jadad, A. (1999). Promoting partnerships: challenges for the Internet age. *British Medical Journal, 319,* 761-764.

Johnson, F. A., & Johnson, C. L. (1976). Role strain in high-commitment career women. *Journal of American Academic Psychoanalysis, 4*(1), 13-36.

Jonas, S. (1984). The case for change in medical education in the United States. *Lancet, 2,* 452-454.

Jones, R. F., & Gold, J. S. (1998). Faculty appointment and tenure policies in medical schools: a 1997 status report. *Academic Medicine, 73,* 212-219.

Jupiter Communications (2000). As quoted in 'Online relief for health care overload', *Financial Post,* Monday May 1st: E1.

Kanter, R. M. (1983). *The change masters.* New York: Simon & Schuster

Kaufman, A. (1998). Leadership and governance. *Academic Medicine, 73*(9) supplement, S11-S15.

Kehrer, B. H. (1976). Factors affecting the incomes of men and women physicians: an exploratory analysis. *Journal of Human Resources, 11*(4), 526-545.

Kets de Vries, M. (1991). *Organizations on the couch.* San Francisco: Jossey-Bass.

Koch, L. W., Pazaki, S. H., & Campbell, J. D. (1992). The first 20 years of nurse practitioner literature: an evolution of joint practice issues. *Nurse Practitioner, 17*(2), 62-71.

Kotter, J. P. (1995). Leading change: why transformation efforts fail. *Harvard Business Review, March-April,* 59-67.

Larkin, M. (1999). US online pharmacies strive for respectability. *Lancet, 354,* 782.

Levinson, W., & Rubenstein, A. (1999). Mission critical: integrating clinician-educators into academic medical centers. *New England Journal of Medicine, 341*(11), 840-843.

Levinson, W., Tolle, S. W., & Lewis, C. (1989). Women in academic medicine combining career and family. *New England Journal of Medicine, 321*(22), 1511-1517.

Levit, E. J. (1973). *Evaluation in continuum of medical education.* Report of the Committee on Goals and Priorities of the National Board of Medical Examiners. Philadelphia, PA.

Levy, S. (1999). Most community pharmacies question value of DTC Rx ads. *Drug Topics, December 6th,* 87.

Lewin, K. (1951). *Field theory in social science.* New York: Harper & Row.

Lewin Group (2000). *The impact of the Medicare Balanced Budget Refinement Act on Medicare payments to hospitals.* Falls Church, VA: American Hospital Association.

Light, D. W. (1988). Toward a new sociology of medical education. *Journal of Health and Social Behavior,* 29(December), 307-322.

Lindberg, M. A. (1998). The process of change: stories of the journey. *Academic Medicine, 73*(9) supplement, S4-S10.

Lindblom, C. E. (1959). The science of "muddling through". *Public Administration Review, 19,* 79-88.

Lorange, P. (1980). *Corporate planning: an executive viewpoint.* Englewood Cliffs, NJ: Prentice Hall.

MacLeod, S. M. (1997). Change and the academic health science centre: 1997 perspective. *ACMC Forum, August,* 3-5.

Macmillan, I. C. (1978). *Strategy formation: political concepts.* St. Paul, MN: West.

Makridakis, S. (1990). *Forecasting, planning and strategy for the 21st century.* New York: Free Press.

March, J. G., & Simon, H. A. (1958). *Organizations.* New York: Wiley.

Mårtenson, D. (1989). Educational development in an established medical school: facilitating and impeding factors in change at the Karolinska Institute. *Medical Teacher, 11*(1), 17-20.

McCormach, C., & Jones, D. (1998). *Building a Web-based education system.* Toronto: Wiley.

McLellan, F. (1998). The Internet. *Lancet, 352*(Supplement II), SII39-SII43.

Medical Post. (1998). National Survey of Doctors. December.

Mennin, S. P., & Kaufman, A. (1989). The change process and medical education. *Medical Teacher, 11*(1), 9-16.

Miller, D. (1979). Strategy, structure and environment: context influences on some bivariate associations. *Journal of Management Studies, 16*(Oct), 294-316.

Miller, D., Droge, C., & Toulouse, J. (1988). Strategic process and content as mediators between organizational context and structure. *Academy of Management Journal, 31*(3), 544-569.

Mintzberg, H., Ahlstrand, B., & Lampel, J. (1998). *Strategy safari: a guided tour through the wilds of strategic management.* New York: Free Press.

Mitchell, A., Pinelli, J., Patterson, C., & Southwell, D. (1993). *Utilization of nurse practioners in Ontario.* Executive Summary (discussion paper). Hamilton, ON: McMaster University School of Nursing.

Mizrahi, T. (1986). *Getting rid of patients: Contradictions in the socialization of physicians.* New Brunswick, NJ: Rutgers University Press.

Mohrman, A. M., Mohrman, A. S., Ledford, G. E., Cummings, T. G., & Lawler, E. E. (1980). *Large-scale organizational change.* San Francisco: Jossey-Bass.

Murray, S. (1998). Separating the wheat from the chaff: evaluating consumer health information on the Internet. *Bibliotheca Medica Canadiana, Summer 19*(4), 142-145.

Myers, I. B. (1962). *Introduction to Type: a description of the theory and application of the Myers-Briggs Type Indicator.* Palo Alto, CA: Consulting Psychologists Press.

Neufeld, V. R., Maudsley, R. F., Pickering, R. J., Walters, B. C., Turnbull, J. F., Spasoff, R. A., Hollomby, D. J., & La Vigne, K. J. (1993). Demand-side medical education: educating future physicians for Ontario. *Canadian Medical Association Journal, 148,* 1471-1477.

Nonaka, I., & Takeuchi, H. (1995). *The knowledge-creating company: How Japanese companies create the dynamics of innovation.* New York: Oxford University Press.

Normann, R. (1977). *Management for growth.* New York: Wiley.

OECD (1999) as quoted by Kettle, J. in Your money or your life. *The Globe & Mail: September 2:* B4.

Osborne, D., & Gaebler, T. (1993). *Reinventing government.* New York: Plume.

Ottawa Citizen. (2000). Billionaire donates $1000M for free online university. Thursday, March 16: A14, columns 2, 3, 4 & 5.

Pardes, H. (1997). The future of medical schools and teaching hospitals in the era of managed care. *Academic Medicine, 72,* 97-102.

Pardes, H. (2000). The perilous state of academic medicine. *Journal of the American Medical Association, 283*(18), 2427-2429.

Parle, J. V., Greenfield, S. M., Skelton, J., Lester, H., & Hobes, F. D. R. (1997). Acquisition of the basic clinical skills in the general practice setting. *Medical Education, 31,* 99-104.

Pellegrino, E. D. (1978). Medical education. *Encyclopedia of Bioethics,* Vol. 2, 863-870. New York: Free Press.

Physicians for the Twenty-First Century: report of the Project Panel on the general professional education of the physician and college preparation for medicine. (1984). Washington, DC: Association of American Medical Colleges.

Pirisi, A. (1999). Patient-directed drug advertising puts pressure on US doctors. *Lancet, 354,* 1887.

PJ (1999). Internet pharmacy. *Pharmaceutical Journal, 263,* 841.

PJ (2000). On-line pharmacy offers NHS dispensing service. *Pharmaceutical Journal, 264,* 201.

Porter, M. E. (1980). *Competitive strategy: Techniques for analyzing industries and competitors.* New York: Free Press.

Powers, L., Parmelle, R. D., & Weisenfelder, H. (1969). Practice patterns of women and men physicians. *Journal of Medical Education, 44,* 481-491.

Pruitt, N. L., Underwood, L. S., & Surver, W. (2000). *BioInquiry: making connections in biology.* New York: Wiley.

Quinn, J. B. (1980). *Strategies for change: Logical incrementalism.* Holmwood: Irwin.

Quinn, J. B. (1982). Managing strategies incrementally. *Omega: International Journal of Management Sciences, 10*(6), 613-627.

Regan-Smith, M. G. (1998). Reform without change: update, 1998. *Academic Medicine, 73*(5), 505-507.

Relman, A. (1980). Here come the women. *New England Journal of Medicine, 302*(22), 1252-1253.

Rhenman, E. (1973). *Organization theory for long-range planning.* London: Wiley.

Rice, R. E., & Richlin, L. (1993). Broadening the concept of scholarship in the professions. In L. Curry & J. F. Wergin (Eds.), *Educating professionals: Responding to new expectations for competence and accountability* (pp. 279-315). San Francisco: Jossey-Bass.

Roddie, I. C. A. (1986). A critique of fashion in medical education: some thoughts on the GPEP Report. *New York State Journal of Medicine, 86,* 421-428.

Saxton, J. F., Blake, D. A., Fox, J. T., & Johns, M. M. E. (2000). The evolving academic health center: strategies and priorities at Emory University. *Journal of the American Medical Association, 283*(18), 2434-2436.

Selnick, P. (1957). *Leadership in administration: A sociological interpretation*. Evanston: Peterson.

Schwartz, P. L., Heath, C. J., & Egan, A. G. (1994). *The art of the possible: Ideas from a traditional medical school engaged in curricular reform*. Dunedin, New Zealand: University of Otago Press.

Science (1993). *Medical Research: Alternative Views*. Letter to the Editor from R. Lamm. American Association for the Advancement of Science (AAAS), 262, December 3: 1497.

Science (1998). News Report. American Association for the Advancement of Science (AAAS), 285, June 26: 2019.

Science (2000) Pedagogy First, Technology Later. American Association for the Advancement of Science (AAAS). 287, January 28: 543.

Science (2000) Free Online University? American Association for the Advancement of Science (AAAS). 287, March 24: 2111.

Senge, P. M. (1990). *The fifth discipline: The art and practice of the learning organization*. New York: Doubleday.

Shahabudin, S. H., & Safiah, N. (1991). Managing the initial period of implementation of educational change. *Medical Teacher, 13*(3), 205-211.

Simon, H. A. (1957). *Administrative behavior*. New York: Macmillan.

Smye, M. (1993). *You don't change a company by memo*. Toronto: Key Porter.

Southgate, L., & Grant, J. (2000). Opportunities and dreams: plans for a networked medical school & foundation course for medicine. Available at http://www.asme.org.uk.

Steiner, G. A. (1979). *Strategic planning: What every manager must know*. New York: Free Press.

Stelfox, H. T., Chua, G., Rourke, K., & Detsky, A. S. (1998). Conflict of interest in the debate over calcium-channel antagonists. *New England Journal of Medicine, 338*, 101-106.

Taub, J. (1997). Drive-Thru U. Higher education for people who mean business. *New Yorker*, October 20th & 27th, 114- 123.

Tosteson, D. C., Adelstein, S. J., & Carver, S. T. (Eds.). (1994). *New pathways to medical education: Learning to learn at Harvard Medical School*. Cambridge, MA: Harvard University Press.

Tuckman, B. W. (1965). Developmental sequences in small groups. *Psychological Bulletin, 63*, 384-399.

Weldon, V. V. (1987). Why the dinosaurs died: Extinction or evolution? *Journal of Medical Education, 62*(February), 109-115.

Wilkins, A. (1989). *Developing corporate character*. San Francisco: Jossey-Bass.

Wilson, A., Fraser, R., McKinley, R. R., Preston-Whyte, E., & Wynn, A. (1996). Undergraduate teaching in the community: can general practice deliver? *British Journal of General Practice, 46*, 457-460.

Wilson, M. (1979). The status of women in medicine: background data. Paper presented at the Mary E. Garrett Symposium at Johns Hopkins University School of Medicine, October 9-10.

Woodward, C. A., Cohen, M. L., & Ferrier, B. M. (1990). Career interruptions and hours practiced: comparison between young men and women physicians. *Canadian Journal of Public Health, 81*, 16-20.

World Health Organization. (1996). *Integration of health care delivery*. WHO Technical Report Series #861. Geneva: WHO.

Zoeller, J. (1999). Rushing the net. *American Druggist, 216*(3), 50-55.

APPENDIX: CHECKLIST FOR CHANGE AGENTS

1. Be very sure you need to implement a large-scale change.
   - Seriously tackle the question of why something needs to change. What is the real problem you are addressing? What are the root causes of that problem?
   - What else could be done to address those issues inside the current structure?
   - Check to see if this sense of needed change is a shared perception. Who is committed to it? Who will help? Who opposes?
   - Know that undertaking any large-scale change will focus the organization on internal matters almost exclusively, which may be counterproductive or dangerous for the organization.
2. Move quickly from a shared sense of need for change to concrete description of possible futures.
   - Define change objectives in terms of the already accepted mission.
   - Set up reflection and deliberation about the mission of the faculty, the school, and the profession. Make this more than a rhetorical exercise.
   - Facilitate articulation and public sharing of beliefs and values.
   - Structure the change process to mirror these virtues.
   - Induce reflection on the relation of the organization's structure and operations with the above avowed values and beliefs.
   - Actively work on "imagine the institution otherwise". This is the "change story".
   - Make these alternate visions concrete. What would be necessary to have each one be actual? All alternative structures under consideration must rapidly become tangible, at least in description, so that people can see the potential "workability" of   the innovation and their exact place in it. Changes implied for vertical hierarchies and horizontal support structures must be made clear. In each possible new scenario: How will individuals and groups make decisions, sustain and continue the change desired, interact with each other and with learners? How will accountability work for individuals, for work products and for results? What support systems will be necessary? What has to change in skill building, performance management systems, and information systems?
   - Design the innovation to be implemented. The change must be do-able with available resources and without performance trade-offs in critical indicators.
3. Broadly define the "community" of involved stakeholders.
   - More than faculty and students are involved in any significant change.
   - Views from interested and affected "outsiders" crucial to the institution are also critical to real innovation.
4. Negotiate for sufficient political support. Structure to protect that support.
   - At least one powerful patron (i.e. the Dean) must be involved.
   - The target change must also be part of the patron's personal agenda.
   - This support of a powerful patron must be visible, and periodically renewed in public for all to see.
   - The patron must be protected:

- Use a structure that allows the power players (the Dean, the Provost, the President) some distance from the specifics of the changes tried.
- Hire or designate a "change leader" who will provide "day to day" direct leadership. This individual must have delegated authority to match this responsibility.
- While continuity is comforting to all involved, the change leader can be changed if he/she proves inept or a poor skill match to requirements.
- Consider cloning your leadership and patrons. The Dean job now has evolved to at least four roles: cheerleader, resource hunter & gatherer, political godfathering, and three types of academic leader (discipline side, research side, and care provision side). Excellent performances in all these roles will be necessary to initiate, sustain and complete any significant change. Some role sharing with other individuals may be helpful both to the incumbent and to the change process.

5. Build the "critical mass" for change. Supportive critical mass is needed in each important stakeholder group: students at each level, basic science faculty, clinical faculty, researchers, administrators, employers, practitioners and funders. The identification and co-optation of an opinion leader in each target constituency is critical to building critical mass.
   - If these opinion leaders are not immediately obvious by observing the behavior of the constituency then conduct a cultural analysis to identify them. Note that there is an important difference between an opinion leader and an elected or appointed leader.
   - Once identified develop these opinion leaders into "change team leaders". If the opinion leader is unwilling, develop one of his/her "lieutenants" (that is one effective way to bring the opinion leader around to supporting the change).
   - A change team leader should be personally fully committed to the change and the change process.
   - A change team leader must dependably defend and advocate for the change and the change process.
   - Negotiate some extra money to pay for this new role on an ongoing basis as long as needed.
   - Structure to hear from and get information to all stakeholder groups.
     - This can be accomplished through the FDI process.
     - With, or more importantly without, the FDI "roll-out" process, invest in and implement a strong two-way communications plan. This might involve newsletters, blast e-mail, telephone trees, town hall meetings, frequent sessions with each stakeholder group or constituency, regular attendance at public events (i.e. lunch in the cafeteria routinely at the same time and same location; all talk to be about the change process and content).

6. Develop internal expertise in necessary areas (capacity building).
   - Develop & operate an effective/efficient secretariat function to regularly "capture the story" and make that available for reflection.
   - Use consultants to bring in expertise as needed, but

- Make sure the consulting contract is constructed around capacity transfer, not dependence
- Use consultants catalytically. Good consultants can help analyze problems, develop new solutions, and bring in new information, new ideas, and different points of view. They can help working groups and communities develop the knowledge, skills and attitudes and the confidence to try new approaches. An experienced consultant can coach leaders (change leaders and their patrons) on how to structure for and support change. Consultants are useful to have a shoulder to cry on in the tough patches and as a scapegoat to fire if blood sacrifice is required.
- Steal ideas with impunity. First investigate thoroughly the up and downsides of any promising idea. Find out what worked and didn't; what they wish they had done; what they learned. If it still looks good, ask the originator for support in importing the idea to your situation. Most people are thrilled to be considered a model.

7. Establish a reward system to recognize individual investment in change.
   - Be creative here. Not all rewards are very expensive.
   - Negotiate interim or experimental, time-limited change in the promotion and tenure process and criteria in order to use these promotions as part of the change process and reward system.
   - Use extra bonus money to carefully reward needed behavior change.
   - Find opportunities to present workshops or presentations on your change process, goals and accomplishments. Use these paid trips outside the school to reward needed behavior and to co-opt opinion leaders. The effects are particularly spectacular if the trip is international.
   - Acknowledge the people behind the behavior, helpful or not. Thank people publicly and privately. Remember birthdays. Write "Thank-you" notes often. Celebrate success: small steps as well as big wins.

8. Manage the fear and despair.
   - No one should delude himself or herself that logic and well-reasoned argument will make the change acceptable or get it implemented.
   - Even if dysfunctional, people are attached to their current systems. The existing processes, procedures, mechanisms are all well-known and well-aligned with existing power structures.
   - Any serious proposal to make a noticeable difference in any aspect of the existing structure will be greeted with suspicion, hostility and defensive aggression.
   - Some of this will be personalized into attacks on you as the individual with the temerity to bring up the new ideas. Your credentials will be attacked. Your credibility will be attacked. Your sanity will be attacked! No wonder the transfer problem is so tough! No wonder most of us give up most of the time.
   - All this negativity is a result of fear and despair that must be actively managed to allow change development, testing and implementation.
   - An important component in the management of fear and despair is to support, teach, and coach faculty, administration and other stakeholders

(including students) in the practical skills and techniques involved in large-scale change.

- A second antidote to fear and despair is having in place the structures (i.e. FDI & a communications plan) that allow all players to have input at all times. Fear is diminished if participants and constituencies have an ongoing and dependable way to revise/reconsider/revamp each piece of the change until the pieces fit, the fear abates and the implementation produces the sought for results.

- Legitimize "research" in the change focus. This means extending a true experimental attitude towards trying different solutions, and hypothesis testing around the questions and problems. With this attitude it is OK to not be entirely successful in the first number of attempts. As long as each effort results in learning and improvement for the next attempt, an experimental attitude will help continue support for the trials.

9. Keep the change fresh and exciting in order to keep the process going.
   - Organizational structures put in place to initiate, sustain and implement change must be flexible and continuously re-created to be responsive to changing needs/fears/demands.
   - Be prepared to change the work structure, the names of committees and the participants on work groups.
   - Change the metaphors, not the direction nor the goals nor the pace.
   - Use formative evaluations, conducted by inside and by outside agents to periodically re-catalyze and re-focus reflection and renewal.

10. Utilize principles of cognitive dissonance to solidify support for the change direction and specifics.
    - Ask wavering or lukewarm individuals to help present overviews on the change at national and international meetings.
    - Tell the change story frequently, repeatedly, in and outside the organization. Cast the story in concrete terms to allow people to imagine themselves in the altered scenario and find that at least tolerable.
    - Create opportunities to "show-off" new ideas, new solutions, and contemplated or actual changes. The more prestigious the setting, the better. National and international venues are best, but even local innovations showcases should be utilized or created. Organize press coverage (facilitate photographs) or publications and display the results prominently.
    - Join formally and participate actively in organizations that support the change you are trying to make. These may be groupings of other similar organizations trying to change (i.e. the Network of Community-Oriented Educational Institutions for Health Sciences, or the Generalists in Medical Education), other organizations beyond the profession dedicated to change and change management or even reform wings of traditional professional organizations. Go yourself and actively encourage broad faculty participation.

11. Larger scale, scope and depth of change make change in any one facet easier. Consider the effects your intended change will have on related bodies or agencies. They may be moving in parallel directions and could bolster local support if tied into your change. The following are usual sources of curricular

change that may have some process or standards improvement project going on that you can incorporate, accelerate, enhance or hitch on to in some way:
- Accreditation systems, criteria, procedures
- Practicum or residency training
- Credentialing systems
- Funding systems.

12. Benchmarks from outside the organization will not be totally applicable or relevant.

Each organization must identify and create its own future with its own resources. The principal utility of outside materials/benchmarks is to act as proof that change is possible and that there are more than the local current practices to consider.

List of Authors

Christina van Barneveld, Measurement and Evaluation, Department of Curriculum Teaching and Learning, Ontario Institute for Students in Education/University of Toronto, 252 Bloor St. W., Rm 11-223, Toronto, Ontario, M5S 1V6, Canada, T: +1 416 367-04783, E: cvanbarneveld@oise.utoronto.ca.

Eta S. Berner, Ed.D., Professor, Health Informatics Program, Department of Health Services Administration, University of Alabama at Birmingham, Birmingham, Alabama, USA, T: +1 205 975-8219, F: +1 205 975-6608, E: eberner@uab.edu.

Carole J. Bland, University of Minnesota Medical School, Department of Family Practice and Community Health, P.O. Box 381, 516 Delaware Street SE, Minneapolis, MN 55455-0392, USA, T: +1 612 624-2072, F: +1 612 624-2525, E: bland001@umn.edu.

Henny P. A. Boshuizen, Ph.D., Associate Professor and Director of Educational Sciences and the Master degree programme on Health Professions Education. Maastricht University, P.O. Box 616, 6200 MD Maastricht, The Netherlands, T: +31 43 388-4035, F: +31 43 388-4575, E: Boshuizen@educ.unimaas.nl.

Sally H. Cavanaugh, Ph.D., Director of Research, EMIG Research Center of York Hospital, 1001 S. George Street, York, Pennsylvania 174405, USA, T: +1 717 851-2223, F: +1 717 851-3470, E: scavanaugh@yorkhospital.edu or shc2@psu.edu.

Sheila W. Chauvin, Director, Office of Educational Research and Services, Associate Professor of Psychiatry, Tulane University School of Medicine, Adjunct Professor of Community Health Sciences, Tulane University School of Public Health and Tropical Medicine, SL6, 1430 Tulane Avenue, New Orleans, LA 70112-2699, USA, T: +1 504 988-6600, F: +1 504 988-6601, E: schauvin@tulane.edu.

Brian E. Clauser, Senior Psychometrician, National Board of Medical Examiners, 3750 Market Street, Philadelphia, PA 19104, USA, T: +1 215 590-9500, F: +1 215 590-9555, E: bclauser@mail.nbme.org.

John Cunnington, Associate Professor, Department of Medicine, McMaster University, 1200 Main St West, Hamilton, Ontario L5N 3Z5, Canada, T: +1 905 521-2100, F: +1 905 521-5053, E: cunningt@mcmaster.ca.

Lynn Curry, Curry Corp, 17 Oakland Avenue, Ottawa, Ontario K1S 2T1, Canada, T: +1 613 232-6708, F: +1 613 232-0038, E: Lynn@CurryCorp.net.

Annie Cushing, Department of Human Science and Medical Ethics, Barts and The London, Queen Mary's School of Medicine and Dentistry, Turner Street, London, E1 2AD, United Kingdom, T: + 44 20 7377-7000 ext. 3047, F: + 44 20 7377-7167, E: A.M.Cushing@mds.qmw.ac.uk.

Eugène, J. F. M. Custers, Ph.D., UMC Utrecht, Onderwijsinstituut, Afdeling Coördinatie Ontwikkeling & Research, Postbus 85060, 3508 AB Utrecht, The Netherlands, T: + 31 030 2532996, F: + 31 030 253 8200, E: e.j.f.m.custers@med.uu.nl.

W. Dale Dauphinee, Executive Director, Medical Council of Canada, P.O. Box 8234 Station T, Ottawa, KIG 3H7, Canada, T: +1 613 521-8787, F: +1 613 521-8831, E: dauphine@mcc.ca.

Wayne K. Davis, formerly Professor of Medical Education, University of Michigan Medical School, 599 Echo Court, Saline, MI 48176, USA.

Diana H. J. M. Dolmans, Ph.D., Educational Psychologist, Department of Educational Development and Research, University of Maastricht, P.O. Box 616, 6200 MD Maastricht, The Netherlands, T: +31 43 388-1107, F: +31 43 388-4140, E: D.Dolmans@educ.unimaas.nl.

Steven M. Downing, Ph.D., Univeristy of Illinois at Chicago, Department of Medical Education, MC 591, College of Medicine, 808 South Wood Street, Chicago, IL 60612-7309, USA, T: +1 773 324-2032, E: smdowning@mindspring.com.

Arthur S. Elstein, Ph.D., Department of Medical Education (m/c 591), University of Illinois at Chicago, 808. S. Wood Street, Chicago, IL 60612-7309, USA, T: +1 312 996-5451, F: +1 312 413-2048, E: aelstein@uic.edu.

Ruth-Marie E. Fincher, Ph.D., Professor of Medicine, Medical College of Georgia, School of Medicine, CB-1847 Augusta, Georgia 30912, USA, T: +1 706 721-3529, F: +1 706 721-7244, E: rfincher@mail.mcg.edu.

Edred A. Flak, M.D., F.R.C.P.C., University of Toronto Faculty of Medicine, Department of Psychiatry, Mount Sinai Hospital, 600 University Avenue, Toronto, Ontario M5G 1X5, Canada, T: +1 416 586-4662, F: +1 416 586-8654, E: eflak@mtsinai.on.ca.

Gregory S. Fortna, M.S.Ed., American Board of Internal Medicine, 510 Walnut Street, Philadelphia, PA 19106-3699, USA, T: +1 215 446-3500, F: +1 215 446-3470, E: sfortna@abim.org.

Alice Z. Frohna, Ph.D., University of Michigan Medical School, Office of Educational Resources and Research, Department of Medical Education, G1111 Towsley Center, Ann Arbor, MI 48109-0201, USA, T: +1 734 641-3306, F: +1 734 936-1641, E: azf@umich.edu.

Larry D. Gruppen, Ph.D., University of Michigan Medical School, Office of Educational Resources and Research, Department of Medical Education, G1111 Towsley Center, Ann Arbor, MI 48109-0201, USA, T: +1 734 763-1153, F: +1 734 936-1641, E: lgruppen@umich.edu.

Robin Guille, Robin Guille American Board of Internal Medicine, 215 Market St. Suite 1700, Philadelphia, PA 19106 – 3699, USA, T: +1 215 446-3581, F: +1 215 446-3476, E: rguille@abim.org.

Ilene B. Harris, Ph.D., University of Minnesota Medical School, Minneapolis, Professor and Director, Office of Education – Educational Development and Research, B611 Mayo, 420 Delaware St. SE, Minneapolis, MN 55455, USA, T: +1 612 625-9497, F: +1 612 626-4200, E: harri001@e.umn.edu.

Brian Hodges, Assistant Professor and Vice-Chair (Education), Department of Psychiatry and The Centre for Research in Education at the University Health Network, University of Toronto, Faculty of Medicine, 200 Elizabeth Street, Eaton South, 1-565, Toronto, Ontario, M5G 2C4, Canada, T: +1 416-340 4451, F: +1 416 340 4198, E: brian.hodges@utoronto.ca.

Hans Asbjørn Holm, M.D., Ph.D., Deputy Secretary General, Norwegian Medical Association, P.O. Box 1152, Sentrum, N-0107 Oslo, Norway, T: + 47 231 09112, F: + 47 231 09100, E: hah@legeforeningen.no.

Brian C. Jolly, University of Sheffield, Department of Medical Education, Coleridge House, Northern General Hospital, Herries Road, Sheffield, S5 7AU, United Kingdom, T: + 44 114 271-5939, F: + 44 114 242-4896, E: b.jolly@sheffield.ac.uk.

Lloyd A. Lewis, Nealing Ave., North Augusta, S. Carolina 29841, USA, T: +1 803 278-1059.

Karen V. Mann, Professor and Director, Division of Medical Education, Clinical Research Centre, Room C-112, Dalhousie University, Halifax, Nova Scotia, B3H 4H7, Canada, T: +1 902 494-1884, F: +1 902 494-2278, E: Karen.Mann@Dal.ca.

William C. McGaghie, Ph.D., Northwestern University Medical School, Office of Medical Education and Faculty Development, 3-130 Ward Building W117, 303 E. Chicago Avenue, Chicago, IL 60611-3008, USA, T: +1 312 503-0174, F: +1 312 503-0840, E: wcmc@northwestern.edu.

Julie J. McGowan, Ph.D., Director and Professor, Knowledge Informatics, Library and Information Resources, 975 W. Walnut Street, (IB-310), School of Medicine, Indiana University, Indianapolis, Indiana 46202, USA, E: jjmcgowa @iupui.edu.

Mathieu R. Nendaz, M.D., M.H.P.E., Faculty Member, Department of Internal Medicine, University of Geneva Hospitals, 1211 Geneva 14, Switzerland, T: +41 22 372-9055, F: +41 22 372-9116, E: Mathieu.Nendaz@hcuge.ch.

David I. Newble, University of Sheffield, Department of Medical Education, Coleridge House, Northern General Hospital, Herries Road, Sheffield, S5 7AU, United Kingdom, T: +44 114 271 5943, F: +44 114 242 4896, E: d.newble@ sheffield.ac.uk.

John Norcini, Senior Vice President for Evaluation & Research, American Board of Internal Medicine, 510 Walnut St, Suite 1410, Philadelphia, PA 19106-3699, USA, T: +1 215 4463500, F: +1 215 4463470, E: jnorcini@abim.org.

Geoff R. Norman, McMaster University, Department of Clinical Epidemiology and Biostatistics, 1200 Main Street West, Health Sciences Centre 2C4, Hamilton, Ontario, L8N 3Z5, Canada, T: +1 905 525-9140, F: +1 905 577-0017, E: norman@mcmaster.ca.

Gordon Page, Professor, Faculty of Medicine, Director, Division of Educational Support and Development, Office of the Co-ordinator, Health Sciences, #400 – 2194 Health Sciences Mall, University of British Columbia, Vancouver, B.C., V6T 1Z6, Canada, T: +1 604 822-6641, F: +1 604 822-2495, E: gpage@ unixg.ubc.ca.

Emil R. Petrusa, Ph.D., Director and Associate Dean of Medical Education, Office of Medical Education Research and Development, Duke University Medical Center, Suite 600, Davison Building, DUMC 3628, Durham, NC 27710, USA, T: +1 919 681-8032, F: +1 919 681-8195, E: petru001@mc.duke.edu.

Glenn Regehr, Ph.D., Associate Director, University of Toronto, Faculty of Medicine, Centre for Research in Education at the University Health Network, IE564-200 Elisabeth Street, Toronto, Ontario, M5G 2C4, Canada, T: +1 416 340-3615, F: +1 416 340-3792, E: g.regehr@utoronto.ca.

Arthur Rothman, Ed.D., Education Office, Department of Medicine, University of Toronto, NSSB S-Wing, Suite 3-805, 190 Elizabeth Street, Toronto, Ontario, M5G 2C4, Canada, T: +1 416 978-4014, F: +1 416 978-4568, E: arthur. rothman@utoronto.ca.

Lambert W. T. Schuwirth, M.D., Ph.D., Department of Educational Development and Research, University of Maastricht, P.O. Box 616, 6200 MD Maastricht, The Netherlands, T: +31 43 388-1129, F: +31 43 338 4140, E: l.schuwirth@ educ.unimaas.nl.

Alan Schwartz, Assistant Professor, Department of Medical Education, Mail Code 591, 808 S. Wood St, 986 CME, University of Illinois at Chicago, Chicago, IL 60612, USA, T: +1 312 996-2070, F: +1 312 413-2048, E: alansz@uic.edu.

Judy A. Shea, Director of the Office of Evaluation and Assessment, Academic Programs Office, University of Pennsylvania, 1232 Blockley Hall, 423 Guardian Drive, Philadelphia, PA 19104-6021, USA, T: +1 215 573-5111, F: +1 215 573-8778, E: sheaja@mail.med.upenn.edu.

Joanne Sinai, M.D., F.R.C.P.C., Lecturer, Department of Psychiatry, University of Toronto, Staff Psychiatrist, Medical Psychiatry Service, St. Michael's Hospital, 30 Bond Street, Toronto, Ontario, Canada, T: +1 416 864-6060, F: +1 416 864-3091, E: j.sinai@utoronto.ca.

Parker A. Small, Jr., M.D., Professor of Pathology, Immunology and Laboratory Medicine, College of Medicine, University of Florida, P.O. Box 100275, Gainesville, Florida, 32610-0275, USA, T: +1 352 392-0686, F: +1 352 392-3324, E: Small@pathology.ufl.edu.

Dame Lesley Southgate, Professor of Primary Care and Medical Education, University College London UK, Centre for Health Informatics and Multiprofessional Education, RFUCMS, 4th Floor, Holborn Union Building, Archway Campus: Highgate Hill, London, N19 3UA, UK, T: +44 20 7288-5209, F: +44 20 7288 3322, E: l.southgate@chime.ucl.ac.uk.

Emanuel Suter, M.D., Professor Emeritus, University of Florida, College of Medicine, 860 Sconset Lane, McLean, Florida, VA 22102, USA, T: +1 703 734-1004, E: esuter@worldnet.att.net.

Richard G. Tiberius, Ph.D., University of Toronto Faculty of Medicine, Centre for Research in Education at the University Health Network, 200 Elizabeth Street, Eaton South 1-583, Toronto, Ontario, M5G 2C4, Canada, T: +1 416 340-4194, F: +1 416 340-3792, E: r.tiberius@utoronto.ca.

Jeff Turnbull, Vice Dean, Undergraduate Medical Education, Assistant Dean, Postgraduate Medical Education, University of Ottawa, Faculty of Medicine, 451 Smyth Road (2042), Ottawa, K1H 8M5, Canada, T: +1 613 562-5800, E: jturnbul@uottawa.ca.,

Cees P.M. Van der Vleuten, Ph.D., Professor and Chair, Department of Educational Research and Development, Maastricht University, P.O. Box 616, 6200 MD Maastricht, The Netherlands, T: +31 43 388-1111, F: +31 43 388-4140, E: c.vandervleuten@educ.unimaas.nl.

Lisa Wersal, University of Minnesota Medical School, Department of Family Practice and Community Health, P.O. Box 381, 516 Delaware Street SE, Minneapolis, MN 55455-0392, USA, T: +1 612 624-2350, F: +1 612 624-2525, E: wers002@umn.edu.

Casey B. White, Assistant Dean for Medical Education, University of Michigan Medical School, 3960 Taubman Library, Ann Arbor, MI 48109, USA, T: +1 734 763-1297, F: +1 734 763-6771, E: bcwhite@umich.edu.

Christel A. Woodward, Ph.D., MacMaster University, Department of Clinical Epidemiology and Biostatistics, 1200 Main Street West, Health Sciences Centre 2C4, Hamilton, Ontario, L8N 3Z5 Canada, T: +1 905 525-9140, F: +1 905 546-5211, E: woodward@mcmaster.ca.

James O. Woolliscroft, M.D., University of Michigan Medical School, M4101 Medical Sciences Building I, Ann Arbor, MI 48109-624, USA, T: +1 734 647-4861, F: +1 734 763-4936, E: wolli@umich.edu.

Subject Index